MR Imaging of Chronic Liver Diseases and Liver Cancer

Editors

KHALED M. ELSAYES
CLAUDE B. SIRLIN

MAGNETIC RESONANCE IMAGING CLINICS OF NORTH AMERICA

www.mri.theclinics.com

Consulting Editors
SURESH K. MUKHERJI
LYNNE S. STEINBACH

August 2021 • Volume 29 • Number 3

ELSEVIER

1600 John F. Kennedy Boulevard • Suite 1800 • Philadelphia, Pennsylvania, 19103-2899

http://www.mri.theclinics.com

MRI CLINICS OF NORTH AMERICA Volume 29, Number 3
August 2021 ISSN 1064-9689, ISBN 13: 978-0-323-77613-4

Editor: John Vassallo (j.vassallo@elsevier.com)
Developmental Editor: Arlene Campos

Magnetic Resonance Imaging Clinics of North America (ISSN 1064-9689) is published quarterly by Elsevier Inc., 360 Park Avenue South, New York, NY 10010-1710. Months of issue are February, May, August, and November. Business and Editorial Offices: 1600 John F. Kennedy Blvd., Ste. 1800, Philadelphia, PA 19103-2899. Customer Service Office: 3251 Riverport Lane, Maryland Heights, MO 63043. Periodicals postage paid at New York, NY and additional mailing offices. Subscription prices are $404.00 per year (domestic individuals), $1037.00 per year (domestic institutions), $100.00 per year (domestic students/residents), $450.00 per year (Canadian individuals), $1063.00 per year (Canadian institutions), $567.00 per year (international individuals), $1063.00 per year (international institutions), $100.00 per year (Canadian students/residents), and $275.00 per year (international students/residents). International air speed delivery is included in all *Clinics* subscription prices. All prices are subject to change without notice. **POSTMASTER:** Send address changes to *Magnetic Resonance Imaging Clinics*, Elsevier Health Sciences Division, Subscription Customer Service, 3251 Riverport Lane, Maryland Heights, MO 63043. Customer Service (orders, claims, online, change of address): Elsevier Health Sciences Division, Subscription **Customer Service, 3251 Riverport Lane, Maryland Heights, MO 63043. Tel:1-800-654-2452 (U.S. and Canada); 314-447-8871 (outside U.S. and Canada). Fax: 314-447-8029. E-mail: journalscustomerservice-usa@elsevier.com (for print support); journalsonlinesupport-usa@elsevier. com (for online support)**.

Reprints. For copies of 100 or more of articles in this publication, please contact the Commercial Reprints Department, Elsevier Inc., 360 Park Avenue South, New York, NY 10010-1710. Tel.: 212-633-3874; Fax: 212-633-3820; E-mail: reprints@elsevier.com.

Magnetic Resonance Imaging Clinics of North America is covered in the *RSNA Index of Imaging Literature, MEDLINE/PubMed (Index Medicus),* and *EMBASE/Excerpta Medica.*

Contributors

CONSULTING EDITORS

SURESH K. MUKHERJI, MD, MBA, FACR
Clinical Professor, Marian University, Director
of Head and Neck Radiology, ProScan
Imaging, Regional Medical Director, Envision
Physician Services, Carmel, Indiana, USA

LYNNE S. STEINBACH, MD, FACR
Emeritus Professor of Radiology on Full Recall,
Department of Radiology and Biomedical
Imaging, University of California, San
Francisco, San Francisco, California, USA

EDITORS

KHALED M. ELSAYES, MD, PhD
Professor, Department of Abdominal Imaging,
The University of Texas MD Anderson Cancer
Center, Houston, Texas, USA

CLAUDE B. SIRLIN, MD
Professor of Radiology, Liver Imaging Group,
Department of Radiology, University of
California, San Diego, San Diego, California,
USA

AUTHORS

MUSTAFA R. BASHIR, MD
Associate Professor of Radiology and
Medicine, Department of Radiology, Duke
University, Durham, North Carolina, USA

AMIR A. BORHANI, MD
Associate Professor of Radiology, Medical
Director of CT, Department of Radiology,
Northwestern University Feinberg School of
Medicine, Chicago, Illinois, USA; Adjunct
Associate Professor of Radiology, University of
Pittsburgh School of Medicine, Pittsburgh,
Pennsylvania, USA

BRIAN T. BRINKERHOFF, MD
Assistant Professor, Department of Pathology,
Oregon Health and Science University,
Portland, Oregon, USA

ROBERTO CANNELLA, MD
Section of Radiology - Department of
Biomedicine, Neuroscience and Advanced
Diagnostics (BiND), University Hospital "Paolo
Giaccone", Department of Health Promotion,
Mother and Child Care, Internal Medicine and
Medical Specialties (PROMISE), University of
Palermo, Palermo, Italy

GUILLERMO CARBONELL, MD
BioMedical Engineering and Imaging Institute,
Department of Diagnostic, Molecular and
Interventional Radiology, Icahn School of
Medicine at Mount Sinai, New York, New York,
USA; Department of Radiology, Virgen de la
Arrixaca University Clinical Hospital, University
of Murcia, Spain

ROBERTA CATANIA, MD
Department of Radiology, Division of
Abdominal Imaging, Northwestern University
Feinberg School of Medicine, Chicago, Illinois,
USA

SILVIA D. CHANG, MD, FRCPC, FSAR
Associate Professor, Department of Radiology,
University of British Columbia, Vancouver
General Hospital, Vancouver, British Columbia,
Canada

VICTORIA CHERNYAK, MD, MS
Professor, Department of Radiology, Beth
Israel Deaconess Medical Center, Boston,
Massachusetts, USA

HAILEY H. CHOI, MD
Assistant Professor of Radiology, Department of Radiology and Biomedical Imaging, University of California, San Francisco, San Francisco, California, USA

KALINA CHUPETLOVSKA, MD
Department of Radiology, University Hospital Saint Ivan Rilski, Sofia, Bulgaria

GUILHERME MOURA CUNHA, MD
Department of Radiology, University of Washington, Seattle, Washington, USA

ANIL DASYAM, MD
Associate Professor of Radiology, Department of Radiology, Abdominal Imaging Division, University of Pittsburgh School of Medicine, Pittsburgh, Pennsylvania, USA

RICHARD K.G. DO, MD, PhD
Associate Attending, Radiology, Memorial Sloan Kettering Cancer Center, Associate Professor, Radiology, Weill Medical College of Cornell University, New York, New York, USA

ROBERT H. EL-MARAGHI, MD, FRCPC
Department of Medical Oncology, Royal Victoria Regional Health Center, University of Toronto, Toronto, Ontario, Canada

MOHAB M. ELMOHR, MD
Resident, Department of Radiology, Baylor College of Medicine, Houston, Texas, USA

KHALED M. ELSAYES, MD, PhD
Professor, Department of Abdominal Imaging, The University of Texas MD Anderson Cancer Center, Houston, Texas, USA

DAVID T. FETZER, MD
Medical Director of Ultrasound, Assistant Professor, Department of Radiology, UT Southwestern Medical Center, Dallas, Texas, USA

KATHRYN J. FOWLER, MD
Liver Imaging Group, Professor, Department of Radiology, University of California, San Diego, San Diego, California, USA

ALICE FUNG, MD
Associate Professor, Department of Diagnostic Radiology, Oregon Health and Science University, Portland, Oregon, USA

ALESSANDRO FURLAN, MD
Department of Radiology, Abdominal Imaging Division, University of Pittsburgh, Pittsburgh, Pennsylvania, USA

SHIVA JAYARAMAN, MD, MESc, FRCSC
Department of Surgery, St. Joseph's Health Centre, University of Toronto, Toronto, Ontario, Canada

AYA KAMAYA, MD
Professor, Department of Radiology, Stanford University, Stanford, California, USA

AVINASH R. KAMBADAKONE, MD
Department of Diagnostic Radiology, Oregon Health and Science University, Portland, Oregon, USA

RONY KAMPALATH, MD
Department of Radiological Sciences, University of California, Irvine, Orange, California, USA

AMAN KHURANA, MD
Assistant Professor, Department of Radiology, University of Kentucky, Lexington, Kentucky, USA

ANIA Z. KIELAR, MD, FRCPC
Joint Department of Medical Imaging, Toronto General Hospital, University of Toronto, Toronto, Ontario, Canada

NAVEEN M. KULKARNI, MD
Department of Radiology, Medical College of Wisconsin, Milwaukee, Wisconsin, USA

ROBERT M. MARKS, MD
Associate Professor, Department of Radiology, Naval Medical Center San Diego, San Diego, California, USA; Department of Radiology, Uniformed Services University of the Health Sciences, Bethesda, Maryland, USA

MISHAL MENDIRATTA-LALA, MD
Associate Professor of Radiology, University of Michigan School of Medicine, Ann Arbor, Michigan, USA

FRANK H. MILLER, MD
Professor of Radiology, Division Chief and Medical Director of MRI, Department of Radiology, Body Imaging Section, Northwestern University Feinberg School of Medicine, Chicago, Illinois, USA

AHMED W. MOAWAD, MD
Department of Imaging Physics, The University of Texas MD Anderson Cancer Center, Houston, Texas, USA

ALI MORSHID, MD
Department of Diagnostic Radiology, The University of Texas Medical Branch, Galveston, Texas, USA

LESLIE W. NELSON, DO
R2 Radiology Resident, Department of Radiology, University of Kentucky, Lexington, Kentucky, USA

COLIN O'ROURKE, MB BCh BAO, FFR (RCSI)
Joint Department of Medical Imaging, Toronto General Hospital, University of Toronto, Toronto, Ontario, Canada

SHUCHI K. RODGERS, MD
Department of Radiology, Clinical Associate Professor of Radiology, Sidney Kimmel Medical College at Thomas Jefferson University, Einstein Healthcare Network, Levy Ground, Philadelphia, Pennsylvania, USA

CARL F. SABOTTKE, MD
Department of Medical Imaging, University of Arizona College of Medicine, Tucson, Arizona, USA

KRISHNA P. SHANBHOGUE, MD
Associate Professor, Department of Radiology, New York University Grossman School of Medicine, New York, New York, USA

AMIT G. SINGAL, MD, MS
UT Southwestern Medical Center, Dallas, Texas, USA

CLAUDE B. SIRLIN, MD
Professor of Radiology, Liver Imaging Group, Department of Radiology, University of California, San Diego, San Diego, California, USA

STEPHANIE SPANN, MD
Assistant Instructor, Department of Radiology, UT Southwestern Medical Center, Dallas, Texas, USA

BRADLEY M. SPIELER, MD
Department of Radiology, Louisiana State University Health Sciences Center, New Orleans, Louisiana, USA

JANIO SZKLARUK, MD, PhD
Professor, Department of Diagnostic Radiology, The University of Texas MD Anderson Cancer Center, Houston, Texas, USA

MYLES T. TAFFEL, MD
Associate Professor, Department of Radiology, New York University Grossman School of Medicine, New York, New York, USA

BACHIR TAOULI, MD, MHA
BioMedical Engineering and Imaging Institute, Department of Diagnostic, Molecular and Interventional Radiology, Icahn School of Medicine at Mount Sinai, New York, New York, USA

NEIL D. THEISE, MD
Professor, Department of Pathology, New York University Grossman School of Medicine, New York, New York, USA

KAREN TRAN-HARDING, MD
Department of Radiological Sciences, University of California, Irvine, Orange, California, USA

JOSEPH H. YACOUB, MD
Associate Professor, Department of Radiology, MedStar Georgetown University Hospital, Washington, DC, USA

VAHID YAGHMAI, MD, MS
Professor and Chair of Radiological Sciences, University of California, Irvine, Orange, California, USA

BENJAMIN M. YEH, MD
Department of Radiology and Biomedical Imaging, UCSF Medical Center, San Francisco, California, USA

Contents

> Effective communication between radiologists and physicians involved in the management of patients with chronic liver disease is paramount to ensuring appropriate and advantageous incorporation of liver imaging findings into patient care. This review discusses the clinical benefits of innovations in radiology reporting, what information the various stakeholders wish to know from the radiologist, and how radiology can help to ensure the effective communication of findings.

> Ultrasound plays a vital role in the evaluation of patients with chronic liver disease and in hepatocellular carcinoma (HCC) surveillance in populations at risk for developing HCC. Semiannual ultrasound for HCC surveillance is universally recommended by all liver societies around the world. Advanced ultrasound techniques, such as elastography and contrast-enhanced ultrasound, offer additional benefits in imaging evaluation of chronic liver disease. Major benefits of ultrasound include its high safety profile and relatively low cost.

> Contrast-enhanced ultrasound (CEUS) is a safe adjunct tool for liver imaging and can be an alternative to computed tomography or MR imaging. CEUS has a proven track record in guiding management for patients with chronic liver disease who need further evaluation of focal liver lesions. CEUS is a dynamic examination with high temporal and spatial resolution. CEUS uses a pure blood pool contrast agent that allows for a unique evaluation of the perfusion kinetics of a region of interest.

> Computed tomography (CT) is often performed as the initial imaging study for the workup of patients with known or suspected liver disease. Our article reviews liver CT techniques and protocols in clinical practice along with updates on relevant CT advances, including wide-detector CT, radiation dose optimization, and

multienergy scanning, that have already shown clinical impact. Particular emphasis is placed on optimizing the late arterial phase of enhancement, which is critical to evaluation of hepatocellular carcinoma. We also discuss emerging techniques that may soon influence clinical care.

MR imaging has become a powerful tool for assessing liver disease and liver cancer; however, it entails complex, time-consuming, and costly protocols. Abbreviated MR imaging (AMRI) is emerging as a simpler, faster, and low-cost alternative to full-abdominal MR imaging protocols. Different AMRI approaches have been tested successfully in hepatocellular carcinoma detection and for assessment of diffuse liver disease. The most accurate, time-effective, and cost-effective protocol as well as the target population need to be defined. Prospective and multicentric studies, exploring different AMRI protocols versus the current standard of reference, should be performed.

Contrast-enhanced MR imaging plays an important role in the evaluation of patients with chronic liver disease, particularly for detection and characterization of liver lesions. The two most commonly used types of contrast agents for liver MR imaging are extracellular agents (ECAs) and hepatobiliary agents (HBAs). In patients with liver disease, the main advantage of ECA-enhanced MR imaging is its high specificity for the diagnosis of progressed HCCs. Conversely, HBAs have an additional excretion mechanism through hepatocyte uptake, which results in high liver-to-lesion contrast and highest sensitivity for lesion detection in the hepatobiliary phase. Emerging data suggest that some features depicted on contrast-enhanced MR imaging are related to tumor biology and can be predictive of patients' prognosis, likely to further expand the role of contrast-enhanced MR imaging in the clinical care of patients with chronic liver disease.

The liver performs many vital functions for the human body. It stores essential vitamins and minerals, such as iron and vitamins A, D, K, and B_{12}. It synthesizes proteins, such as blood clotting factors, albumin, and glycogen, as well as cholesterol, carbohydrates, and triglycerides. Additionally, it acts as a detoxifier, metabolizing and helping to clear alcohol, drugs, and ammonia. Typical MR imaging protocols for liver imaging include T2-weighted, chemical shift imaging, and precontrast and postcontrast T1-weighted sequences. This article discussed MR imaging of diffuse liver diseases and their typical imaging findings.

In the background of chronic liver disease, hepatocellular carcinoma develops via a complex, multistep process called hepatocarcinogenesis. This article reviews the causes contributing to the process. Emphasis is made on the imaging manifestations of the pathologic changes seen at many stages of hepatocarcinogenesis, from regenerative nodules to dysplastic nodules and then to hepatocellular carcinoma.

The Liver Imaging Reporting and Data System (LI-RADS) is a comprehensive system for standardizing the lexicon, technique, interpretation, reporting, and data collection of liver imaging. Developed specifically for assessment of liver observations in patients at risk for hepatocellular carcinoma (HCC), LI-RADS classifies hepatic observations on the basis of the probability of their being HCC, from LR-1 (definitely benign) to LR-5 (definitely HCC). This article discusses the technical requirements, major features, and ancillary features of and a systematic approach for using the LI-RADS diagnostic algorithm, with special emphasis on MR imaging.

Locoregional therapy (LRT) for hepatocellular carcinoma can be used alone or with other treatment modalities to reduce rates of progression, improve survival, or act as a bridge to cure. As the use of LRT expands, so too has the need for systems to evaluate treatment response, such as the World Health Organization and modified Response Evaluation Criteria In Solid Tumors systems and more recently, the Liver Imaging Reporting and Data System (LI-RADS) treatment response algorithm (TRA). Early validation results for LI-RADS TRA have been promising, and as research accrues, the TRA is expected to evolve in the near future.

Hepatocellular carcinoma (HCC) is the most common liver malignancy associated with chronic liver disease. Nonhepatocellular malignancies may also arise in the setting of chronic liver disease. The imaging diagnosis of non-HCC malignancies may be challenging. Non-HCC malignancies in patients with chronic liver disease most commonly include intrahepatic cholangiocarcinoma and combined hepatocellular-cholangiocarcinoma, and less commonly hepatic lymphomas and metastases. On MR imaging, non-HCC malignancies often demonstrate a targetoid appearance, manifesting as rim arterial phase hyperenhancement, peripheral washout, central delayed enhancement, and peripheral restricted diffusion. When applying the Liver Imaging Reporting and Data System algorithm, observations with targetoid appearance are categorized as LR-M.

MRI is an important problem-solving tool for accurate characterization of liver lesions. Chronic liver disease alters the typical imaging characteristics and complicates liver imaging. Awareness of imaging pitfalls and technical artifacts and ways to mitigate them allows for more accurate and timely diagnosis.

MAGNETIC RESONANCE IMAGING CLINICS OF NORTH AMERICA

VISIT THE CLINICS ONLINE!
Access your subscription at:
www.theclinics.com

PROGRAM OBJECTIVE
The goal of *Magnetic Resonance Imaging Clinics of North America* is to keep practicing physicians up to date with current clinical practice by providing timely articles reviewing the state of the art in patient care.

TARGET AUDIENCE
All practicing physicians and healthcare professionals who provide patient care utilizing findings from Magnetic Resonance Imaging.

LEARNING OBJECTIVES
Upon completion of this activity, participants will be able to:
1. Review research/clinical topics related to imaging of diffuse liver diseases.
2. Discuss benefits of the LI-RADS treatment response algorithm in the assessment of liver lesions.
3. Recognize new developments in the assessment of liver diseases using artificial intelligence (AI) models.

ACCREDITATION
The Elsevier Office of Continuing Medical Education (EOCME) is accredited by the Accreditation Council for Continuing Medical Education (ACCME) to provide continuing medical education for physicians.

The EOCME designates this journal-based CME activity enduring material for a maximum of 14 *AMA PRA Category 1 Credit*(s)™. Physicians should claim only the credit commensurate with the extent of their participation in the activity.

All other healthcare professionals requesting continuing education credit for this enduring material will be issued a certificate of participation.

DISCLOSURE OF CONFLICTS OF INTEREST
The EOCME assesses conflict of interest with its instructors, faculty, planners, and other individuals who are in a position to control the content of CME activities. All relevant conflicts of interest that are identified are thoroughly vetted by EOCME for fair balance, scientific objectivity, and patient care recommendations. EOCME is committed to providing its learners with CME activities that promote improvements or quality in healthcare and not a specific proprietary business or a commercial interest.

The planning committee, staff, authors and editors listed below have identified no financial relationships or relationships to products or devices they or their spouse/life partner have with commercial interest related to the content of this CME activity:
Mustafa R. Bashir, MD; Amir A. Borhani, MD; Brian T. Brinkerhoff, MD; Roberto Cannella, MD; Guillermo Carbonell, MD; Silvia D. Chang, MD, FRCPC, FSAR; Regina Chavous-Gibson, MSN, RN; Hailey H. Choi, MD; Kalina Chupetlovska, MD; Guilherme Moura Cunha, MD; Anil Dasyam, MD; Richard K.G. Do, MD, PhD; Mohab M. Elmohr, MD; Khaled M. Elsayes, MD, PhD; Kathryn J. Fowler, MD; Alice Fung, MD; Shiva Jayaraman, MD, MESc, FRCSC; Rony Kampalath, MD; Aman Khurana, MD; Ania Z. Kielar, MD, FRCPC; Pradeep Kuttysankaran; Robert M. Marks, MD; Mishal Mendiratta-Lala, MD; Frank H. Miller, MD; Ahmed W. Moawad, MD; Ali Morshid, MD; Leslie W. Nelson, DO; Colin O'Rourke, MB BCh BAO, FFR (RCSI); Shuchi K. Rodgers, MD; Carl F. Sabottke, MD; Krishna P. Shanbhogue, MD; Stephanie Spann, MD; Bradley M. Spieler, MD; Janio Szklaruk, MD, PhD; Myles T. Taffel, MD; Neil D. Theise, MD; Karen Tran-Harding, MD; John Vassallo; Joseph H. Yacoub, MD; Vahid Yaghmai, MD, MS.

The planning committee, staff, authors and editors listed below have identified financial relationships or relationships to products or devices they or their spouse/life partner have with commercial interest related to the content of this CME activity:
Roberta Catania, MD: Research support: Siemens Healthineers

Victoria Chernyak, MD, MS: Consultant/advisor: Bayer AG

Robert H. El-Maraghi, MD, FRCPC: Consultant/advisor: AstraZeneca, Bristol-Myers Squibb Company, Eisai, Novartis AG, Pfizer, Inc

David T. Fetzer, MD: Research support: Bracco Diagnostic, Philips Healthcare, Siemens Healthineers

Alessandro Furlan, MD: Research support: ENDRA Life Sciences Inc.; Royalties/Patents: Elsevier

Aya Kamaya, MD: Royalties: Elsevier

Avinash R. Kambadakone, MD: Research support: GE Healthcare, Philips Healthcare

Naveen M. Kulkarni, MD: Consultant/advisor: GE Healthcare

Amit G. Singal, MD, MS: Consultant/advisor: Bayer AG, Exact Sciences Corporation, FUJIFILM Wako Diagnostics USA Corporation, Glycotest, Grail, Roche

Claude B. Sirlin, MD: Consultant/advisor: Blade Therapeuitics, Boehringer Ingelheim, Epigenomics AG; Stock ownership: Livivos, Inc

Bachir Taouli, MD, MHA: Consultant/advisor: Bayer AG, Guerbet; Research support: Bayer AG, Regeneron Pharmaceuticals, Inc, Takeda Pharmaceutical Company Limited

Benjamin M. Yeh, MD: Speaker's bureau: Canon Medical Systems USA Inc, GE Healthcare, Philips Healthcare; Consultant/advisor: GE Healthcare; Stock ownership: Nextrast, Inc; Research support: GE Healthcare, Guerbet, Philips Healthcare

UNAPPROVED/OFF-LABEL USE DISCLOSURE

The EOCME requires CME faculty to disclose to the participants:

1. When products or procedures being discussed are off-label, unlabelled, experimental, and/or investigational (not US Food and Drug Administration [FDA] approved); and

2. Any limitations on the information presented, such as data that are preliminary or that represent ongoing research, interim analyses, and/or unsupported opinions. Faculty may discuss information about pharmaceutical agents that is outside of FDA-approved labelling. This information is intended solely for CME and is not intended to promote off-label use of these medications. If you have any questions, contact the medical affairs department of the manufacturer for the most recent pre-scribing information.

TO ENROLL

To enroll in the *Magnetic Resonance Imaging Clinics of North America* Continuing Medical Education program, call customer service at 1-800-654-2452 or sign up online at http://www.theclinics.com/home/cme. The CME program is available to subscribers for an additional annual fee of USD 281.00.

METHOD OF PARTICIPATION

In order to claim credit, participants must complete the following:

1. Complete enrolment as indicated above.
2. Read the activity.
3. Complete the CME Test and Evaluation. Participants must achieve a score of 70% on the test. All CME Tests and Evaluations must be completed online.

CME INQUIRIES/SPECIAL NEEDS

For all CME inquiries or special needs, please contact elsevierCME@elsevier.com.

Foreword

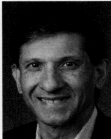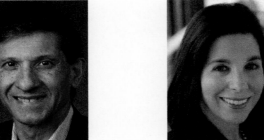

Suresh K. Mukherji, MD, MBA, FACR   Lynne S. Steinbach, MD, FACR

Consulting Editors

The diagnosis and management of liver disease are still considered a clinical challenge and one that warrants both clinical and imaging evaluation. MR imaging has become an essential tool for diagnosing a variety of liver diseases, including chronic liver disorders and hepatic neoplasms. This issue of *Magnetic Resonance Imaging Clinics of North America* is specifically devoted to hepatic imaging, and we are thrilled to have Drs Khaled Elsayes and Claude Sirlin be our Guest Editors.

This wonderful issue has articles focused on MR, CT, and ultrasound for hepatic imaging. There are articles devoted to hepatocellular carcinoma (HCC), including surveillance imaging, chronic liver disease, diffuse liver disease, liver transplantation, LI-RADS (Liver Reporting and Data System), treatment response, and artificial intelligence...to name a few.

We would like to personally thank all the article authors for their outstanding contributions. These are world-renowned experts who continue to advance the field of hepatic imaging. Their content is superb, and the images are dazzling! We would also like to thank Drs Khaled Elsayes and Claude Sirlin for coediting this issue. We have had the privilege of knowing both of these individuals for many years, and are both delighted and honored to have them guest edit this important issue. Thanks to all for creating this state-of-the-art "tour de force" issue focused on hepatic imaging!

Suresh K. Mukherji, MD, MBA, FACR
Marian University
ProScan Imaging
Envision Physician Services
Carmel, IN, USA

Lynne S. Steinbach, MD, FACR
Department of Radiology and
Biomedical Imaging
University of California, San Francisco
505 Parnassus
San Francisco, CA 9413-0628, USA

E-mail addresses:
sureshmukherji@hotmail.com (S.K. Mukherji)
lynne.steinbach@ucsf.edu (L.S. Steinbach)

https://doi.org/10.1016/j.mric.2021.05.016
1064-9689/21/

Preface
MR Imaging of Chronic Liver Diseases and Liver Cancer

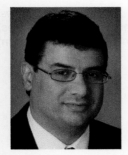 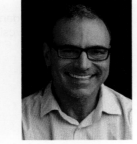

Khaled M. Elsayes, MD, PhD   Claude B. Sirlin, MD
Editors

Since its invention almost five decades ago, MR imaging has become an indispensable tool for diagnosing liver diseases, particularly chronic diseases and liver cancer. Nevertheless, the diagnosis and management of liver diseases are still considered a clinical challenge, one that warrants systematic research. This issue of *Magnetic Resonance Imaging Clinics of North America*, for which we are honored to serve as guest editors, highlights cutting-edge research and future directions in MR imaging of chronic liver diseases and liver cancer.

The top radiology experts featured in this issue work to continually advance noninvasive imaging as an integral component in liver disease management. The initial role of radiology in establishing the diagnosis of chronic liver disease and liver cancer is emphasized, as well as how imaging can provide guidance for hepatologists, oncologists, and surgeons in treating their patients.

One of the highlights of this issue is the article on advanced protocols and techniques for imaging liver diseases and cancer with both MR imaging and computed tomography. Following that are several articles about the role of imaging in hepatocellular carcinoma (HCC), including the use of ultrasonography for HCC surveillance, the correlation between radiology and pathology in

assessing hepatocarcinogenesis, the application of MR imaging to assign LI-RADS (Liver Reporting and Data System) categories reflecting the relative probability of HCC, and evaluating HCC treatment response after locoregional therapy.

The issue also features the use of MR imaging in non-HCC malignancies, chronic liver disease, diffuse liver disease, and liver transplantation. The accurate interpretation of imaging is difficult, even for experienced radiologists, so we have included an article about common errors and misinterpretations in the imaging of chronic liver disease and how to avoid such problems.

The last article in this issue is about applying artificial intelligence (AI) in the imaging of chronic liver disease. AI shows promise for assisting radiologists in interpreting and reporting diagnostic imaging. We believe that it will eventually be integrated into routine radiology practice and will have a significant impact on liver disease management.

We want to express our gratitude to our outstanding contributors for their excellent articles and more broadly for their dedication to the continued advancement of medical imaging. To the readers, we hope you enjoy this issue and find it as educational as anticipated. Finally, we would like to thank the *Magnetic Resonance*

Magn Reson Imaging Clin N Am 29 (2021) xvii–xviii
https://doi.org/10.1016/j.mric.2021.05.015
1064-9689/21/© 2021 Published by Elsevier Inc.

Imaging Clinics of North America committee for offering us the opportunity to serve as guest editors for this issue.

Khaled M. Elsayes, MD, PhD
Department of Abdominal Imaging
The University of Texas MD Anderson
Cancer Center
Houston, TX, USA

Claude B. Sirlin, MD
Liver Imaging Group
Department of Radiology
University of California, San Diego
408 Dickinson Street
San Diego, CA 92103-8226, USA

E-mail addresses:
KMElsayes@mdanderson.org (K.M. Elsayes)
csirlin@ucsd.edu (C.B. Sirlin)

Chronic Liver Disease and Liver Cancer
What the Hepatologists, Oncologists, and Surgeons Want to Know from Radiologists

Colin O'Rourke, MB BCh BAO, FFR (RCSI)[a], Shiva Jayaraman, MD, MESc, FRCSC[b],
Robert H. El-Maraghi, MD, FRCPC[c], Amit G. Singal, MD, MS[d],
Ania Z. Kielar, MD, FRCPC[a],*

KEYWORDS

- Chronic liver disease • Liver cancer • Radiology • Oncologists • Hepatologists • Surgeons
- LI-RADS

KEY POINTS

- Clear communication between specialties in medicine is associated with better patient outcomes.
- Understanding what each specialty requires in imaging reports helps to improve radiologist consistency and report quality.
- Participation in multidisciplinary conference allows for the exchange of key imaging findings, creation of communication opportunities between, specialties and a feedback mechanism for peer-learning opportunities in radiology.

INTRODUCTION

Chronic liver disease affects 1.5 billion people globally, and accounts for 3.5% of all deaths worldwide.[1] Hepatocellular carcinoma (HCC), one of the major complications of cirrhosis, is the fourth leading cause of cancer-related death worldwide and one of the fastest increasing causes of cancer-related mortality in the United States. The strongest risk factor for HCC is the presence of cirrhosis, and more than 90% of HCCs occur in the setting of chronic liver disease.

HCC is a unique malignancy in that its diagnosis relies predominantly on imaging, without the need for histologic confirmation in many, if not most, cases. Given the central importance of imaging to HCC diagnosis, there has been great emphasis on accurate interpretation and consistent reporting of imaging findings for patients in whom there is a clinical concern of HCC. The diagnosis of HCC is one of few malignancies where therapeutic decisions rely predominantly on imaging, without need for biopsy in every case.

The Liver Imaging and Reporting Data System (LI-RADS) is a living document first published and endorsed by the American College of Radiology (ACR) and is updated on a regular cycle. After the first release in 2011, official updates took place in 2014, 2017, and 2018.[2,3] The 2018 updates coincided with adoption of LI-RADS into version 2018 of the American Association for the Study of Liver Disease guidelines.[4] All evidence-based updates to the LI-RADS document have been evaluated and vetted by radiologists, with direct input from hepatologists and liver surgeons, who are members of the LI-RADS steering committee.

[a] Department of Medical Imaging, Toronto General Hospital, University of Toronto, 200 Elizabeth Street, Toronto, ON M5G 2C4, Canada; [b] Department of Surgery, St. Joseph's Health Centre, University of Toronto, 30 The Queensway Suite 221 SSW, Toronto, ON M6R 1B5, Canada; [c] Department of Medical Oncology, Royal Victoria Regional Health Center, University of Toronto, 201 Georgian Drive Barrie, Toronto, ON L4M 6M2, Canada; [d] UT Southwestern Medical Center, 2201 Inwood Road #920, Dallas, TX 75235, USA
* Corresponding author.
E-mail address: ania.kielar@uhn.ca

Magn Reson Imaging Clin N Am 29 (2021) 269–278
https://doi.org/10.1016/j.mric.2021.05.001
1064-9689/21/© 2021 Elsevier Inc. All rights reserved.

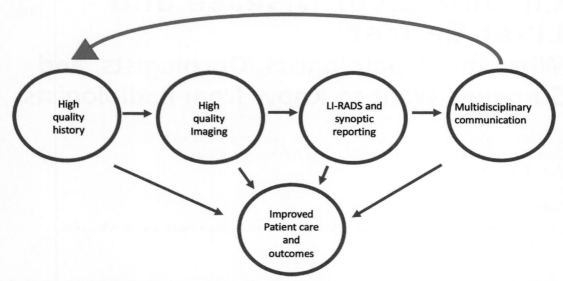

Fig. 1. The various steps involved in patient imaging and management.

The importance of communication between radiologists and key stakeholders, including clinicians and surgeons, is paramount to ensuring appropriate and effective incorporation of liver imaging findings into patient care [**Fig. 1**]. In addition to improving direct communication, when used consistently, application of the LI-RARDS in radiology reports can allow for more robust multicenter research that will lead to ongoing improvements of this system. This review discusses the benefits of innovations in radiology reporting to the clinical decision process, the patient experience, the cost of imaging, and the overall contributions to the health of the population. Future directions, including the use of artificial intelligence, are reviewed.

THE CURRENT STATE OF THE LIVER IMAGING AND REPORTING DATA SYSTEM IN THE WORLD

The need for the standardization and classification in liver imaging became clear to a group of radiologists in 2006 during a meeting of hepatologists and surgeons at the University of California San Diego, which drew attention to problems in both interpretation and at interdisciplinary communication of computed tomography and MRI findings. In brief, it was identified that clinicians and surgeons often did not understand the radiologic findings because of their lack of descriptive clarity, many times using different words for the same concept or the same words for different findings, generating a lot of confusion.[2,5]

The main goals of LI-RADS are to apply consistent terminology, decrease variability in image interpretation, and improve the clarity of communication. There is a growing body of evidence that structured reporting improves the quality and value of a radiologist's major work product, namely, the radiology report.[6–9] Additionally, the ACR Economics Committee on Value Based Payments recommended that radiologists not only transition to structured reporting, but in particular, move onto disease-specific reports.[10] This transition was further supported when the American Association for the study of Liver Disease began including LI-RADS in its practice guidelines in 2018.

Currently in North America, the Organ Procurement Transplant Network requires that all imaging studies of potential HCC in liver transplant candidates be reviewed by radiologists in transplant centers, even if they were performed and initially interpreted at another site.[11–13] Tania Rahman and colleagues[13] have shown that reinterpretations at a transplant center were more likely to use a scoring system such an LI-RADS, more likely to characterize a lesion as definite HCC, and more likely to be considered comprehensive and easy to understand. Furthermore, the differing interpretations predicted a change in clinical management in 50% of cases, including the avoidance of potentially risky and unnecessary biopsies,[13] whereas Flusberg and colleagues[12] have suggested that universal use of LI-RADS would eliminate the need for complete re-interpretation owing to the availability of standardized reports.

Currently, several other systems exist worldwide for diagnosing HCC by imaging and for determining subsequent patient management. These include recommendations by the Organ Procurement Transplant Network, the European Society of Gastrointestinal and Abdominal Radiology, and the European Association for the Study of the Liver.[14] The reasons that these alternative guidelines have not adopted LI-RADS are multifactorial, including language barriers, adversity to change, and the perceived complexity of LI-RADS guidelines. The recent European Association for the Study of the Liver guidelines regarding the management of HCC, presented at the European Association for the Study of the Liver Annual Meeting in April 2018 in Paris, have stated that the LI-RADS is not validated prospectively in all its major features and is therefore not accepted by the European Society for the Study of the Liver.[5]

In Germany, Ringe and colleagues[15] found that even though there was a clear trend toward using structured reporting systems such as LI-RADS, implementation has so far been met with limited success. They found that knowledge and application of LI-RADS varied greatly depending on specialty and professional experience, as well as whether an individual was associated with either a clinical or an academic background, with participants from larger hospitals tending to be more familiar with LI-RADS. They also identified that the perceived complexity of the LI-RADS system and a potential language barriers may be possible reasons that it has not been adopted into guidelines universally.[15] Of note, the ACR LI-RADS manual has been translated into 9 languages by the LI-RADS International Working Group. Alenazi and colleagues[16] surveyed 152 physicians worldwide involved in the care of patients at high risk for HCC, where they tried to identify reasons for LI-RADS not being implemented globally. More than two-thirds of participants (69%) believed radiologists are not adapting LI-RADS or using it inconsistently (47%), with 36% reporting a preference for alternative guidelines.[16]

The use and implementation of LI-RADS worldwide is a constantly evolving process that will require ongoing prospective research, updating of the algorithms, and delivering education from groups such as the LI-RADS Outreach & Education Group and the Society of Abdominal Radiology Disease Focused Panel.[17]

WHAT CLINICIANS WANT TO KNOW

There are many physicians involved in the care of patients at high risk for developing HCC. These include surgeons (eg, hepatobiliary surgeons, transplant surgeons), gastroenterologists, hepatologists, oncologists, general internists, interventional radiologists, pathologists, and family physicians. The type of treatment a patient receives and the response to treatment are discussed at a hepatobiliary or HCC-specific multidisciplinary case conference. Although many of the stakeholders involved in a patient's care will have common things they need to know, certain points of information are particular to their specialty. Again, in the study published by Alenazi and colleagues[16] physicians in various specialties and in different work settings (eg, academic hospital and private practice) were asked about their preferences regarding radiology reports related to HCC. The groups surveyed included hepatologists, transplant surgeons, internal medicine specialists, and other physicians, including primary practice physicians. Results were broken down by specialty as well as work environment. Overall, there was significant approval for use of LI-RADS when reporting imaging in patients at risk for HCC, with almost 90% preferring LI-RADS over other systems or nonstandardized reporting.

INFORMATION RELEVANT TO SURGEONS

The opportunities for cure in HCC involve surgical extirpation via either resection or liver transplantation. When surgeons review imaging reports, they depend on reliable confirmation of the diagnosis of HCC. Historically, this confirmation was performed by describing the degree of arterial enhancement and venous or delayed washout alone. With the adoption of LI-RADS, radiologists should report both major and minor characteristics that alter their risk assessment for the presence of HCC as well as report an overall LI-RADS category. By extension, they will also want to ensure that benign or other malignant causes for imaging findings have been ruled out. Once a diagnosis of HCC is established, accurate tumor staging is required, including the number of definite HCC lesions, the tumor diameter for each HCC, and the presence of vascular invasion (LI-RADS tumor-in-vein) or metastatic disease. An accurate assessment of tumor burden has implications for treatment decisions, including eligibility for curative therapies.

Surgical resection is typically reserved for unifocal lesions and nonmetastatic to either lymph nodes nor to distant sites, so the presence of satellite lesions or multifocality is important to know when considering resection. Imaging demonstrating small satellite lesions around a dominant lesion are not considered multifocal HCC. Although multifocal disease usually precludes resection, such patients may still be candidates for liver transplantation as per the Milan Criteria, or other transplant criteria. Similarly, local ablative therapies have the best efficacy for lesions less than 3 cm in maximum diameter, so accurate reporting of the tumor diameter can determine the choice of local ablative therapy versus alternatives.

For a lesion to be considered locally resectable, it is essential that the lesion can be resected to negative margins while preserving sufficient liver parenchyma for the future liver remnant. A suitable future liver remnant volume will depend on factors related to the condition of the liver such as the presence of cirrhosis or nonalcoholic fatty liver disease. Either cirrhosis or nonalcoholic fatty liver disease may limit the extent of liver resection possible; therefore, an accurate description of the precise location and size of the index lesion is essential. In addition to the quality and quantity of the remaining hepatic parenchyma, it is important to know the relationship of the tumor to the portal pedicles and the hepatic venous outflow tracts. If the future liver remnant has an inadequate blood supply and biliary drainage, or if there is insufficient drainage of blood through the hepatic veins, surgery is not possible. Finally, the presence or absence of major vascular invasion is important. Major vascular invasion is a contraindication to resection. The presence of portal hypertension or hepatic decompensation can have implications for immediate treatment decisions, as well as the risk of complications. Surgical resection is reserved for patients with Child A cirrhosis without portal hypertension, so presence of these imaging features would typically preclude resection. The tolerance for portal hypertension in part depends on the extent of the planned resection and expected future liver remnant. Laparoscopic limited resection may be possible in a patient with mild portal hypertension, whereas a major resection (eg, right or left lobectomy) would be restricted to those without significant portal hypertension at baseline.

INFORMATION RELEVANT TO HEPATOLOGISTS

Hepatologists are interested in the imaging features of chronic liver disease and the characteristics of liver observations. Background liver features such as iron and fat deposition should be mentioned and quantified, sometimes utilizing techniques such as a Ferriscan or those developed by the University of Rennes in the case of iron deposition.[18]

Signs of portal hypertension are important, including splenomegaly, ascites, venous varices, and a recanalized paraumbilical vein. Because transplantation is the definitive therapy for chronic liver disease, an assessment of tumor burden is particularly important. Patients listed for transplant are only eligible for Model for End-Stage Liver Disease exception points if they have a T2 HCC, that is, 2 cm or greater. Similarly, those exceeding the Milan Criteria (1 lesion ≤5 cm or 2–3 lesions ≤3 cm, without vascular invasion or distant metastases) must be downstaged to within the Milan Criteria by locoregional therapy before Model for End-Stage Liver Disease exception points can be applied.[19]

Beyond initial tumor burden, an assessment of the treatment response to surgical, locoregional, or systemic therapies is important for subsequent treatment decisions. With an expanding landscape of treatment options, patients who fail 1 line of therapy are often quickly transitioned to an alternative treatment option. For example, patients who are treated with locoregional therapy who exhibit progressive disease can be considered for systemic therapy, even if the tumor remains localized to the liver. This factor is a potential shortcoming of the LI-RADS treatment response categorization, because it is lesion specific and may not give a broader sense of progressive disease versus partial response, because these are both categorized as LR-TR viable. Therefore, it can often be helpful if radiology reports explicitly comment on if lesions seem to have partial response versus progressive disease in cases with viable tumor after treatment.

INFORMATION RELEVANT TO INTERVENTIONAL RADIOLOGISTS

Interventional radiologists perform many of the treatment options for liver-directed therapy, such as radiofrequency ablation, microwave ablation, cryoablation, ethanol ablation, chemoembolization, and radioembolization. The type of liver-directed therapy is usually decided at multidisciplinary case conferences, with the tumor size, location, and number all contributing to the decision. The presence of heat sinks and the identification of nearby structures that may be susceptible to injury (eg, colon next to the liver being evaluated for radiofrequency of microwave ablation) is also important.[20]

Small or peripheral HCCs are more commonly treated with ablation techniques, including radiofrequency ablation and microwave ablation, whereas larger HCCs will be more suitable to endovascular treatments. Hepatic arterial anatomy will be of interest before endovascular treatments such as chemoembolization and radioembolization to aid in procedural planning. A knowledge of hepatic arterial anatomy, including important variants, such as a replaced right hepatic artery, is essential for the planning of catheter-based interventions.

Interventional radiologists will be interested in both the response to locoregional treatment of HCC and complications associated with chronic liver disease. The use of the LI-RADS treatment response algorithm can help to provide standard reporting for various types of locoregional therapy.[20] An imaging evaluation of an area previously treated with locoregional therapy will dictate whether a patient requires further treatment rather than standard imaging follow-up (**Fig. 2**).

With regard to chronic liver disease, interventionalists perform procedures such as variceal embolization, transjugular intrahepatic portosystemic shunt, and balloon occluded retrograde transvenous obliteration. For patients being considered for this type of intervention, a detailed description of the venous anatomy is required before the appropriate procedure is performed. The patency of the portal vein, the location of venous varices and venous shunting, along with the presence of ascites, are all important factors in deciding what intervention will benefit the patient.

INFORMATION RELEVANT TO MEDICAL AND RADIATION ONCOLOGISTS

Medical oncologists will work within the multidisciplinary group to determine if identified HCCs can be managed via a localized approach such as surgery, interventional radiology, or stereotactic body radiation therapy versus those that may be multifocal or metastatic and not amenable to such treatment. For those who do undergo locoregional treatment, determining the initial success and ongoing response is critical with regard to the timing of additional therapeutic interventions. For those with more advanced disease, a medical oncologist will be interested in the presence of metastases, such as locoregional lymphadenopathy, distant lymphadenopathy, and bone metastases so it can guide the timing and determination of response to systemic therapy. Importantly, the LI-RADS treatment response algorithm is currently designed for patients receiving locoregional therapy only; therefore, it is important to be aware that it should currently not be applied to patients receiving systemic therapy.

Radiation oncologists are also commonly involved in the care of patients with HCC and there is increasing use of stereotactic body radiation therapy, either with or without systemic therapy as an additional treatment option. HCC treated with stereotactic body radiation therapy has been shown to demonstrate persistent arterial phase hyperenhancement for at least 12 months after stereotactic body radiation therapy, which does not necessarily indicate a viable neoplasm. Future updates of the LI-RADS treatment response algorithm will take this into account in a more systematic way, as new data emerge in the literature. For the current algorithm, often radiologists report this as LR-TR equivocal because they cannot accurately assess for the presence of residual viable neoplasm within this timeframe.[21]

INFORMATION RELEVANT TO FAMILY PRACTITIONERS AND FAMILY PHYSICIANS

Although the majority of patients at high risk of developing HCC will be under the care of a hospital-based physician and be followed-up with

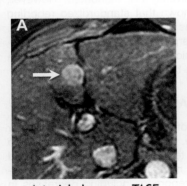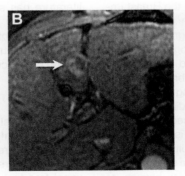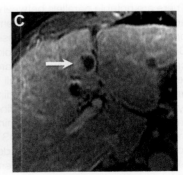

Arterial phase pre-TACE

Arterial phase 1-mo post-TACE

PV phase MR 1-mo post-TACE

Fig. 2. A 64-year-old man with ethanol-induced cirrhosis underwent transarterial chemoembolization (TACE). (*A*) Pretreatment hyperenhancing appearance. (*B*) At 1 month after TACE. (*C*) At 3 months after TACE there is still some degree of nodular enhancement of the HCC, indicating viable disease. This information is important for interventional radiologists as well as the treating team to determine the best management option for this patient.

an HCC-specific multidisciplinary case conference, it remains important that the family physician be familiar with and understand the nomenclature of the LI-RADS algorithm. This practice may help them to guide patient management and follow-up imaging so as to ensure that patients proceed with their planned treatment or surveillance pathway. Many patients return to their family physician to seek advice or question why they are having certain diagnostic tests or treatment; familiarity with the LI-RADS algorithm will aid family physicians to reassure and help provide supportive advice to their patients. Having specific recommendations in radiology reports, which also specify the recommended type and frequency of follow-up, may help to ensure that best practices are followed. In the study by Alenazi and colleagues,[16] the majority of physicians who are not surgeons and particularly those working outside an academic institution preferred to receive specific management recommendations (as provided in LI-RADS reports).

FEEDBACK FROM THOSE WHO RECEIVE OUR REPORTS

Getting feedback and input about what should go into a report from our colleagues who receive these radiology reports is very important and will help to ensure the reports remain relevant to surgeons and clinicians. As in radiology, changes are ongoing in other specialties, including new therapies and interventions. Therefore, to ensure ongoing high-quality reports, yearly surveys or feedback forms can be considered.[22]

GENERAL AND UNIVERSAL COMMUNICATIONS

There are notable parallels between the Breast Imaging Reporting and Data System (BI-RADS) in breast imaging and the general design of LI-RADS. Both implement standard terminology, have a 5-category system, and have standard management recommendations. In BI-RADS, all breast findings are included in this system, including various subtypes of cancers as well as benign findings, although the exact diagnosis is not determined from imaging.[20] In contradistinction, LI-RADS is applied only to adult patients at risk for HCC. Additional caveats exist as well; for example, this system should not be used in patients who have vascular causes of cirrhosis such as Budd-Chiari syndrome or cardiac cirrhosis (eg, post-Fontan procedure) because the imaging appearance of benign vascular lesions and HCC overlap.[14] These causes of chronic liver disease are rare and, to preserve the high specificity of imaging diagnosis of HCC, it was determined that

these small groups of patients should not have the LI-RADS criteria applied at the time of image interpretation.

Another difference between BI-RADS and LI-RADS is that BI-RADS depends almost entirely on biopsy to make the final diagnosis, especially for malignant lesions, whereas HCC can be diagnosed solely on imaging characteristics. LI-RADS has a few additional categories in the diagnostic categories, including LR-NC (noncategorizable), which indicates that the imaging quality or patient factors may have led to imaging quality that is not sufficient for assigning a final LI-RADS category.[23] There is also a separate tumor-in-vein category that has been created. The presence of enhancing material within either a hepatic or portal vein indicates the presence of tumor extension into the vessels, portends a worse clinical outcome for patients, and limits therapeutic options. This information is crucial for surgeons and hepatologists in management and decision-making and, therefore, has been felt to be of sufficient importance to have its own diagnostic category (**Fig. 3**). LI-RADS also has a category called LR-M (malignant).[23] Given that LI-RADS was specifically designed to assess the imaging characteristics of HCC, patients may still have other types of malignancies that develop in the liver. These include cholangiocarcinoma as well as metastases from other primaries. If an observation does not have the imaging characteristics expected for HCC, the LR-M category should be applied because the diagnosis often requires biopsy and the treatment options are very different than those for HCC.[24]

BI-RADS have become mandated for use in imaging reports and is required internationally as a feature of accreditation. Other systems, including LI-RADS are currently not mandated. However, literature has shown that standardized reporting systems such as TI-RADS (for thyroid nodules), PI-RADS (for interpreting prostate MRI) are important for communication standardization and maintaining evidence-based information.[25]

RADIOLOGIST ADDING VALUE

The major goal of a radiology report is to deliver timely, accurate, and actionable information to the patient care team and the patient. Structured reporting offers multiple advantages over traditional free-text reporting, including decreases in diagnostic errors, greater comprehensiveness, adherence to national consensus guidelines, revenue capture, data collection, and research.[12] Various technological innovations in dictation systems can enhance integration of structured reporting into everyday clinical practice.

60 yr   old with EtOH cirrhosis

| Arterial phase | PVP | Delayed Phase |

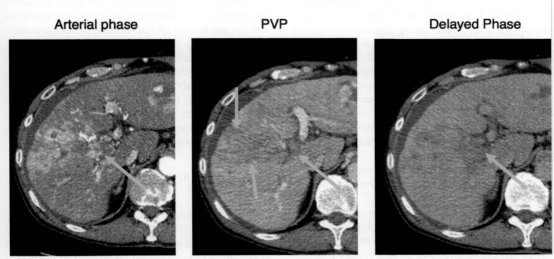

Fig. 3. One of key roles of radiologists is to identify tumor in vein as this changes management. Bland thrombus versus tumor in vein can be challenging to differentiate and small branch tumor-in-vein is also difficult. Tumor thrombus usually shows connection to an invading tumor, enhancement on a computed tomography scan and MRI with diffusion restriction. It also may expand the vessel lumen, which is less common than with bland thrombus. PVP, portal venous phase.

KEY INFORMATION TO INCLUDE IN THE RADIOLOGY REPORTING TEMPLATES

There are a number of institutions that have implemented synoptic reports for imaging, including specific ones for reporting in patients at risk for HCC. There are different versions available for download from various websites, including the ACR LI-RADS website.[3]

Key information for inclusion in a synoptic report includes the following:
a) Number and size of HCC, when present.
b) The size measurement is on the axial plane, in the longest dimension, using the same plane and imaging area as previously, if there are previous for comparison.
c) The segment(s) of liver involved.
d) Whether there is tumor thrombus or bland thrombus in the hepatic or portal veins.
e) The imaging characteristics (specifically the major imaging features).
f) The final LI-RADS category.

When an observation is identified, ideally the series and image number should be included for each observation. This practice allows for easier follow-up as well as a more efficient evaluation at a multidisciplinary case conference.

By encouraging all radiologists to report imaging using these templates, all key information is readily available for radiologists presenting cases at a multidisciplinary case conference. Tt also allows for more concrete provision of feedback to reporting radiologists if a discrepancy is subsequently identified.

ROLE OF RADIOLOGISTS AT MULTIDISCIPLINARY CASE CONFERENCES

Radiologists often perform a central role at multidisciplinary case conferences. They show and describe the imaging related to each patient and may sometimes serve as time keepers to ensure all patient issues are discussed in the time provided. Proximity to vessels for surgical planning versus locoregional therapy is often discussed at the multidisciplinary case conference. Discussion about need for biopsy or if patient should go straight to intervention/local therapy based on LR-4 category. They may also be asked if there are ancillary features that may help in decision-making.

Discussions at multidisciplinary case conferences often include technical issues with imaging quality that may affect accuracy. Based on this need, surgeons may ask how confident is the radiologist of their LI-RADS category if there are technical issues. The quality of imaging is key to ensuring the visualization of key findings related to HCC, especially in the late arterial phase. Patients who cannot hold their breath or have large volume ascites can have a poor quality of MRI. As a result, this particular group of patients may have better image quality with computed tomography scans, given that it has faster temporal image acquisition. However, many ancillary features related to the imaging observations are only evaluable on MRI; therefore, this modality may be the desired imaging in some cases (**Fig. 4**). Discussions related to these general topics can take place at multidisciplinary case conference to ensure that future patient imaging requests take into account these patient factors, thereby increasing the likelihood of obtaining diagnostic quality images.

Challenges in reporting postlocoregional therapy for HCC led to the development of LI-RADS tumor response algorithm in 2017.[26] Differences exist in expected appearances for various time points after each therapy. The combination of therapies over the years highlights the importance of providing a comprehensive clinical history and underscores the importance of 2-way communication with the radiologist. Without an appropriate clinical history, imaging is more challenging and sometimes impossible to interpret. Similarly, patients being assessed after yttrium-90 therapy for HCC are challenging and more research is needed for better understanding of the temporal changes including appearance of treated rather than viable tumor.

Some of the challenging issues that have been identified at multidisciplinary case conferences include the lack of an appropriate history provided to the reporting radiologists regarding prior interventions. This factor can make otherwise straightforward cases challenging to interpret and lead to errors. It is important to remember that opportunities arise for feedback from multidisciplinary case conference findings and the resulting decisions to the radiologists who created the original report in the form of peer-learning opportunities.[26]

FUTURE INCORPORATION OF ARTIFICIAL INTELLIGENCE

Artificial intelligence is a growing field with many near future applications in radiology, including standard report generation in HCC.[27] Information about an observation can be extracted from MRI and computed tomography imaging, including the temporal data after contrast enhancement to help identify major imaging features and integrate them to determine the optimal LI-RADS category. Although this type of information is not yet in mainstream use in clinical practice, it has the potential to increase the accuracy of

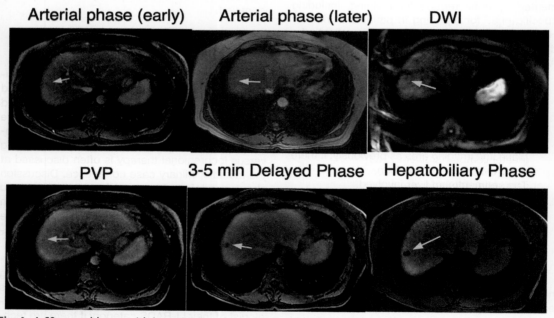

Fig. 4. A 60-year-old man with hepatitis C cirrhosis. There a hypointense observation in segment 7/8 on the arterial phase, which seems to have a subtle capsule in the portal venous phase (PVP) and is hypointense to the parenchyma on PVP. It is 9 mm in size. Given its size and major imaging characteristics, this would be classified as LR-3. However the hypointensity on delayed imaging after gadoxetic acid is an ancillary finding in favor of malignancy; therefore, this lesion could be categorized as LR-4. DWI, diffusion-weighted imaging.

the final diagnosis and help with future improvements of LI-RADS. The use of deep learning models for the assessment of tumor response is also underway using meta-data of expected imaging findings.[28]

SUMMARY

LI-RADs was created by radiologists as well as clinicians and surgeons and designed as a living document that is updated on a regular basis, based on available published evidence. This system was created to be used by all radiologists in all work settings to ensure that all clinicians, regardless of specialty, could speak the same language. Furthermore, standard terminology and reporting templates both help to improve communication between specialties and between medical centers, as well as in ongoing research, with the ultimate goal of improving future patient care.

CLINICS CARE POINTS

- There are many stakeholders involved in the care of patients at high risk for developing HCC, including clinicians, surgeons, and pathologists. Clear communications between specialties in medicine is associated with better patient outcomes.

- The use of a standardized reporting template such as LI-RADS helps to apply consistent terminology, decrease variability in image interpretation, and improve the clarity of communication.

- The major goal of a radiology report is to deliver timely, accurate, and actionable information to the patient care team and the patient. Structured reporting offers multiple advantages over traditional free-text reporting, including fewer diagnostic errors, greater comprehensiveness, adherence to national consensus guidelines, revenue capture, data collection, and research.

DISCLOSURE

The authors have nothing to disclose.

REFERENCES

1. Moon AM, Singal AG, Tapper EB. Contemporary Epidemiology of Chronic Liver Disease and Cirrhosis. Clin Gastroenterol Hepatol 2020;18(12):2650–66.

2. Sirlin CB. The LI-RADS adventure—a personal statement. Abdom Radiol 2018;43:1–2.

3. LI-RADS Web Application. Available: http://lirads.net/. Accessed: October 10, 2020.

4. Marrero JA, Kulik LM, Sirlin CB, et al. Diagnosis, staging, and management of hepatocellular carcinoma: 2018 practice guidance by the American Association for the Study of Liver Diseases. Hepatology 2018;68(2):723–50.

5. Renzulli M, Clemente A, Brocchi S, et al. LI-RADS: a great opportunity not to be missed. Eur J Gastroenterol Hepatol 2019;31(3):283–8.

6. Weiss DL, Langlotz CP. Structured reporting: patient care enhancement or productivity nightmare? Radiology 2008;249(3):739–47.

7. Brook OR, Brook A, Vollmer CM, et al. Structured reporting of multiphasic CT for pancreatic cancer: potential effect on staging and surgical planning. Radiology 2015;274(2):464–72.

8. Schwartz LH, Panicek DM, Berk AR. Improving Communication of through Structured Reporting. Radiology 2011;260(1):174–81.

9. Goldberg-Stein S, Walter WR, Amis ES, et al. Implementing a Structured Reporting Initiative Using a Collaborative Multistep Approach. Curr Probl Diagn Radiol 2017;46:295–9.

10. Boland GW, Glenn L, Goldberg-Stein S, et al. Report of the ACR's Economics Committee on Value-Based Payment Models. J Am Coll Radiol 2017;14(1):6–14.

11. Wald C, Russo MW, Heimbach JK, et al. New OPTN/UNOS policy for liver transplant allocation: standardization of liver imaging, diagnosis, classification, and reporting of hepatocellular carcinoma. Radiology 2013;266(2):376–82.

12. Flusberg M, Ganeles J, Ekinci T, et al. Impact of a structured report template on the quality of CT and MRI reports for hepatocellular carcinoma diagnosis. J Am Coll Radiol 2017;14(9):1206–11.

13. Tania Rahman W, Hussain HK, Parikh ND, et al. Reinterpretation of outside hospital MRI abdomen examinations in patients with cirrhosis: is the OPTN mandate necessary? Am J Roentgenol 2016;207(4):782–8.

14. Kielar AZ, Chernyak V, Bashir MR, et al. LI-RADS 2017: an update. J Magn Reson Imaging 2018;47(6):1459–74.

15. Ringe KI, Gut A, Grenacher L, et al. LI-RADS in the year 2020 – are you already using it or still considering? RöFo - Fortschritte auf dem Gebiet der Röntgenstrahlen und der Bildgeb. Verfahren 2020;193(2):186–93.

16. Alenazi AO, Elsayes KM, Marks RM, et al. Clinicians and surgeon survey regarding current and future versions of CT/MRI LI-RADS. Abdom Radiol (NY) 2020;45(8):2603–11.

17. Elsayes KM, Kielar AZ, Elmohr MM, et al. White paper of the Society of Abdominal Radiology

hepatocellular carcinoma diagnosis disease-focused panel on LI-RADS v2018 for CT and MRI. Abdom Radiol (NY) 2018;43(10):2625–42.

18. Castiella A, Alústiza JM, Emparanza JI, et al. Liver iron concentration quantification by MRI: are recommended protocols accurate enough for clinical practice? Eur Radiol 2011;21(1):137–41.

19. Mazzaferro V, Regalia E, Doci R, et al. Liver transplantation for the treatment of small hepatocellular carcinomas in patients with cirrhosis. N Engl J Med 1996;334(11):693–9.

20. Zhu F, Rhim H. Thermal ablation for hepatocellular carcinoma: what's new in 2019. Chin Clin Oncol 2019;8(6):58.

21. Mendiratta-Lala M, Masch W, Shankar PR, et al. Magnetic resonance imaging evaluation of hepatocellular carcinoma treated with stereotactic body radiation therapy: long term imaging follow-up. Int J Radiat Oncol Biol Phys 2019;103(1):169–79.

22. McMenamy J, Rosenkrantz AB, Jacobs J, et al. Use of a referring physician survey to direct and evaluate department-wide radiology quality improvement efforts. J Am Coll Radiol 2015;12(11):1223–5.

23. Mitchell DG, Bruix J, Sherman M, et al. LI-RADS (Liver Imaging Reporting and Data System): summary, discussion, and consensus of the LI-RADS Management Working Group and future directions. Hepatology 2015;61(3):1056–65.

24. Kim MY, Joo I, Kang HJ, et al. LI-RADS M (LR-M) criteria and reporting algorithm of v2018: diagnostic values in the assessment of primary liver cancers on gadoxetic acid-enhanced MRI. Abdom Radiol (NY) 2020;45(8):2440–8.

25. An JY, Unsdorfer KML, Weinreb JC. BI-RADS, C-RADS, CAD-RADS, LI-RADS, Lung-RADS, NI-RADS, O-RADS, PI-RADS, TI-RADS: reporting and data systems. Radiogr A Rev Publ Radiol Soc North Am Inc 2019;39(5):1435–6.

26. Shi W, Kuang S, Cao S, et al. Deep learning assisted differentiation of hepatocellular carcinoma from focal liver lesions: choice of four-phase and three-phase CT imaging protocol. Abdom Radiol (NY) 2020; 45(9):2688–97.

27. Giordano S, Takeda S, Donadon M, et al. Rapid automated diagnosis of primary hepatic tumour by mass spectrometry and artificial intelligence. Liver Int 2020;40(12):3117–24.

28. Morshid A, Elsayes KM, Khalaf AM, et al. A machine learning model to predict hepatocellular carcinoma response to transcatheter arterial chemoembolization. Radiol Artif Intell 2019;1(5):e180021.

Role of Ultrasound for Chronic Liver Disease and Hepatocellular Carcinoma Surveillance

Hailey H. Choi, MD[a], Shuchi K. Rodgers, MD[b], Aman Khurana, MD[c],
Leslie W. Nelson, DO[c], Aya Kamaya, MD[d],*

KEYWORDS

- Ultrasound • HCC surveillance • Chronic liver disease • Ultrasound elastography
- Hepatocellular carcinoma

KEY POINTS

- Ultrasound plays a key role in the evaluation of chronic liver disease, which includes assessment for fibrosis and cirrhosis, hepatic vasculature, and portal hypertension.
- The goal of ultrasound surveillance is to detect preclinical hepatocellular (HCC) at an early stage, when it can be potentially cured to improve survival.
- Semiannual ultrasound HCC surveillance is recommended by all liver societies worldwide.
- Ultrasound surveillance has many advantages, is well tolerated by most patients without adverse effects of intravenous contrast administration, and has very few limitations.

INTRODUCTION

Chronic liver disease can result from many etiologies, including chronic hepatitis B and C viral infections (HBV, HCV), metabolic disease, such as nonalcoholic fatty liver disease (NAFLD), nonalcoholic steatohepatitis (NASH), and excessive alcohol use. Persistent inflammation of the liver leads to the deposition of fibrotic scar tissue, eventually culminating in cirrhosis. Complications of cirrhosis include portal hypertension, hepatic decompensation, variceal bleeding, and hepatocellular carcinoma (HCC) development. Ultrasound plays a vital role in evaluating patients with chronic liver disease to offer prognostic information, and subsequently to monitor disease severity and detect portal hypertension. Furthermore, ultrasound screens patients who are at risk for HCC. In this article, we highlight the role of ultrasound in the evaluation of chronic liver disease and HCC surveillance and summarize major advantages and limitations of ultrasound.

ROLE FOR ULTRASOUND IN CHRONIC LIVER DISEASE

Ultrasound plays a crucial role in the evaluation and management of chronic liver disease. Ultrasound can evaluate the hepatic parenchyma for echogenicity and surface nodularity, liver fibrosis, vessel patency, and manifestations of portal hypertension. Notably, NAFLD and NASH have

[a] Department of Radiology and Biomedical Imaging, University of California San Francisco, 1001 Potrero Avenue Building 5 Room 1X57, San Francisco, CA 94110, USA; [b] Department of Radiology, Sidney Kimmel Medical College at Thomas Jefferson University, Einstein Healthcare Network, Levy Ground, 5501 Old York Road, Philadelphia, PA 19141, USA; [c] Department of Radiology, University of Kentucky, 800 Rose Street, HX 316, Lexington, KY 40536, USA; [d] Department of Radiology, Stanford University, 300 Pasteur Drive H1307, Stanford, CA 94305, USA
* Corresponding author.
E-mail address: kamaya@stanford.edu

Magn Reson Imaging Clin N Am 29 (2021) 279–290
https://doi.org/10.1016/j.mric.2021.05.005

steadily increased in prevalence over the past 3 decades,[1] with NAFLD and NASH affecting 25% and 2% to 5% of the general population in 2016, respectively.[2] Other major etiologies of chronic liver disease include chronic HBV and HCV, and alcohol-related liver disease (ALD).[3] Evolution from NAFLD to NASH rests on a complex interplay between liver cells and pathologic signals from the gut and adipose tissues.[4] Persistent inflammation and fibrogenesis can lead to cirrhosis. Although NAFLD progresses to cirrhosis less predictably and at a slower rate than HCV, and has a lower risk of HCC compared with HCV, cirrhosis, or alcoholic cirrhosis, the sheer number of patients affected by NAFLD results in a greater number of patients with eventual NASH-induced cirrhosis and potential HCC development.[5]

Chronic HBV and HCV are 2 important etiologies of chronic liver disease worldwide. HBV is highly prevalent in Asia-Pacific and sub-Saharan regions, whereas HCV is more evenly distributed. Globally, HBV involves 3.5% of the world's population, and HCV 1%.[6] Unlike HCV, HBV integrates itself into the host DNA and may be directly implicated in HCC pathogenesis.[7] HCV infection alters lipid metabolism, and is associated with coexisting NAFLD.[8] Although new antiviral regimens are more widely available and can result in cure, persistent infection with HCV can lead to cirrhosis. ALD is another major cause of liver disease and cirrhosis-related mortality worldwide.[3] Its prevalence has ranged from 0.8% to 1% over the past 3 decades.[1] The by-products of alcohol metabolism result in increased fat accumulation and inflammation in the liver and ultimately cirrhosis.[9]

Evaluation of Fibrosis and Cirrhosis

Persistent and chronic inflammation from chronic liver disease leads to the accumulation of fibrosis and eventually to cirrhosis. Ultrasound findings of cirrhosis include heterogeneous and coarse echotexture of the liver, nodular contour of the hepatic surface best seen with high-frequency transducer (**Fig. 1**), lobar redistribution with caudate and left hepatic lobe hypertrophy, and relative reduction in the size of the right hepatic lobe.[10] Although these findings are suggestive of cirrhosis, interobserver variability may lead to variable sensitivity.[10] Fibrosis staging is a key factor in determining disease prognosis and surveillance and treatment strategies.[11,12] Although liver biopsy with histologic evaluation is the gold standard for fibrosis diagnosis and staging,[13] it is an invasive procedure with risk of potentially serious complications such as hemorrhage, vasovagal response, infection, pneumothorax, and

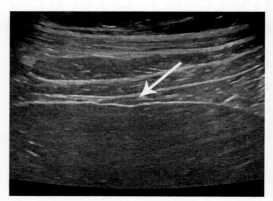

Fig. 1. Ultrasound image of the right liver surface using a high-frequency transducer in a 72-year-old woman with fatty liver disease reveals subtle surface nodularity (*arrow*), compatible with cirrhosis.

even death.[14,15] Furthermore, liver biopsy is subject to sampling error due to the small liver sample obtained.[16] Because of these reasons, noninvasive imaging-based methods of fibrosis evaluation, including ultrasound shear wave elastography and magnetic resonance elastography, are increasingly used.

Imaging-based ultrasound shear wave elastography (point shear wave elastography pSWE and 2D-SWE) is available on most conventional ultrasound machines and uses acoustic radiation force impulse (ARFI) to create shear waves within the visualized portion of the liver.[17] Ultrasound measures the speed of the resulting shear waves, which propagate perpendicular to the ARFI. This shear wave speed estimates Young's modulus, a measure of tissue elasticity. pSWE interrogates a single point of interest, while 2D-SWE evaluates multiple focal zones, resulting in a broader region of interest.[17] Real-time grayscale imaging ensures assessment of a homogeneous part of the liver parenchyma, free of vessels and masses (**Fig. 2**).[12] Ultrasound elastography accurately identifies advanced fibrosis and cirrhosis (area under the receiver operating characteristic curve of 0.88 and 0.91, respectively[18]). Thus, patients with advanced fibrosis and cirrhosis, who are at high risk of developing HCC and portal hypertension complications, can be identified, closely monitored, and treated.

Vessel Patency

As chronic liver disease progresses to cirrhosis, intrahepatic vascular resistance increases and portal blood flow into the liver decreases.[19] In addition to many other factors, such as imbalances in the hemostasis mechanism, this stagnant blood flow

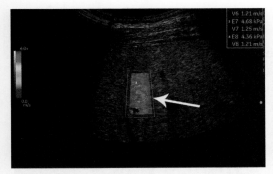

Fig. 2. Ultrasound elastography in a 37-year-old man with NAFLD. Grayscale ultrasound imaging via an intercostal approach allows accurate placement of the elastogram (*arrow*) within a homogeneous area of the right liver. Elastogram reveals low stiffness. Shear wave speed and Young's modulus are measured (*circle*).

increases the risk for developing venous thrombosis. In advanced cirrhosis, the risk of portal venous thrombosis (PVT) increases,[20] and ultrasound is often the first-line imaging modality for evaluation.[20] Ultrasound findings of PVT include echogenic material obstructing the lumen of the portal vein with complete or partial absence of flow on Doppler imaging.[21] Contrast-enhanced ultrasound (CEUS) can differentiate thrombus from stagnant portal vein flow that is too slow to detect by traditional Doppler interrogation.[22] Ultrasound also distinguishes benign thrombus from malignant tumor in vein, by demonstrating internal vascularity (eg, arterial waveforms) and/or contrast enhancement at CEUS (**Figs. 3** and **4**).[23]

Doppler ultrasound can also be used to evaluate the hepatic veins and arteries. Patency of the hepatic veins can be easily assessed with color Doppler, thereby excluding the diagnosis of Budd-Chiari syndrome as a potential cause of hepatic decompensation. Spectral Doppler can be used to assess hepatic venous waveforms that may be altered in chronic liver disease; decreased liver compliance caused by fibrotic, inflammatory, or fatty changes in the liver can result in dampening of the normally triphasic hepatic waveforms.[24] With cirrhosis and portal hypertension, hepatic arterial flow increases via the hepatic arterial buffer response to compensate for the relatively diminished portal venous inflow.[24,25] In patients awaiting liver transplantation, hepatic arterial evaluation is important to exclude preexisting hepatic arterial pathology, such as celiac artery atherosclerosis or median arcuate ligament syndrome, which may compromise the hepatic allograft and require correction before transplant.[26]

Evaluation for Portal Hypertension

Ultrasound detects stigmata of portal hypertension and associated morphologic changes of the liver. Normal portal venous flow is characterized by continuous hepatopetal flow toward the liver with peak velocities of 20 to 40 cm/s.[24] Portal hypertension occurs when the intrahepatic resistance exceeds the passive pressure of the spleen and splanchnic portal venous return, and can result in the following: low portal vein velocity less than 16 cm/s, dilated main portal vein (13 mm or greater in diameter), reversal of portal vein flow direction (eg, flow in a hepatofugal direction), and increase in portosystemic collaterals.[27] The latter 2 findings are pathognomonic for portal hypertension.[10] Common portosystemic collaterals include

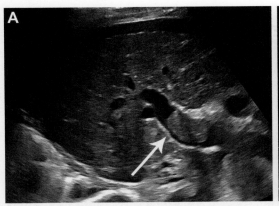
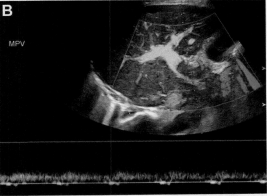

Fig. 3. 57-year-old man with chronic HBV. Grayscale imaging (*A*) of the main portal vein reveals echogenic thrombus (*arrow*) nearly occluding the vessel lumen. Color and spectral Doppler interrogation (*B*) demonstrates low-resistance arterial vascularity within the thrombus, consistent with tumor in vein. New thrombus in vein, whether tumor in vein or bland thrombus, qualifies an HCC surveillance ultrasound examination as US-3, Positive, and further diagnostic evaluation with a multiphase contrast-enhanced imaging study is recommended.

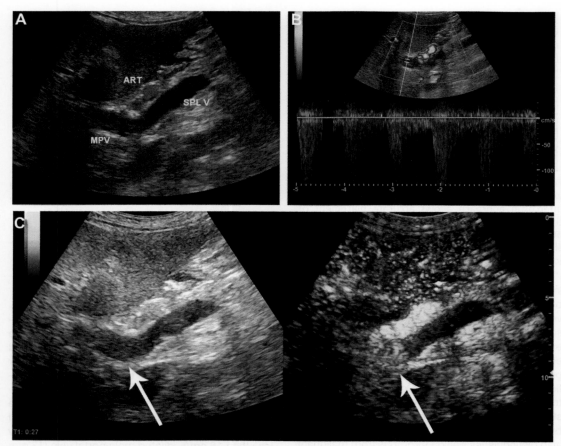

Fig. 4. Tumor in vein in a 73-year-old man with newly diagnosed HCC. (*A*) Grayscale image at the porta hepatis reveals echogenic thrombus within the main portal vein (MPV). Splenic vein (SPLV) and common hepatic artery (ART) are adjacent. (*B*) Spectral Doppler interrogation reveals arterial waveforms within the echogenic area of the portal vein compatible with tumor thrombus. (*C*) CEUS was performed. In the arterial phase at 27 seconds following contrast injection, there is avid enhancement of the portal vein (*arrows*), and nonenhancement of the splenic vein. Findings are diagnostic for tumor in vein in the portal vein and bland thrombus in the splenic vein.

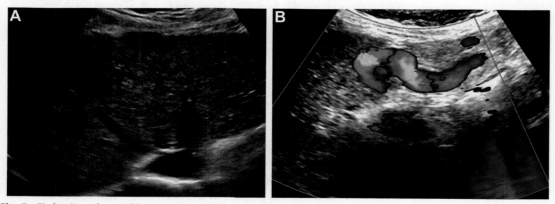

Fig. 5. Cirrhosis and portal hypertension with recanalized paraumbilical vein. Transverse grayscale image of the left hepatic lobe (*A*) demonstrates coarse hepatic echotexture and surface nodularity compatible with cirrhosis. Color Doppler image of the falciform ligament in the left lobe (*B*) demonstrates flow within a large recanalized paraumbilical vein, specific for portal hypertension.

recanalized paraumbilical veins or perisplenic varices (**Fig. 5**).[28] Splenomegaly and ascites are other features of portal hypertension and decompensated cirrhosis, respectively, that are easily diagnosed with ultrasound. Although the presence of one or more features can confirm the diagnosis of portal hypertension, these imaging features individually have moderate sensitivity, particularly in the setting of compensated cirrhosis.[10]

ULTRASOUND IN HEPATOCELLULAR CARCINOMA SCREENING AND SURVEILLANCE

HCC is cancer of the hepatocytes. HCC is the sixth most common cause of cancer but the second leading cause of cancer-related death in the world.[29] HCC typically only occurs in patients with chronic liver disease, with the most common risk factors including HBV (with or without cirrhosis), HCV cirrhosis, and alcoholic cirrhosis.[30] Due to the sheer numbers of people developing NASH worldwide, this is an additional increasing etiology of cirrhosis that can lead to an increased risk of HCC.[30]

As HCC is so prevalent and lethal, proper screening and surveillance of at-risk patients improves survival.[31–37] The goal of screening and surveillance is to detect HCC at an early stage, when cure is potentially achievable either with local therapy or with liver transplantation. Semiannual surveillance has been shown to be the optimal imaging interval for detection of HCC.[31,38–41]

In the context of HCC, screening is the term used for the application of a diagnostic test to the population at risk, but without any reason to suspect already having the disease. Surveillance is the repeated application of the same diagnostic test at a defined time interval.

The decision to offer cancer screening to an asymptomatic population is contingent on the following criteria[42]:

1. The disease is an important health problem
2. There is an identifiable target population
3. Treatment of occult disease is advantageous to treatment of symptomatic disease
4. Screening test is cost-effective and affordable
5. The test is acceptable to the population and provider
6. There are standardized recall procedures
7. There is an acceptable level of accuracy

Ultrasound fulfills the preceding criteria and has proven to be the best test for detecting HCC.[31,38–41] In patients who are not ideal ultrasound candidates, transplant candidates, or patients who have current or prior HCC, alternative imaging methods for HCC screening such as contrast-enhanced computed tomography (CT) or MRI may be considered.[31] Of note, CEUS has not been validated in the screening and

Table 1
Comparison of major hepatology societies' recommendations for HCC surveillance in at-risk populations

Etiology of Liver Disease	JSH 2019	APASL 2019	KLCSG-NCC 2018	EASL 2018	AASLD 2018	LI-RADS 2017
Non-cirrhotic HBV carriers	+	+[a]	+	+[b]	+[b]	+[a]
Chronic HCV	+	−	+	−	−	−
HCV with severe (bridging) liver fibrosis	+	−	+	+[c]	−	−
Cirrhosis	+	+	+	+	+	+
Child-Pugh C cirrhosis	−	−	−	−	−	−
Child-Pugh C cirrhosis awaiting liver transplant	−	−	−	+[d]	+[d]	+[d]

Abbreviations: +, HCC surveillance is recommended; −, HCC surveillance is not recommended. AASLD, American Association for the Study of Liver Diseases; APASL, Asian Pacific Association for the Study of the Liver; EASL, European Association for the Study of the Liver; HBV, hepatitis B virus; HCV, hepatitis C virus; JSH, Japan Society of Hepatology; KLCSG-NCC, Korean Liver Cancer Study Group – National Cancer Center; LI-RADS, Liver Imaging Reporting And Data System.
 [a] Surveillance recommended for subgroups of HBV carriers: Asian man older than 40, Asian woman older than 50, those with family history of HCC, African and/or North American black individuals (older than 20 per APASL).[39,50]
 [b] EASL recommends surveillance in non-cirrhotic patients with HBV at intermediate or high risk, depending on PAGE-B score ≥ 10 (Platelet, Age, Gender, hepatitis B).[41]
 [c] EASL states weak recommendations for surveillance in patients with advanced fibrosis of any etiology[41].
 [d] For cirrhotic patients awaiting liver transplantation, surveillance is recommended, although there is no society consensus guideline on modality or time interval.

surveillance setting and currently is used for characterization (rather than detection) of focal liver lesions.

Current Guidelines

All major hepatology societies worldwide recommend ultrasound surveillance for HCC at 6-month intervals[31,38–41] (**Table 1**). This recommendation is based on multiple studies, including 2 randomized controlled trials in patients with chronic hepatitis in China that demonstrated significant survival benefits,[35,43] and dates back to 2003.[44] All societies recommend ultrasound, with or without tumor markers such as alpha fetoprotein (AFP), at 6-month intervals. Asian societies[38–40] recommend ultrasound with AFP; whereas the European and American societies recommend using ultrasound for screening and surveillance but do not make firm recommendations regarding AFP. All societies emphasize that chronic HBV infection and cirrhosis are major risk factors to warrant regular surveillance. Target populations for HCC surveillance vary slightly depending on regional preferences, reflecting differences in the etiology of chronic liver disease and management strategies. For example, there is a higher incidence of HBV infection in Asian countries; Japanese and Korean liver societies both recommend surveillance for all non-cirrhotic patients with HBV,[38,40] whereas the other societies only recommend surveillance for specific subgroups of HBV carriers.[31,39,41] Although there is some evidence suggesting that alcohol and NAFLD impact the development of HCC,[39,45] stronger evidence is needed to recommend surveillance for these individuals who have risk factors but have not yet progressed to cirrhosis.

American College of Radiology Ultrasound Liver Imaging Reporting and Data System

The American College of Radiology (ACR) introduced the Ultrasound Liver Imaging Reporting

Table 2
Summary of HCC surveillance ultrasound examination interpretation and reporting, per ACR US LI-RADS

Ultrasound Category	
US-1, Negative	No evidence of HCC: • No focal observations OR • Definitely benign observation. Management: return to ultrasound surveillance in 6 mo.
US-2, Subthreshold	Focal observation <10 mm in diameter that is not definitely benign. Management: short-interval 3–6 month follow-up ultrasound.
US-3, Positive	• Focal observation ≥ 10 mm that is not definitely benign OR • Geographic area of parenchymal distortion OR • New thrombus in vein Management: Multiphase contrast-enhanced CT, MRI, or CEUS
Visualization Score	
VIS-A, No or minimal limitations	• No limitations OR • Limitations are unlikely to affect examination sensitivity
VIS-B, Moderate limitations	Limitations may obscure small masses <10 mm. Examples include moderately heterogeneous liver parenchyma, moderate sound beam attenuation, or cases where some portions (<50%) of liver or liver/diaphragm interface are not well visualized.
VIS-C, Severe limitations	Limitations significantly lower examination sensitivity, where larger masses ≥ 10 mm may be obscured. Examples include severe parenchymal heterogeneity, severe sound beam attenuation, or cases where large portions (>50%) of the liver or liver/diaphragm interface are not visualized.

Abbreviations: ACR, American College of Radiology; CEUS, contrast-enhanced ultrasound; CT, computed tomography; US LI-RADS, Ultrasound Liver Imaging Reporting and Data System.
Adapted from ACR US LI-RADS Core Document[46]

and Data System (US LI-RADS) in 2017.[46] It provides guidelines for standardized imaging technique, interpretation, and next step recommendations for screening and surveillance ultrasound examinations in patients at risk for developing HCC. Imaging should be performed in a standard fashion, optimizing ultrasound scan parameters to image the entire liver.[47,48] Each examination is assigned an ultrasound category and a visualization score (**Table 2**). The ultrasound category summarizes the findings of the examination and directs next steps in management. There are 3 possible ultrasound categories: US-1 is a negative examination, in which there is no evidence of HCC (**Fig. 6**A); the recommendation is to return to ultrasound surveillance in 6 months. US-2 denotes a subthreshold examination, in which a focal observation less than 10 mm is

detected (**Fig. 6**B). A short-interval follow-up ultrasound in 3 to 6 months is recommended to detect any change; when the observation reaches the threshold size of 10 mm, it is considered US-3, or Positive, and a multiphase contrast-enhanced CT, MRI or CEUS is recommended. US-3 defines a positive examination. Findings that can lead to a positive examination include a focal observation at least 10 mm in diameter, a geographic area of parenchymal distortion, or a new thrombus in a vein (**Fig. 6**C, see **Figs 3** and **4**). All 3 scenarios prompt further evaluation with multiphase contrast-enhanced CT, MRI, or CEUS. These ultrasound categories are now incorporated into the 2018 American Association for the Study of Liver Diseases guidelines.[31]

The visualization score is a concept that is unique to US LI-RADS. The visualization score is

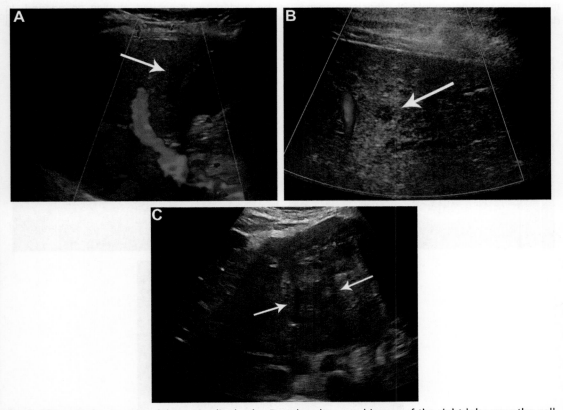

Fig. 6. Ultrasound categories. (*A*) Longitudinal color Doppler ultrasound image of the right lobe near the gallbladder shows a geographic region of relatively decreased echogenicity (*arrow*), against a background of hyperechoic liver parenchyma, consistent with focal fatty sparing, a benign finding. The remainder of the examination was normal, and it was categorized as US-1, Negative. (*B*) Transverse ultrasound image of the left lobe of the liver demonstrates a <1 cm in diameter hypoechoic observation (*arrow*), consistent with a US-2, Subthreshold examination, and short-interval follow-up ultrasound in 3 to 6 months is recommended. (*C*) Transverse ultrasound image of the left lobe of the liver reveals a large area of parenchymal distortion, without identifiable portal triads, with areas of refractive edge shadowing (*arrows*) due to infiltrative HCC. The examination was categorized as US-3, Positive.

analogous to the breast density categories with Breast Imaging Reporting and Data System, and conveys the expected level of sensitivity of the test but does not alter management. There are 3 possible visualization scores: VIS-A refers to an examination with no or minimal limitations: the liver is seen entirely or near-entirely. VIS-B, or moderate limitations, can result from parenchymal heterogeneity, sound beam attenuation or suboptimal acoustic windows, such that small masses (<10 mm) or small portions of the liver are obscured. VIS-C, or severe limitations, are felt to significantly lower the examination's sensitivity such that the sensitivity for large masses (>2 cm) may be obscured or difficult to delineate from the background liver (**Fig. 7**). This may result from marked parenchymal heterogeneity, sound beam attenuation, or poor acoustic windows, where large portions of the liver (>50%) are obscured. In the cases of suboptimal visualization, the decision to supplement with other imaging modalities may be made on an individual basis,

weighing risks, benefits, added costs, and potential adverse effects. Based on a multi-institutional review of US LI-RADS performance, only a small percentage (4.2%) fall into the VIS-C category.[49]

Advantages and Limitations for Ultrasound Surveillance

Numerous advantages of using ultrasound for screening and surveillance for HCC meet the World Health Organization criteria for a screening test. Ultrasound is well tolerated and can be performed at the patient's bedside or in the operating room, and even if the patient cannot lay flat (**Fig. 8**). Ultrasound is completely noninvasive, as it does not require an intravenous catheter. Furthermore, patients with renal insufficiency can safely undergo ultrasound without nephrotoxic iodinated or gadolinium intravenous contrast. Elastography, fat quantification, and CEUS can be added to ultrasound studies as needed. In interventional radiology, ultrasound is useful to

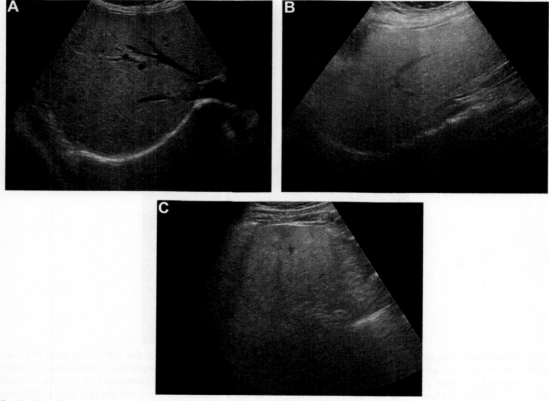

Fig. 7. Visualization scores. (*A*) The right liver is visualized in its entirety (VIS-A) on this transverse ultrasound image in a patient with chronic HCV and early cirrhosis. (*B*) Longitudinal image of the right hepatic lobe shows increased parenchymal echogenicity due to steatosis, which moderately limits the detection for HCC (VIS-B). The diaphragm is visualized almost entirely. (*C*) Severely limited visualization (VIS-C) due to significant sound beam attenuation, which leads to visualization of less than 50% of the diaphragm.

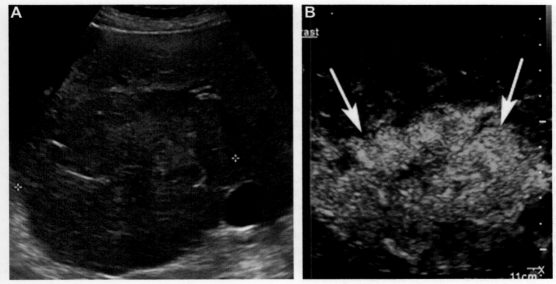

Fig. 8. CEUS LR-5 in a 70-year-old woman with cryptogenic cirrhosis and a liver observation on screening ultrasound. (*A*) A transverse ultrasound image shows a large area of architectural distortion (between calipers) in the right lobe of the liver. Patient was unable to lay flat due to hepatohydrothorax and could not undergo CT/MRI. CEUS shows arterial phase hyperenhancement of the nodule (*arrows* in *B*, 13 seconds), with mild, late washout (not shown), characterized as CEUS LR-5. (Images reprinted with permission from Clinical Liver Disease [Rodgers SK, Fetzer DT, Kono Y. Using LI-RADS with Contrast-Enhanced Ultrasound. Clinical Liver Disease 2021; 17(3):154-158. doi: 10.1002/cld.1077.])

guide procedures and biopsy, as it offers real-time, dynamic guidance without exposing the patient and operator to ionizing radiation. Doppler ultrasound assesses the hepatic vasculature and provides physiologic information, including portal flow direction, without the need for intravenous contrast (**Fig. 9**). Spectral waveform analysis can detect signs of right heart failure, portal hypertension, and arterial inflow problems. Certain artifacts encountered on CT/MRI (motion, streak, or beam-hardening artifact, pulsation artifact) are entirely avoided on ultrasound. Arterial-portal shunts or perfusional abnormalities are completely avoided on ultrasound; when these findings are present on contrast-enhanced CT/MRI examinations, it can lead to unnecessary follow-up studies.

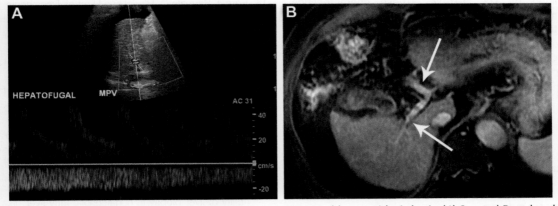

Fig. 9. Reversed direction of flow in the portal vein in a 73-year-old man with cirrhosis. (*A*) Spectral Doppler ultrasound evaluation of the MPV reveals reversed flow within the MPV, away from the liver (hepatofugal). Venous waveform is detected below the baseline, directed away from the ultrasound transducer (and hepatic parenchyma). (*B*) Contrast-enhanced MRI 3 weeks prior demonstrates contrast opacified portal veins at the hepatic hilum (*arrows*). Although the portal veins are patent, the direction of flow cannot be ascertained on MRI.

A distinct advantage over CT is the lack of ionizing radiation in ultrasound and MRI. Last, ultrasound is more cost-effective compared with CT and MRI.

The disadvantages of ultrasound are few. The most critical limitation is the operator dependency of ultrasound. A quality ultrasound department requires continual oversight and training of ultrasound technologists. Certain patients may not be conducive to ultrasound evaluation. MRI/CT offers a larger field of view and optimal imaging evaluation in patients with marked liver heterogeneity, severe steatosis, large body habitus, or when the liver is obscured by bowel gas, ascites, or rib shadows. Specific advantages of CT include a short examination time, making CT well tolerated by patients, and advanced imaging techniques in spectral/dual energy CT. Additional benefits of MRI include functional and advanced imaging techniques (elastography, diffusion-weighted imaging, iron quantification, proton density fat fraction), as well as higher soft tissue contrast compared with ultrasound and CT.

SUMMARY

Ultrasound is the primary imaging modality in the initial evaluation and continued monitoring of patients with chronic liver disease. Many etiologies of chronic liver disease can lead to cirrhosis and associated complications, such as portal hypertension, hepatic decompensation, and HCC. Advanced ultrasound technologies such as ultrasound shear wave elastography and CEUS can offer valuable additional diagnostic information, such as liver fibrosis grading and focal liver lesion characterization. For HCC surveillance, semiannual ultrasound is the universally recommended imaging modality in at-risk populations, as outlined by US LI-RADS. These characteristics make ultrasound invaluable in the imaging evaluation of the patient with chronic liver disease.

CLINICS CARE POINTS

- Ultrasound is an essential imaging modality in the setting of chronic liver disease.
- Chronic liver disease patients who are at risk for developing HCC should undergo ultrasound surveillance every 6 months.

DISCLOSURE

H.H. Choi, A. Khurana, L.W. Nelson, S.K. Rodgers: No disclosures. A. Kamaya: Book royalties, Elsevier.

REFERENCES

1. Younossi ZM, Stepanova M, Younossi Y, et al. Epidemiology of chronic liver diseases in the USA in the past three decades. Gut 2020;69(3):564.
2. Younossi ZM, Koenig AB, Abdelatif D, et al. Global epidemiology of nonalcoholic fatty liver disease-Meta-analytic assessment of prevalence, incidence, and outcomes. Hepatology 2016;64(1):73–84.
3. Asrani SK, Devarbhavi H, Eaton J, et al. Burden of liver diseases in the world. J Hepatol 2019;70(1):151–71.
4. Pierantonelli I, Svegliati-Baroni G. Nonalcoholic fatty liver disease: basic pathogenetic mechanisms in the progression from NAFLD to NASH. Transplantation 2019;103(1):e1–13.
5. Mahady SE, George J. Predicting the future burden of NAFLD and NASH. J Hepatol 2018;69(4):774–5.
6. World Health Organization. Global hepatitis report, 2017 [Internet]. 2017. p. 1–83. Available at: https://www.who.int/hepatitis/publications/global-hepatitis-report2017/en/. Accessed November 21, 2020.
7. Di Bisceglie AM. Hepatitis B and hepatocellular carcinoma. Hepatology 2009;49(SUPPL. 5):S56.
8. Lonardo A, Loria P, Adinolfi LE, et al. Hepatitis C and steatosis: a reappraisal. J Viral Hepat 2006;13(2):73–80.
9. Ceni E, Mello T, Galli A. Pathogenesis of alcoholic liver disease: role of oxidative metabolism. World J Gastroenterol 2014;20(47):17756–72.
10. Procopet B, Berzigotti A. Diagnosis of cirrhosis and portal hypertension: imaging, non-invasive markers of fibrosis and liver biopsy. Gastroenterol Rep 2017;5(2):79–89.
11. Lai M, Afdhal NH. Liver fibrosis determination. Gastroenterol Clin North Am 2019;48(2):281–9.
12. Barr RG, Wilson SR, Rubens D, et al. Update to the Society of Radiologists in Ultrasound Liver Elastography Consensus Statement. Radiology 2020;296(2):263–74.
13. Berg T, Sarrazin C, Hinrichsen H, et al. Does noninvasive staging of fibrosis challenge liver biopsy as a gold standard in chronic hepatitis C? Hepatology 2004;39(5):1456–7.
14. Tian G, Kong D, Jiang T, et al. Complications after percutaneous ultrasound-guided liver biopsy: a systematic review and meta-analysis of a population of more than 12,000 patients from 51 cohort studies. J Ultrasound Med 2020;39(7):1355–65.
15. Chi H, Hansen BE, Tang WY, et al. Multiple biopsy passes and the risk of complications of percutaneous liver biopsy. Eur J Gastroenterol Hepatol 2017;29(1):36–41.
16. Ratziu V, Charlotte F, Heurtier A, et al. Sampling variability of liver biopsy in nonalcoholic fatty liver disease. Gastroenterology 2005;128(7):1898–906.
17. Sigrist RMS, Liau J, Kaffas A El, et al. Ultrasound elastography: review of techniques and clinical applications. Theranostics 2017;7(5):1303–29.

18. Hu X, Qiu L, Liu D, et al. Acoustic Radiation Force Impulse (ARFI) elastography for non-invasive evaluation of hepatic fibrosis in chronic hepatitis B and C patients: a systematic review and meta-analysis. Med Ultrason 2017;19(1):23–31.

19. Harding DJ, Perera MTPR, Chen F, et al. Portal vein thrombosis in cirrhosis: controversies and latest developments. World J Gastroenterol 2015;21(22): 6769–84.

20. Mantaka A, Augoustaki A, Kouroumalis EA, et al. Portal vein thrombosis in cirrhosis: diagnosis, natural history, and therapeutic challenges. Ann Gastroenterol 2018;31(3):315–29.

21. Sacerdoti D, Serianni G, Gaiani S, et al. Thrombosis of the portal venous system. J Ultrasound 2007; 10(1):12–21.

22. Chawla YK, Bodh V. Portal vein thrombosis. J Clin Exp Hepatol 2015;5(1):22–40.

23. Tarantino L, Ambrosino P, Di Minno MND. Contrast-enhanced ultrasound in differentiating malignant from benign portal vein thrombosis in hepatocellular carcinoma. World J Gastroenterol 2015;21(32): 9457–60.

24. Iranpour P, Lall C, Houshyar R, et al. Altered Doppler flow patterns in cirrhosis patients: an overview [Internet]. Ultrasonography. Korean Society of Ultrasound in Medicine; 2015. p. 3–12.

25. Park HS, Desser TS, Jeffrey RB, et al. Doppler ultrasound in liver cirrhosis: correlation of hepatic artery and portal vein measurements with model for end-stage liver disease score. J Ultrasound Med 2017; 36(4):725–30.

26. Horrow MM, Huynh MHL, Callaghan MM, et al. Complications after liver transplant related to preexisting conditions: diagnosis, treatment, and prevention. Radiographics 2020;40(3):895–909.

27. Barr RG. Ultrasound of diffuse liver disease including elastography. Radiol Clin North Am 2019; 57(3):549–62.

28. Singal AK, Ahmad M, Soloway RD. Duplex Doppler ultrasound examination of the portal venous system: an emerging novel technique for the estimation of portal vein pressure. Dig Dis Sci 2010;55(5): 1230–40.

29. Fitzmaurice C, Akinyemiju TF, Al Lami FH, et al. Global, regional, and national cancer incidence, mortality, years of life lost, years lived with disability, and disability-adjusted life-years for 29 cancer groups, 1990 to 2016 a systematic analysis for the global burden of disease study global burden of disease cancer collaboration. JAMA Oncol 2018;4(11): 1553–68.

30. McGlynn KA, London WT. The global epidemiology of hepatocellular carcinoma: present and future. Clin Liver Dis 2011;15(2):223–43.

31. Marrero JA, Kulik LM, Sirlin CB, et al. Diagnosis, staging, and management of hepatocellular

carcinoma: 2018 practice guidance by the American Association for the Study of Liver Diseases. Hepatology 2018;68(2):723–50.

32. Amit S, Jorge AM. Screening for hepatocellular carcinoma. Gastroenterol Hepatol (N Y) 2008;4(3): 201–8.

33. Chen JG, Parkin DM, Chen QG, et al. Screening for liver cancer: results of a randomised controlled trial in Qidong, China. J Med Screen 2003;10(4):204–9.

34. Yeh YP, Hu TH, Cho PY, et al. Evaluation of abdominal ultrasonography mass screening for hepatocellular carcinoma in Taiwan. Hepatology 2014;59(5): 1840–9.

35. Zhang B-H, Yang B-H, Tang Z-Y. Randomized controlled trial of screening for hepatocellular carcinoma. J Cancer Res Clin Oncol 2004;130(7): 417–22.

36. Choi DT, Kum HC, Park S, et al. Hepatocellular carcinoma screening is associated with increased survival of patients with cirrhosis. Clin Gastroenterol Hepatol 2019;17(5):976–87.e4.

37. Mittal S, Kanwal F, Ying J, et al. Effectiveness of surveillance for hepatocellular carcinoma in clinical practice: a United States cohort. J Hepatol 2016; 65(6):1148–54.

38. Kokudo N, Takemura N, Hasegawa K, et al. Clinical practice guidelines for hepatocellular carcinoma: The Japan Society of Hepatology 2017 (4th JSH-HCC guidelines) 2019 update. Hepatol Res 2019; 49(10):1109–13.

39. Omata M, Cheng AL, Kokudo N, et al. Asia–Pacific clinical practice guidelines on the management of hepatocellular carcinoma: a 2017 update. Hepatol Int 2017;11(4):317–70.

40. Park JW, Lee JS, Suh KS, et al. 2018 Korean Liver Cancer Association-National Cancer Center Korea practice guidelines for the management of hepatocellular carcinoma. Gut Liver 2019;13(3):227–99.

41. Galle PR, Forner A, Llovet JM, et al. EASL clinical practice guidelines: management of hepatocellular carcinoma. J Hepatol 2018;69(1):182–236.

42. WHO Regional Office for Europe. Screening programmes: a short guide. Increase effectiveness, maximize benefits and minimize harm [Internet]. 2020. Available at: https://apps.who.int/iris/bitstream/handle/10665/330829/9789289054782-eng.pdf. Accessed November 21, 2020.

43. Yang B, Zhang B, Xu Y, et al. Prospective study of early detection for primary liver cancer. J Cancer Res Clin Oncol 1997;123(6):357–60.

44. Bruix J, Sherman M, Llovet JM, et al. Clinical management of hepatocellular carcinoma. Conclusions of the Barcelona-2000 EASL conference. J Hepatol 2001;35(3):421–30.

45. Cholankeril G, Patel R, Khurana S, et al. Hepatocellular carcinoma in non-alcoholic steatohepatitis:

current knowledge and implications for management. World J Hepatol 2017;9:533–43.

46. American College of Radiology. Ultrasound LI-RADS v2017 [Internet]. Available at: https://www.acr.org/Clinical-Resources/Reporting-and-Data-Systems/LI-RADS/Ultrasound-LI-RADS-v2017. Accessed November 21, 2020.

47. American College of Radiology. ACR–AIUM–SPR–SRU practice parameter for the performance of an ultrasound examination of the abdomen and/or retroperitoneum [Internet]. Available at: https://www.acr.org/-/media/ACR/Files/Practice-Parameters/US-Abd-Retro.pdf. Accessed November 21, 2020.

48. Choi HH, Rodgers SK, Fetzer DT, et al. Ultrasound Liver Imaging Reporting and Data System (US LI-RADS): an overview with technical and practical applications. Acad Radiol 2020. https://doi.org/10.1016/j.acra.2020.06.004.

49. Millet JD, Kamaya A, Choi HH, et al. ACR ultrasound liver reporting and data system: multicenter assessment of clinical performance at one year. J Am Coll Radiol 2019;16(12):1656–62.

50. Heimbach JK, Kulik LM, Finn RS, et al. AASLD guidelines for the treatment of hepatocellular carcinoma. Hepatology 2018;67(1):358–80.

Contrast-Enhanced Ultrasound in Chronic Liver Diseases

Stephanie Spann, MD, David T. Fetzer, MD*

KEYWORDS

- Contrast-enhanced ultrasound • Microbubbles • CEUS LI-RADS • Focal liver lesions • HCC

KEY POINTS

- Contrast-enhanced ultrasound (CEUS) is an extremely safe examination that can be used to further characterize focal liver lesions, particularly in patients with chronic liver disease and when contrast-enhanced computed tomography or MR imaging is contraindicated or suboptimal.
- Ultrasound-specific contrast agents are pure intravascular agents that allow for a unique evaluation of the vascularity of focal liver lesions.
- CEUS offers real-time viewing and continuous imaging with high temporal and spatial resolution and high signal-to-background and can be used for same-day trouble shooting, in the inpatient or outpatient setting.

INTRODUCTION

Contrast-enhanced ultrasound (CEUS) is a modality with a long, successful, world-wide track record and is gaining acceptance in the United States. CEUS allows for continuous, real-time imaging that can be easily performed within the inpatient or outpatient setting, either immediately following a "noncontrast" ultrasound (US) examination, as a troubleshooting tool, or as a primary diagnostic modality. In patients with chronic liver disease, CEUS can be used for characterization of observations and is particularly useful when contrast-enhanced computed tomography (CT) or MR imaging is contraindicated or suboptimal. In this chapter, a short introduction to CEUS is provided, the use of CEUS in patients with chronic liver disease is discussed, and key differences between CEUS and MR imaging relevant to this patient population are highlighted.

Contrast Agent

Ultrasound-specific contrast agents (UCAs), commonly referred to as microbubble contrast, consist of small particles of poorly dissolvable fluorocarbon gas encased by a lipid or protein shell. These particles are slightly smaller than red blood cells (approximately 5 μm), small enough to pass through capillary beds although too large to diffuse into the extravascular space, allowing UCAs to function as pure intravascular (blood pool) agents when injected intravenously. Vessels containing these microbubbles become highly echogenic during real-time imaging, allowing for assessment of vascularity down to the capillary level and perfusion characteristics of an interrogated region of interest. UCAs are rapidly cleared from the body (half-life 5–8 minutes); the gas core diffuses into the alveolar spaces and is exhaled, whereas components of the shell are processed by the reticuloendothelial system.

Department of Radiology, UT Southwestern Medical Center, 5323 Harry Hines Boulevard, E6-230-BF, Dallas, TX 75390-9316, USA
* Corresponding author.
E-mail address: David.Fetzer@UTSouthwestern.edu
Twitter: @DTFetzer (D.T.F.)

Magn Reson Imaging Clin N Am 29 (2021) 291–304
https://doi.org/10.1016/j.mric.2021.05.006
1064-9689/21/

Importantly, there is no renal clearance, and this enables a user to administer multiple doses during a single examination, and there is no practical absolute dose limit.[1]

Safety Profile

UCAs are considered extremely safe. Mild side effects such as headache, nausea, dysgeusia, chest pain/discomfort, and dizziness have rarely been reported (1% or less), with these symptoms resolving completely without medical intervention. Very few anaphylactoid reactions have been reported, occurring in less than 1 out of 10,000 patients. Furthermore, there is no evidence of nephrotoxicity, cardiotoxicity, or hepatotoxicity, essentially eliminating the need to obtain laboratory findings before the procedure (aside from a urine pregnancy test, when applicable).[2,3]

Contraindications

Although microbubbles are considered low-risk contrast agents, UCAs should be used with caution in certain situations. Although there is no known cross-reactivity with other radiological contrast agents, patients should be screened for prior hypersensitivity reactions specifically to UCAs. Relative contraindications include acute coronary syndrome or clinically unstable ischemic cardiac disease, worsening or unstable congestive heart failure, or serious ventricular arrhythmias.[4,5] CEUS is not currently clinically approved for use during pregnancy or breastfeeding due to the lack of safety data, although preliminary studies suggest that CEUS may be safely used.[5–8]

Contrast-Enhanced Ultrasound Compared with MR Imaging

There are many benefits as well as drawbacks of CEUS compared with MR imaging, as summarized in **Table 1**. Understanding these pros and cons can help a provider choose which modality may be more appropriate for each individual patient and situation.[9,10]

PROTOCOL/PROCEDURE
Technique for Contrast Administration

Before administering a UCA, a "precontrast" US should be performed to evaluate the liver. This allows for detection of findings of cirrhosis or portal hypertension, which may influence the interpretation of CEUS imaging findings. In addition, precontrast imaging helps ensure optimized visualization of the target observation. Preferably, a CEUS examination is performed with transducer oriented along the axis of respiratory movement to ensure

---

Table 1
Benefits and drawbacks of contrast-enhanced ultrasound

Characteristics of Contrast-Enhanced Ultrasound (CEUS)	
Benefits	**SAFETY PROFILE** • Very few contraindications; • Very low contrast allergy rate; • High patient tolerance. No need for sedation; • Rapid contrast clearance. Can reinject multiple times if necessary. No absolute dose limit. **IMAGING** • High temporal resolution. Inherent real-time viewing and continuous imaging essentially eliminates risk of contrast mistiming; • High spatial resolution; • High signal-to-background using contrast-specific imaging mode. **WORKFLOW** • Same-day evaluation of findings identified during screening/surveillance ultrasound; • No laboratory screening needed (aside from pregnancy test, when applicable); • Imaging possible during patient's free breathing; • Portable. Can be performed in emergency department, operation room, and intensive care units.
Drawbacks	**LIMITATIONS** • Some areas of liver may be obscured by ribs, lung, or bowel gas; • Poor visualization of some deep targets due to poor penetration in obesity, fatty liver. **TARGETED EXAMINATION** • Evaluates fewer observations per examination (usually one nodule per contrast injection); • Not usually appropriate for complete disease staging. **AVAILABILITY** • Not yet universally available in the United States;

(continued on next page)

Table 1
(continued)

Characteristics of Contrast-Enhanced Ultrasound (CEUS)

- Contrast-specific software and skilled sonographer needed.
ACCEPTANCE
- CEUS LI-RADS not universally embraced by all clinicians, societies, and guidelines at this time;
- Not yet recognized by OPTN for transplant evaluation;
- Not yet recommended by LI-RADS for treatment response evaluation.

Abbreviations: LI-RADS, liver imaging, reporting and data system; OPTN, organ procurement and transplantation network.

the observation remains in plane during respiration (minimizing out-of-plane motion). A 23-gauge or larger diameter venous line is typically placed within the left antecubital vein, although a central line can be used as long as there is no filter. Smaller gauge catheters should be used with caution, as the shear forces experienced during bolus injection through a kinked or narrow catheter may result in microbubble destruction and poor enhancement. Typically a 1 to 2 mL/s bolus of the UCA is injected followed by a 5 to 10 mL saline bolus to flush the small volume. A 3-way stopcock is often used to allow administration of the UCA followed by the flush in rapid succession.[11,12]

Time Points for Imaging

An on-cart timer is activated at the initiation of the saline flush and displayed on the US images—this should be easily visible to allow for precise timing of image acquisition and accurate interpretation of temporal perfusion changes during retrospective review of the acquired images. The typical vascular phases captured during a CEUS examination of the liver mimics a multiphasic CT or MR imaging,[9,13] as shown in **Table 2**.

Imaging Technique

Unlike iodinated or gadolinium-based contrasts that are unchanged by the imaging acquisition technique, the physical property of the UCAs is inherently affected by the insonated US pulse. Microbubbles are not only strong reflectors due to their gas core but they also oscillate in response to US pulse insonation, at frequencies dependent on the primary frequency transmitted by the US machine (fundamental frequency). This oscillation allows microbubbles to act as local US transmitters. When insonated at low pressure, the microbubble oscillation (compression and rarefaction) is linear, producing signals at the same fundamental frequency. At slightly higher pressures, the microbubbles undergo nonlinear rarefaction, producing strong harmonics of the fundamental frequency. These differences in response between the microbubbles and surrounding soft tissues facilitate a unique imaging mode that combines pulse inversion, amplitude modulation, and harmonic filtering, allowing for tissue signal to be completely subtracted during real-time imaging, isolating signal from microbubbles ("contrast-only" image). A CEUS study is often performed in

Table 2
Postcontrast timing, image viewing, and capture

Phase[a]	Viewing	Image Capture
Arterial (10–20 s to 30–45 s)	Continuous	Cine clip from arrival of first bubble to peak liver parenchymal enhancement (up to 60 s)
Portal venous (30–45 s to 2 min)	60 s, 90 s, and 120 s, limiting viewing to approximately 5–10 s	At least one representative image per time point; can obtain short, <5 s cine clips
Late/delayed (2 min to 4–6 min, until unequivocal washout of observation or clearance of microbubbles from parenchyma)	Every 60 s thereafter, limiting viewing to approximately 5–10 s	At least one representative image per time point; can obtain short, <5 s cine clips

[a] Initiation of saline flush is time zero.

a dual display mode that presents the standard grayscale image alongside the contrast-only image, facilitating anatomic orientation.[14]

A related unique aspect of this microbubble-US interaction occurs at even higher pressures. The pulse power used during normal grayscale and Doppler imaging destabilizes the lipid shell, resulting in rapid collapse of the microbubbles and destruction of the microbubble-related signal.[15] Thus, contrast imaging requires low power (low mechanical index) imaging, inherent in the contrast mode discussed earlier. However, microbubbles can be purposefully destroyed, facilitating unique clinical uses. For example, the sonographer can accelerate microbubble clearance from the blood pool and target organ, reducing the time between injections. Similarly, a short series of high-power pulses (a "flash" or "burst") can purposely destroy all bubble-related signal within the field of view, and the pattern of contrast wash-in can be reimaged. This "reperfusion" technique can be used to repeatedly image the pattern of early enhancement without the need for addition injections and facilitates perfusion analysis.

APPLICATIONS
Focal Liver Lesions in Low-Risk Patients

A focal liver lesion in a low-risk patient is fairly common, with a prevalence of approximately 15% in some studies.[16] Although some liver lesions such as simple hepatic cyst have a classic benign appearance, many liver lesions remain indeterminate on grayscale US. Despite the fact that most incidental liver lesions in low-risk patients are benign, definitive characterization is often desired by the patient or their physician. Fortunately, CEUS performs well in the differentiation of benign from malignant focal liver lesions.

One of the most important differentiating features is the presence of washout. Malignant lesions nearly universally demonstrate washout relative to the adjacent liver, whereas benign lesions usually remain isoenhancing or hyperenhancing. Therefore, the lack of washout often is the initial step for differentiating benign versus malignant causes.[13] Then, once a benign cause is suspected, the pattern of arterial phase enhancement is used to provide additional specificity. Examples of a few classic enhancement patterns of benign lesions are detailed in **Table 3**.[12]

Focal Liver Lesions in High-Risk Patients

An important application of CEUS is the definitive characterization of observations identified in patients at risk for hepatocellular carcinoma (HCC). Often, nodules or other observations are detected

Table 3
Enhancement pattern of benign liver lesions

Hemangioma	Peripheral discontinuous nodular enhancement with contrast puddling, resulting in progressive centripetal fill-in. This may occur rapidly or slowly. Fewer hemangiomas will demonstrate complete fill-in compared with CT and MR imaging. Rarely, hemangiomas may show late washout (**Fig. 1**).
Focal Nodular Hyperplasia	Radiating pattern of enhancement with centrifugal fill-in from a central nidus (spoke-wheel pattern). No washout is expected (**Fig. 2**).
Adenoma	Arterial phase hyperenhancement classically beginning peripherally with rapid filling from the periphery inwards. There is sustained enhancement on delayed imaging. Similar to CT and MR imaging, some adenomas may show washout (**Fig. 3**).

during an abdominal US performed for HCC screening/surveillance. CEUS allows for better characterization of focal liver lesions compared with grayscale or Doppler US alone.

Contrast-enhanced ultrasound liver imaging, reporting and data system

The Liver Imaging, Reporting and Data System (LI-RADS) includes an algorithm specific for liver imaging by CEUS.[17] The CEUS LI-RADS algorithm, endorsed by the American College of Radiology, is similar to CT/MR imaging LI-RADS, describing the technique, interpretation, and recommended management of focal observations evaluated in patients at risk for developing HCC. Key features will be highlighted here, along with key differences between CEUS LI-RADS and CT/MR imaging LI-RADS. For instance, CEUS LI-RADS is based on a nodule visible on grayscale US (nodule-based), whereas CT/MR imaging LI-RADS is observation based (**Fig. 4**).

Major imaging features In CEUS LI-RADS, only 2 major imaging features are considered: nonrim arterial phase hyperenhancement (APHE) and

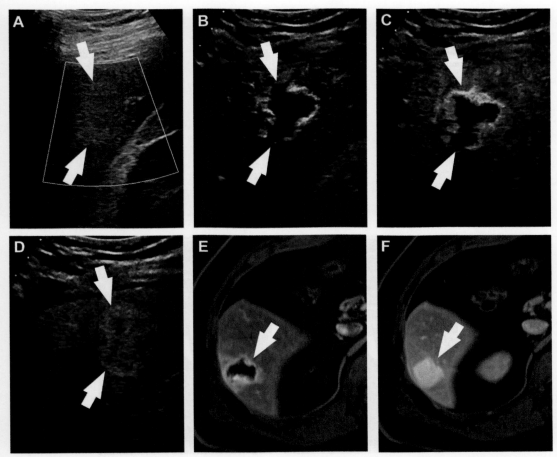

Fig. 1. Hemangioma. A 63-year-old man with a history of prostate and renal cancer found to have a hepatic mass on initial staging CT. Grayscale US image with color Doppler (*A*) shows a subtle, hyperechoic lesion (*arrows*) without significant hypervascularity. Contrast-only images during the early arterial phase (13 seconds) (*B*), late arterial (24 seconds) (*C*) and late (2 minutes, 29 seconds) (*D*) phases show peripheral nodular discontinuous enhancement and centripetal fill-in, consistent with a hemangioma. MR imaging from the same patient shows continuous rim of arterial phase hyperenhancement (*E*), although with complete fill-in by the delayed phase (*F*). The continuous imaging in CEUS allows the early peripheral discontinuous enhancement to be captured.

washout. Unlike with CT/MR imaging LI-RADS, capsule appearance is not a feature in CEUS LI-RADS, due to the differences in perfusion dynamics between UCAs (pure blood pool agents) and CT/MR imaging agents, which diffuse into the interstitial spaces to create the tumor capsule appearance that may be seen by these modalities.

Arterial phase hyperenhancement In order for a lesion to be characterized with APHE, the lesion must be unequivocally higher in echogenicity relative to the liver during the arterial phase. Although this is generally diffuse, partial enhancement is adequate for this characterization as long as it is not rimlike nor peripheral and discontinuous (the latter is a diagnostic feature of hemangioma,

CEUS LR-1). CEUS is especially useful in detecting arterial phase hyperenhancement, as US imaging is continuous, compared with multiphasic CT or MR imaiging where the timing is fixed and the peak arterial phase hyperenhancement may be missed.[18]

Washout, onset, and degree The pure intravascular nature of the UCA combined with the high temporal resolution and continuous scanning capabilities of US allows for the detection of subtle washout that multiphasic CT or MR imaging may not be as sensitive at detecting due to the limited time points of imaging and contrast kinetics.[18] Unlike in CT/MR imaging LI-RADS where simply the presence of washout is evaluated, for CEUS LI-RADS, both the timing of the onset of washout

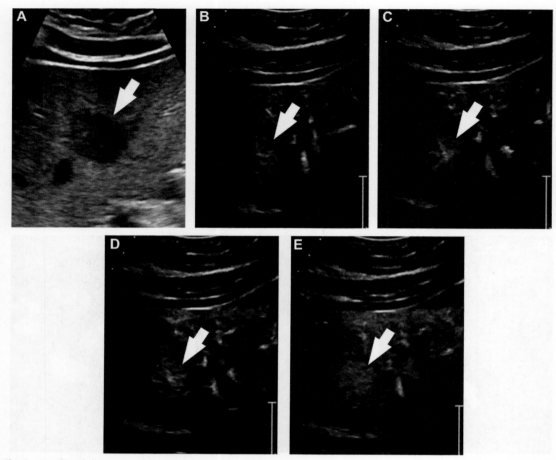

Fig. 2. Focal nodular hyperplasia (FNH). A 44-year-old man with an incidental liver lesion. Grayscale US image of a right upper quadrant US performed for abdominal pain (*A*) shows a rounded hypoechoic nodule (*arrow*). Contrast-only images in the arterial phase at 12 seconds (*B*), 13 seconds (*C*), and 14 seconds (*D*) demonstrate a spoke-wheel pattern of enhancement from a central nidus (*arrow*) with complete centrifugal fill-in at 17 seconds (*E*), consistent with an FNH. The high temporal resolution, spatial resolution, and signal-to-background of CEUS allow for this specific enhancement pattern to be captured.

(early or late) and the degree of washout (mild or marked) are 2 separate features that help to characterize a hepatic nodule. Washout is defined as the time in seconds after injection at which washout (decreased echogenicity relative to liver) is first detected:

- *Early washout*—occurs before 60 seconds
- *Late washout*—occurs at or after 60 seconds

The degree of washout is characterized by subjectively comparing the echogenicity of the nodule relative to adjacent liver during the portal venous and late phases:

- *Marked washout*—nearly devoid of enhancement ("punched-out") within 2 mins of contrast injection

- *Mild washout*—less enhancing than liver, although not devoid. Mild washout will generally progress slowly to marked washout in a later phase, therefore marked washout is only relevant if detected within the first 2 minutes[17]

Ancillary features When compared with CT/MR imaging LI-RADS, there are fewer ancillary imaging features in CEUS LI-RADS. Ancillary features that favor malignancy include the following:

- *Definite growth*—defined as unequivocal spontaneous increase in nodule size and is the CEUS correlate to "threshold growth" used with CT/MR imaging LI-RADS; this favors malignancy, not HCC in particular.

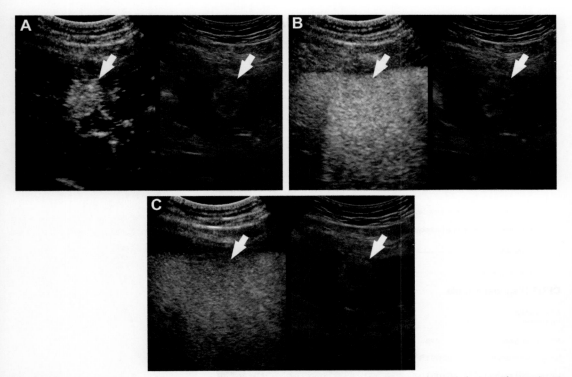

Fig. 3. Adenoma. A 23-year-old man with quadriparesis found to have an enlarging hepatic lesion. The patient's condition precluded breath-holding, compromising characterization on CT and MR secondary to motion artifact. Side-by-side CEUS images with contrast-only panel (*left*) and grayscale panel (*right*) in the arterial phase at 15 seconds (A) show a nonspecific, heterogeneous pattern of arterial phase hyperenhancement (*arrows*). At 63 seconds (B) the lesion is isoechoic relative to background liver. No washout is evident by 4 minutes (C). The lack of washout is highly predictive of a benign cause, whereas the nonspecific enhancement pattern suggests an adenoma.

Research regarding absolute or percent threshold cutoffs is currently underway;

- *Nodule-in-nodule architecture*—defined as the presence of a smaller inner nodule within and having different imaging features than the larger outer nodule. In cirrhosis, this suggests HCC;
- *Mosaic architecture*—defined as the presence of randomly distributed internal nodules or compartments, usually with different imaging features. This also favors HCC.

In addition, there are ancillary features that favor benignity, which include

- *Size stability*—benignity is favored if there is no significant change in the nodule size greater than or equal to 2 years, in the absence of treatment;
- *Size reduction*—if the lesion unequivocally spontaneously decreases in size over time, this also suggests a benign process.[17]

Example lesions characterized by using the CEUS LI-RADS algorithm are provided in **Figs. 5–8**.

LR-M features Not all hepatic nodules in an at-risk patient are hepatocellular carcinoma, as intrahepatic cholangiocarcinoma (iCC) and metastasis may also be encountered. Similar to CT/MR imaging LI-RADS, CEUS LI-RADS describes features that, if present, characterize LR-M, high probably of malignancy although not specific for HCC. These features include

- *Rim enhancement* (followed by any washout)
- *Early washout* (<60 seconds)
- *Marked washout* (within 2 minutes)

Diagnostic accuracy of contrast-enhanced ultrasound liver imaging, reporting and data system A focal hepatic lesion characterized as CEUS LR-5 has been shown to have excellent positive predictive value for the diagnosis of HCC (>95% specificity, equivalent to CT/MR imaging

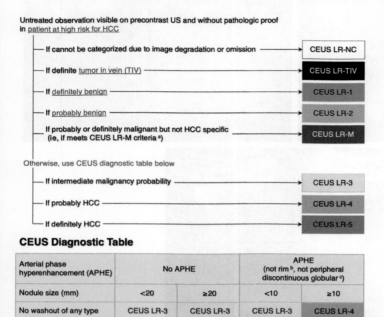

CEUS LI-RADS v2017 ESSETIALS
(For CEUS with Pure Blood Pool Agents)

Untreated observation visible on precontrast US and without pathologic proof in <u>patient at high risk for HCC</u>

If cannot be categorized due to image degradation or omission	CEUS LR-NC
If definite <u>tumor in vein (TIV)</u>	CEUS LR-TIV
If <u>definitely benign</u>	CEUS LR-1
If <u>probably benign</u>	CEUS LR-2
If probably or definitely malignant but not HCC specific (ie, if meets CEUS LR-M criteria [a])	CEUS LR-M

Otherwise, use CEUS diagnostic table below

If intermediate malignancy probability	CEUS LR-3
If probably HCC	CEUS LR-4
If definitely HCC	CEUS LR-5

CEUS Diagnostic Table

Arterial phase hyperenhancement (APHE)	No APHE		APHE (not rim [b], not peripheral discontinuous globular [c])	
Nodule size (mm)	<20	≥20	<10	≥10
No washout of any type	CEUS LR-3	CEUS LR-3	CEUS LR-3	CEUS LR-4
Late and mild washout	CEUS LR-3	CEUS LR-4	CEUS LR-4	CEUS LR-5

a. CEUS LR-M criteria – any of following:
- rim APHE, followed by washout (regardless of onset or degree) **OR**
- early (<60 s) washout **OR**
- marked washout (<2 min)

b. rim APHE followed by any washout **indicates CEUS LR-M**
c. peripheral discontinuous globular APHE indicates hemangioma (CEUS LR-1)

If unsure about the presence of any major feature: characterize that feature as absent

Fig. 4. CEUS LI-RADS essentials algorithm (Reprinted with permission, American College of Radiology).

LI-RADS LR-5); this is in part due to the CEUS LI-RADS algorithm inclusion of the LR-M category that helps prevent the misdiagnosis of non-HCC malignancies as HCC. This potential misdiagnosis, most commonly attributed to iCC, has more recently been reported to be as low as 4.4% when applying the CEUS LI-RADS LR-M criteria. Because the management and prognosis of iCC is significantly different from HCC, distinguishing these 2 entities remains critical.[19,20]

Differentiating Nonperfused Structures from Perfused Tissues

Given the exquisite signal-to-background ratio provided by CEUS, and the pure intravascular nature of microbubbles, this technique can be used to definitively differentiate nonperfused structures from lesions with internal vascularity. For example, hepatic abscesses may demonstrate overlapping features with a hypoenhancing liver mass on CT and MR imaging. CEUS will demonstrate complete absence of enhancement within liquefied components, indicating lack of internal flow within an abscess cavity. In addition, given the excellent spatial resolution of US, CEUS can be used to differentiate necrosis from perfused tissue within a hepatic mass; this is especially useful for biopsy planning in order to target viable portions of a mass to obtain samples with more cellularity for conclusive histologic diagnosis (**Fig. 9**).[21]

Differentiating Bland Thrombus from Tumor-in-Vein

Similarly, CEUS has been shown to be useful in differentiating bland from malignant in intravascular tissue. Thrombus, regardless of cause, may seem similar on grayscale and color Doppler US and can even be challenging to characterize on

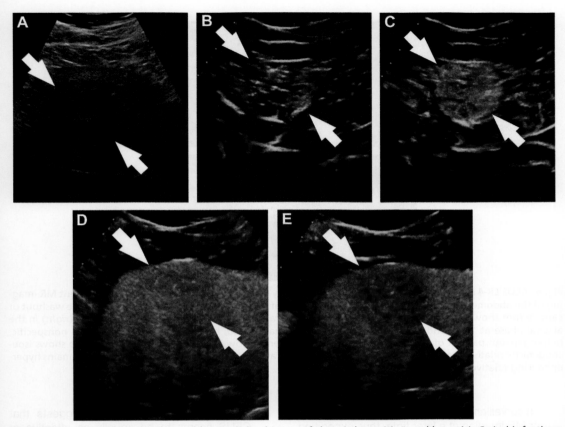

Fig. 5. CEUS LR-5 nodule. A 62-year-old man with a history of chronic hepatitis B and hepatitis C viral infections, found to have a focal hypoechoic liver nodule on screening US (*arrows, A*). Contrast-only image in the arterial phase at 12 seconds (*B*) and 13 seconds (*C*) shows a nonspecific, heterogeneous pattern of arterial phase hyperenhancement. At 122 seconds (*D*) the nodule shows late (>1 min) and mild washout, more evident in the late phase at 4 minutes, 9 seconds (*E*). CEUS performed the same day allowed for immediate nodule characterization—in this case, CEUS LR-5, definitive for HCC. Patient underwent a left lateral hepatectomy with pathology confirming well-differentiated hepatocellular carcinoma.

CT and MR imaging. At CEUS, occlusive bland thrombus will not enhance after UCA administration, appearing as a tubular signal void. For nonocclusive thrombus, determining the arrival time of the microbubbles can help differentiate between bland and tumor thrombus. When there is unequivocal enhancing soft tissue within a vein, with microbubbles arriving at the time of hepatic arterial enhancement, tumor-in-vein can be diagnosed with a high degree of accuracy. However, if the enhancement occurs several seconds after the hepatic artery opacifies, this is favored to represent flow within the patent portions of the portal vein in the setting of nonocclusive bland thrombus[22,23] (**Fig. 10**).

Evaluating for Active Extravasation

CEUS can also be used to evaluate for active hemorrhage in the postprocedural or trauma setting.

Because a UCA functions as a pure blood pool agent, if microbubbles are seen in the peritoneal or retroperitoneal space, outside the confines of a solid organ or vessel, this is diagnostic for active extravasation[24] (**Fig. 11**).

ADDITIONAL APPLICATIONS AND FUTURE DIRECTIONS

A significant amount of CEUS-related research is ongoing, exploring the many possible applications of UCAs. A few examples are provided here:

- Screening US has long been used in patients with chronic liver disease to detect observations suspicious for HCC. Once identified, these observations often require definitive workup with multiphasic CT or MR imaging. However, CEUS may allow a radiologist to immediately characterize a lesion identified

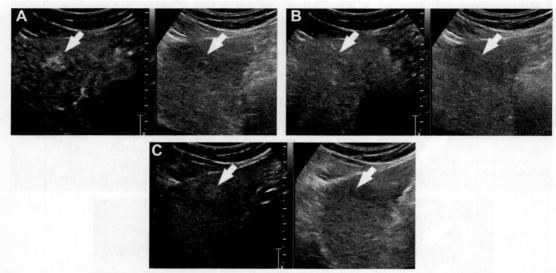

Fig. 6. CEUS LR-4 nodule. A 70-year-old man with a history of hepatitis C–related cirrhosis with recent MR imaging of the abdomen demonstrating interval enlargement of an LR-3 lesion, although without definite washout or capsule (not shown). Side-by-side CEUS images with contrast-only panel (*left*) and grayscale panel (*right*) in the arterial phase at 16 seconds (*A*) shows a 1.5 cm poorly marginated, hypoechoic nodule exhibiting nonspecific, heterogeneous pattern of arterial phase hyperenhancement (*arrows*). At 32 seconds (*B*) the nodule shows isoechogenicity relative to the adjacent liver. In the late phase at 5 minutes, 28 seconds (*C*) the nodule remains hyperenhancing relative to liver. CEUS LR-4, probably HCC.

on surveillance US, instead of waiting for a CT or MR imaging at a later time, thus expediting a patient's workup.[25]

- Many uses of CEUS in liver intervention have been reported. For instance, the addition of UCA has shown superior diagnostic tissue yield during US-guided biopsy and increased success rates in percutaneous ablation.[26]
- CEUS performs well in the evaluation of treatment response following local-regional therapies. Ongoing research suggests that CEUS seems to be equally as effective at evaluating treatment response, and potentially at earlier timepoints, compared with CT or MR imaging.[27]
- A specific UCA that targets Kupffer cells is currently available outside the United States. This agent allows for a delayed phase of imaging similar to hepatobiliary agents in MR imaging, with normally functioning liver

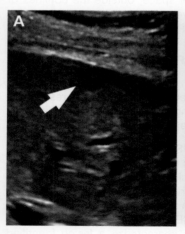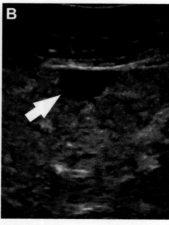

Fig. 7. CEUS LR-1 nodule. A 57-year-old man with chronic hepatitis C, high viral load, and elevated liver function tests found to have a focal hypoechoic subcapsular liver nodule on grayscale US (*arrows, A*). Contrast-only image in the late arterial phase at 35 seconds (*B*) shows the nodule to be completely devoid of enhancement, consistent with a hepatic cyst. CEUS LR-1, benign. This same-day CEUS study allowed for immediate characterization, alleviating patient anxiety and limiting use of unnecessary follow-up imaging and other resources.

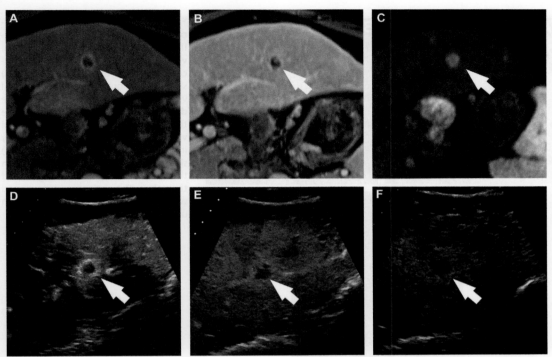

Fig. 8. CEUS LR-M nodule. A 66-year-old man with hepatitis C–related cirrhosis without a known primary cancer, found to have numerous hepatic observations with imaging features not typical of HCC, characterized as LR-M on prior MR. A representative observation in the left lobe (*arrows*), with rim-enhancement in the arterial phase (*A*), lack of fill-in in the delayed phase (*B*), and hyperintense signal on diffuse-weighted image (*C*). US-guided biopsy was requested. Contrast-only image in the late arterial phase at 18 seconds (*D*) shows rim arterial-phase hyperenhancement, without fill-in at 60 seconds (*E*). In the late phase at 3 minute (*F*), the lesion seems washed-out. CEUS LR-M, malignancy, not specific for HCC. Biopsy revealed poorly differentiated carcinoma. Based on immunostain profile, the origin of the tumor could not be confirmed with certainty, although HCC was considered less likely.

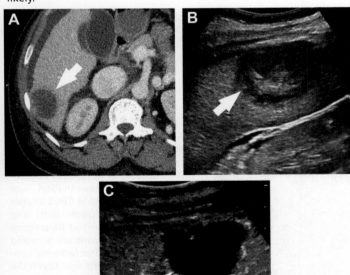

Fig. 9. Abscess. A 49-year-old patient with a history of cirrhosis who presented with persistent fevers, abdominal pain, and elevated alpha-fetoprotein. Image from a single-phase CT image in the portal-venous phase (*A*) demonstrates an indeterminate 4.3 cm mass within hepatic segment VI (*arrow*). Grayscale US demonstrates a hypoechoic, heterogenous subcapsular mass with posterior acoustic enhancement (*B*). Biopsy was requested. Contrast-only image in the late arterial phase at 57 seconds (*C*) shows a completely avascular lesion, consistent with a fluid-filled cavity, concerning for abscess given the clinical presentation. Percutaneous drainage obtained frankly purulent material, from which methicillin-resistant *Staphylococcus aureus* (MRSA) was cultured.

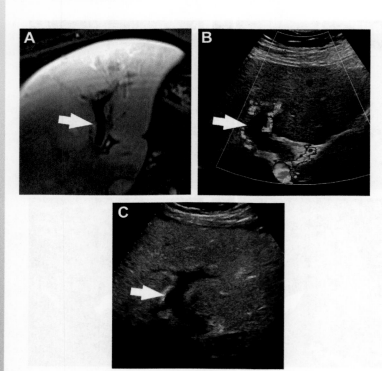

Fig. 10. Bland thrombus. A 54-year-old patient with untreated diverticulitis found to have extensive portal vein thrombus on MR imaging. Post-contrast T1-weighted image (*A*) shows thrombus filling the left portal vein (*arrows*). Color doppler US image demonstrates hypoechoic occlusive thrombus within the main portal vein (*B*). Representative contrast-only image in the portal-venous phase (*C*) shows complete lack of contrast in the portal vein, confirming bland thrombus. The patient was diagnosed with septic thrombophlebitis from untreated diverticulitis.

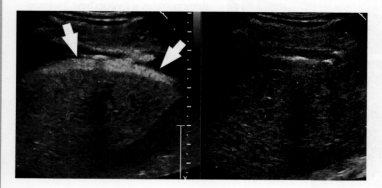

Fig. 11. Active extravasation. A 74-year-old man with cirrhosis presented for biopsy of a suspicious liver observation. Because of postbiopsy abdominal pain, CEUS examination was performed. Side-by-side CEUS images with contrast-only panel (*left*) and grayscale panel (*right*) at 63 seconds show extrahepatic contrast admixed with perihepatic ascites (*arrows*), confirming active hemorrhage. Given the pure blood-pool nature of US contrast agents, microbubbles remain in the space in which they are injected. Extravascular contrast that had been injected intravenously confirms extravasation. The patient was treated conservatively although monitored closely, without additional complications.

demonstrating contrast accumulation and nonhepatocellular structures showing contrast washout. Research into the utility in chronic liver disease imaging is ongoing, and future version of CEUS LI-RADS is expected to incorporate this agent.[28,29]

SUMMARY

CEUS is a valuable modality, offering many benefits applicable to liver imaging, including in the setting of chronic liver disease. CEUS is quickly proving to have numerous clinical uses, particularly in the diagnosis of focal liver lesions suspicious for HCC. In at-risk patients, CEUS can diagnose HCC with the same level of specificity as CT and MR imaging, can provide same-day characterization of focal liver lesions identified during surveillance US, and is especially useful when CT or MR is indeterminate or contraindicated.

CLINICS CARE POINTS

- CEUS is a proven modality for the characterization of focal liver lesions, particularly when multiphasic contrast-enhanced CT or MR imaging is contraindicated or suboptimal.

- US-specific contrast agents are incredibly safe, with few contraindications. Microbubbles function as a pure blood pool agent, allowing for the evaluation of perfusion within a region of interest, without contamination by extravascular, interstitial accumulation of contrast. Nonenhancing structures and vascularized tissue can be easily distinguished.

- CEUS allows for real-time viewing and continuous imaging with high temporal and spatial resolution, nearly eliminating concerns regarding contrast timing and respiratory motion. However, a contrast-specific imaging mode is required, a skilled user is often needed, and typically only a small number of lesions can be interrogated at a time.

- Although not universally embraced at this time, CEUS LI-RADS, endorsed by the American College of Radiology, is a standardized algorithm similar to CT/MR imaging LI-RADS, allowing for the definitive characterization of HCC in at-risk patients.

DISCLOSURE

D. Fetzer: Research agreements, Philips Healthcare and Siemens Healthineers. S. Spann: None.

REFERENCES

1. Kaspar M, Partovi S, Aschwanden M, et al. Assessment of microcirculation by contrast-enhanced ultrasound: a new approach in vascular medicine. Swiss Med Wkly 2015;145:w14047.
2. Piscaglia F, Bolondi L, Italian Society for Ultrasound in M, et al. The safety of Sonovue in abdominal applications: retrospective analysis of 23188 investigations. Ultrasound Med Biol 2006;32(9):1369–75.
3. Hu C, Feng Y, Huang P, et al. Adverse reactions after the use of SonoVue contrast agent: characteristics and nursing care experience. Medicine (Baltimore) 2019;98(44):e17745.
4. Appis AW, Tracy MJ, Feinstein SB. Update on the safety and efficacy of commercial ultrasound contrast agents in cardiac applications. Echo Res Pract 2015;2(2):R55–62.
5. Lumason [package insert]. Monroe Township (NJ): Bracco Diagnostics Inc; 2016.
6. Schwarze V, Marschner C, Negrão de Figueiredo G, et al. Single-Center Study: evaluating the diagnostic performance and safety of Contrast-Enhanced Ultrasound (CEUS) in pregnant women to assess hepatic lesions. Ultraschall Med 2020;41(1):29–35.
7. Windrim R, Kingdom J, Jang HJ, et al. Contrast enhanced ultrasound (CEUS) in the prenatal evaluation of suspected invasive placenta percreta. J Obstet Gynaecol Can 2016;38(10):975–8.
8. Schwarze V, Froelich MF, Marschner C, et al. Safe and pivotal approaches using contrast-enhanced ultrasound for the diagnostic workup of non-obstetric conditions during pregnancy, a single-center experience. Arch Gynecol Obstet 2021;303(1):103–12.
9. Pang EHT, Chan A, Ho SG, et al. Contrast-enhanced ultrasound of the liver: optimizing technique and clinical applications. Am J Roentgenol 2017; 210(2):320–32.
10. Ranganath PG, Robbin ML, Back SJ, et al. Practical advantages of contrast-enhanced ultrasound in abdominopelvic radiology. Abdom Radiol (NY) 2018; 43(4):998–1012.
11. Dietrich CF, Averkiou M, Nielsen MB, et al. How to perform Contrast-Enhanced Ultrasound (CEUS). Ultrasound Int Open 2018;4(1):E2–15.
12. Burrowes DP, Medellin A, Harris AC, et al. Contrast-enhanced US approach to the diagnosis of focal liver masses. RadioGraphics 2017;37(5):1388–400.
13. Yang HK, Burns PN, Jang HJ, et al. Contrast-enhanced ultrasound approach to the diagnosis of focal liver lesions: the importance of washout. Ultrasonography 2019;38(4):289–301.

14. Phillips P, Gardner E. Contrast-agent detection and quantification. Eur Radiol 2004;14(Suppl 8):P4–10.

15. Qin S, Caskey CF, Ferrara KW. Ultrasound contrast microbubbles in imaging and therapy: physical principles and engineering. Phys Med Biol 2009;54(6):R27–57.

16. Kaltenbach TE, Engler P, Kratzer W, et al. Prevalence of benign focal liver lesions: ultrasound investigation of 45,319 hospital patients. Abdom Radiol (NY) 2016;41(1):25–32.

17. American College of Radiology Committee on LI-RADS (Liver) Contrast-Enhanced Ultrasound Liver Imaging Reporting and Data System.2017.

18. Jang HJ, Kim TK, Burns PN, et al. CEUS: an essential component in a multimodality approach to small nodules in patients at high-risk for hepatocellular carcinoma. Eur J Radiol 2015;84(9):1623–35.

19. Li F, Li Q, Liu Y, et al. Distinguishing intrahepatic cholangiocarcinoma from hepatocellular carcinoma in patients with and without risks: the evaluation of the LR-M criteria of contrast-enhanced ultrasound liver imaging reporting and data system version 2017. Eur Radiol 2020;30(1):461–70.

20. Terzi E, Iavarone M, Pompili M, et al. Contrast ultrasound LI-RADS LR-5 identifies hepatocellular carcinoma in cirrhosis in a multicenter restropective study of 1,006 nodules. J Hepatol 2018;68(3):485–92.

21. Zhou JH, Shan HB, Ou W, et al. Contrast-enhanced ultrasound improves the pathological outcomes of US-guided core needle biopsy that targets the viable area of anterior mediastinal masses. Biomed Res Int 2018;2018:9825709.

22. Danila M, Sporea I, Popescu A, et al. Portal vein thrombosis in liver cirrhosis - the added value of contrast enhanced ultrasonography. Med Ultrason 2016;18(2):218–33.

23. Tarantino L, Ambrosino P, Di Minno MN. Contrast-enhanced ultrasound in differentiating malignant from benign portal vein thrombosis in hepatocellular carcinoma. World J Gastroenterol 2015;21(32):9457–60.

24. Miele V, Piccolo CL, Galluzzo M, et al. Contrast-enhanced ultrasound (CEUS) in blunt abdominal trauma. Br J Radiol 2016;89(1061):20150823.

25. Lyshchik A, Kono Y, Dietrich CF, et al. Contrast-enhanced ultrasound of the liver: technical and lexicon recommendations from the ACR CEUS LI-RADS working group. Abdom Radiol (NY) 2018;43(4):861–79.

26. Malone CD, Fetzer DT, Monsky WL, et al. Contrast-enhanced US for the interventional radiologist: current and emerging applications. Radiographics 2020;40(2):562–88.

27. Zheng SG, Xu HX, Liu LN. Management of hepatocellular carcinoma: the role of contrast-enhanced ultrasound. World J Radiol 2014;6(1):7–14.

28. Suzuki K, Okuda Y, Ota M, et al. Diagnosis of hepatocellular carcinoma nodules in patients with chronic liver disease using contrast-enhanced sonography: usefulness of the combination of arterial- and kupffer-phase enhancement patterns. J Ultrasound Med 2015;34(3):423–33.

29. Maruyama H, Sekimoto T, Yokosuka O. Role of contrast-enhanced ultrasonography with Sonazoid for hepatocellular carcinoma: evidence from a 10-year experience. J Gastroenterol 2016;51(5):421–33.

Computed Tomography Techniques, Protocols, Advancements, and Future Directions in Liver Diseases

Naveen M. Kulkarni, MD[a], Alice Fung, MD[b], Avinash R. Kambadakone, MD[c], Benjamin M. Yeh, MD[d],*

KEYWORDS

- Liver • CT • CT technique • Late arterial phase • Dual-energy CT

KEY POINTS

- Attention to technique for the late arterial phase is critical for evaluation of possible arterial phase hyperenhancing lesions.
- Delayed phase imaging provides superior assessment of washout compared with portal venous phase imaging.
- CT technology is advancing rapidly.

INTRODUCTION

Computed tomography (CT) is often chosen for the initial workup of focal and diffuse liver disease because it is well tolerated, the images have few artifacts, and the entire abdomen and pelvis can be imaged quickly within a single breath hold.[1] In the past decade, CT technology has advanced rapidly such that most modern scanners have the capability to image with wide-detector arrays, low kilovoltage (kVp) settings, iterative reconstruction, dual-energy CT (DECT), and now deep learning image reconstructions.[2] Attention to imaging parameters is now more important than ever for optimal evaluation of liver disease.

GENERAL TECHNIQUE CONSIDERATIONS
Hardware

Multidetector row CT has become the norm such that modern CT scanners typically have 4 to 64 detector rows that allow large z-axis coverage in a single rotation with isotropic resolution (down to 0.5 mm).[3] Premium CT scanners offer even wider detectors with up to 320 detector rows that cover up to 16 cm in the z-axis and fast gantry rotation times down to 0.25 seconds.[3] Such scanners include Revolution Apex, General Electric Healthcare; Force, Siemens; and Aquilion ONE Vision, Canon. Scanning in the axial mode eliminates artifacts that are associated with the helical scanning technique,[4] but should be performed with caution in the liver so as to not exclude portions of the organ.

CT systems with wide-detector configuration are at disadvantage from increased scatter, heel effect, cone beam artifacts, and the trade-off between spatial resolution and image noise owing to the large cone angle that may impact low contrast resolution. To compensate for such negative effects on image quality, some CT manufacturers have introduced advanced 3D antiscatter grids.[5] Although wide-detector systems have shown encouraging results in cardiovascular applications, its value in other applications such as liver imaging needs to be established.

[a] Department of Radiology, Medical College of Wisconsin, 9200 W Wisconsin Avenue, Milwaukee, WI 53226, USA; [b] Department of Radiology, Massachusetts General Hospital, White 270, 55 Fruit Street, Boston, MA 02114, USA; [c] Department of Diagnostic Radiology, Oregon Health & Science University, SW Sam Jackson Park Road, L-340, Portland, OR 97239, USA; [d] Department of Radiology and Biomedical Imaging, UCSF Medical Center, 505 Parnassus Avenue, San Francisco, CA 94143-0628, USA
* Corresponding author.
E-mail address: Benjamin.Yeh@ucsf.edu

Magn Reson Imaging Clin N Am 29 (2021) 305–320
https://doi.org/10.1016/j.mric.2021.05.002

Scan times of less than one second can minimize motion in patients who are not cooperative or unable to hold breath and decrease radiation exposure.[3,4] Wide-detector CT systems permit protocols to image the entire liver (in axial mode) at multiple time points during the early/late arterial phase, which may potentially detect more hypervascular liver lesions than single arterial phase scans.[6] Wide-detector scanners also allow whole-liver dynamic perfusion imaging, which is not feasible on CT systems with limited z-axis coverage.[7]

Radiation Dose Considerations

The need to limit the radiation dose at CT to as low as reasonably allowable is universally recognized, particularly for multiphase examinations, which are required for most dedicated liver scans.[8] Despite the need to limit radiation exposure, an essential guiding principle is that CT images must be diagnostic to be useful.[5] Radiation dose tracking software is used at many institutions to flag CT scans that are obtained with unexpectedly high doses. Generally, these scans are obtained in patients with morbid obesity and are justified, but monitoring helps reduce inadvertent over-radiation and allows for follow-up of affected patients.

Radiation dose is proportional to the tube current (mA). Modern CT scanners allow for automatic tube current modulation (ATCM) along the z-axis based on patient density on the scout image to achieve a acceptable target noise level.[9] Use of ATCM may reduce radiation dose by up to 50% compared with fixed mA.[10]

Radiation dose is exponentially reduced at lower kVp settings.[11] When the tube current is held constant, lowering the tube potential from 120 to 100 kVp or 120 to 80 kVp may reduce the dose by 33% and 65%, respectively.[12,13] Reduced kVp settings also increase the attenuation of iodine contrast by up to 70% (**Fig. 1**). Although the low kVp technique can be applied in thinner adults while maintaining acceptable image noise, its application to large patients is commonly limited owing to noise and owing to excessive attenuation of low-energy X rays by thick body parts.[14] In fact, for patients with severe obesity, high kVp settings (140 or 150 kVp) are frequently needed to achieve sufficient X-ray penetration for diagnostic scans. New CT systems with high-output X-ray tubes partially overcome the X-ray attenuation concerns of lower kVp, and automated kVp selection may assist in choosing appropriate kVps for patients of different sizes.[12,15]

Powerful X-ray tubes have also been developed that help exploit the benefits of low kVp technique in patients across different body habitus, including large patients, with some high-end tubes capable of providing tube current up to 1800 mA even at 70/80 kVp settings.[3] Although one may perceive that higher tube power means a higher dose to the patient, high tube power allows for using a stronger prefiltration by using dedicated prefilters to remove excessively low-energy photons from the beam that would contribute disproportionately to the patient dose but not to image quality.[15]

Iterative reconstruction has further enabled radiation dose reduction by reducing CT image noise. In conjunction with other approaches, iterative reconstructions has enabled radiation dose reduction of up to 75% while maintaining acceptable image noise and quality (see **Fig. 1**). However, one should be cautious with aggressive radiation dose reduction as several recent studies have demonstrated that low contrast lesion detection is not maintained at moderate to large levels of dose reduction and can limit the detection and characterization of hypodense hepatic lesions such as liver metastases, particularly for subcentimeter lesions.[13,16,17]

LIVER CT TECHNIQUE

Although CT is generally considered to be nonoperator dependent and robust, careful attention to imaging technique remains crucial for optimal detection and characterization of liver pathologies. **Table 1** describes general CT and contrast parameters for multiphase liver CT.

Unlike for angiographic imaging that can be obtained with small doses of accurately timed contrast material to opacify the arteries, optimal liver imaging generally requires robust contrast enhancement of the entire hepatic vasculature (the artery, the portal vein, and hepatic veins) and liver parenchyma, which can only be consistently acquired by rapid injection of relatively large doses of intravenous (IV) contrast material. Use of adequately large IV contrast doses is particularly important for multiphase imaging for detection and characterization of liver lesions including metastases and hepatocellular carcinoma (HCC). It is valuable to use the same kVp setting for all phases of a liver examination so that Hounsfield unit (HU) values are directly comparable between phases.

Noncontrast Phase

The noncontrast (precontrast) phase serves as a baseline for determining the extent of liver lesion enhancement with IV contrast and is useful to

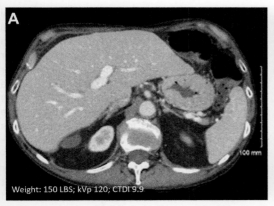
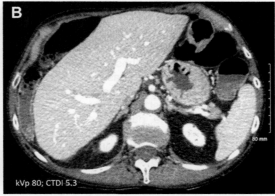

Weight: 150 LBS; kVp 120; CTDI 9.9

kVp 80; CTDI 5.3

Fig. 1. Low kVp technique. Contrast-enhanced portal venous phase images of a patient acquired at (*A*) 120 kVp and (*B*) 80 kVp setting (3 months apart). By use of 80-kVp and iterative reconstruction technique (ASiR-V), almost 50% radiation dose reduction was achieved with minimal increase in image noise and with improved contrast attenuation.

Table 1
Basic recommendations for liver CT imaging[19,23]

Parameters	Recommendation	Rationale
CT Scanner Configuration	≥ 8-row multidetector CT	Enables rapid acquisition for multiphase imaging Enables thinner slices
Slice Thickness	2–5 mm	Limits volume averaging Improves detection of small lesions. Reduces noise compared with thinner slices
Multiplanar Reformats	Coronal and sagittal planes for arterial and portal venous phases	Improves anatomic assessment Improves lesion characterization Improves assessment for recurrence or residual disease along periphery of observations
Contrast Dose	Weight-based dosing at 1.5–2 mL/kg body weight to achieve 521–647 mg I/kg Maximum dose of 63–70 g of iodine in large patients	Allows for ideal maximum hepatic enhancement of at least 50 HU[20] Individualizes dosing. Maximum hepatic enhancement is inversely related to body weight. Larger patients have larger plasma and interstitial fluid volumes, diluting the contrast dose[19]
Contrast Concentration	≥300 mg I/mL	Provides a reasonable volume when adjusted for the appropriate contrast dose
Injection Rate	5 mL/s if possible	Increases magnitude of arterial enhancement[23] Increases temporal separation of arterial and portal venous phases[23]
Saline Flush	20–50 mL at the same injection rate as contrast. For the test bolus, use the same amount and rate of saline flush as for the diagnostic bolus.	Improves contrast enhancement[23] Increases efficiency of contrast use[23]

assess background liver disease such as steatosis. For certain tumors such as neuoroendocrine metastases, the noncontrast CT is often the best phase to compare scan-to-scan tumor size. For HCC evaluation, the precontrast phase helps identify subtle areas of arterial phase hyperenhancement.[18,19] Some institutions use lower radiation dose for the noncontrast phase than for the postcontrast phase. If the patient has undergone locoregional treatment, the precontrast phase is valuable to distinguish iodized oil staining, blood, and proteinaceous material from true arterial phase hyperenhancement.[20] Nevertheless, controversy exists for its use in assessing focal liver lesions. For CT imaging of treatment-naive HCC, the inclusion of a noncontrast phase is optional by Liver Imaging Reporting and Data System and other HCC staging standards.

Postcontrast Phases

IV contrast plays a critical role in detection and characterization of focal liver lesions. Although the portal venous phase is sufficient for detection of hypovascular liver metastases, the late arterial and delayed phases are most important for evaluation of hypervascular tumors including HCC. Multiple factors govern the quality of multiphase liver CT.[21] While portal venous phase parenchymal enhancement is mainly related to the iodine dose as delineated by contrast medium volume and iodine concentration, the quality of late arterial images depends on rapid contrast injection and accurate scan timing.[22]

Late Arterial Phase

Achieving an optimal late arterial phase scan is critical for detection of hypervascular liver lesions, such as HCC. The late arterial phase shows hypervascular lesions against a minimally enhanced liver parenchyma and is characterized by excellent hepatic arterial enhancement with good portal vein enhancement, but no forward enhancement of the hepatic veins[23,24] (Fig. 2). In comparison, the early arterial phase shows enhancement of hepatic arteries without significant contrast in portal or hepatic veins and generally does not show hypervascular lesions well.[23] Because the late arterial phase is well established for the detection of arterial phase hyperenhancing lesions, we use the term arterial phase to specifically refer to the late arterial phase in our article.

Unlike MRI and ultrasound (US), which allow multiple arterial phase images to be acquired without a radiation dose penalty, CT imaging requires accurate scan delay timing to capture a single optimal arterial phase consistently. Unlike the other phases of enhancement (noncontrast, portal venous, and delayed phases), the late arterial phase occurs in a brief moment—mistiming can render a liver CT scan insufficient for HCC or other hyperenhancing lesion detection and staging. For this reason, we recommend that late arterial phase scan protocols should be patient specific (Tables 2–4) and use rapid bolus injections of large contrast material doses followed by a rapid bolus injection of saline to flush contrast agents into general circulation.[25] Fixed scan delays do not account for interindividual comorbidities or catheter placement issues that often profoundly affect contrast arrival time in the liver. We recommend the test-bolus method that aims for an optimal scan but is more time-consuming or the bolus-tracking method that aims for a good scan and is more automated. Both of these patient-specific methods monitor the abdominal aorta every 1 to 2 seconds with low mA technique and have proven robust in clinical practice.

Given the relative importance of the late arterial phase, some practices use a higher radiation dose to achieve lower image noise for this critical phase than for other phases of a liver CT examination.

Portal Venous Phase

The portal venous phase of CT liver imaging typically occurs at 60 to 90 seconds after the start of IV contrast injection and is characterized by full enhancement of portal veins and hepatic arteries, forward enhancement of hepatic veins, and bright liver parenchymal enhancement. This phase of contrast optimally displays hypovascular metastases and biliary abnormalities[26,27] and may be better than the arterial phase in detecting residual disease enhancement after arterial embolization for the treatment of HCC.[28] Washout in HCC may be seen in this phase, but is often better seen in the delayed phase (Fig. 3). Timing of the portal venous phase is more forgiving than for the arterial phase, but erring on slightly late acquisition (80 seconds) may be better than acquisition that is too early. When using a timing bolus for the arterial phase, the optimal portal venous phase scan delay may also be calculated[29,30] (Table 4).

Delayed Phase

The delayed phase, also known as the equilibrium phase, is obtained at 3 to 5 minutes after contrast injection. During this phase, contrast has equilibrated between the intravascular and interstitial water of the liver, such as in areas of liver fibrosis. The delayed phase is the optimal phase for detection of washout, capsule appearance, and mosaic architecture of HCC, particularly in lesions smaller

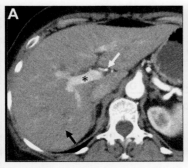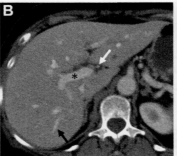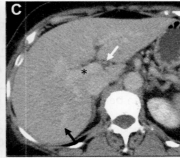

Fig. 2. Multiphase liver CT protocol for HCC. Late arterial (*A*), portal venous (*B*), and equilibrium (*C*) phases. The hepatic late arterial phase is when the hepatic artery (*white arrows*) is fully enhanced with good portal vein (*asterisk*) enhancement, but without visible antegrade hepatic vein enhancement (*black arrows*). During the portal venous phase, the hepatic arteries, portal veins, and hepatic veins are all well enhanced. During the equilibrium phase, also known as the delayed phase, the contrast enhancement of all vessels is uniform and contrast has largely equilibrated with the interstitial space of the liver parenchyma.

than 2 cm (see **Fig. 3**).[26,27,31–33] Multiple studies have shown that the use of the delayed phase increases the detection of and confidence in the diagnosis of HCC and increases the rate of detection of hypovascular tumors and cholangiocarcinomas.[26,27,31–33]

DUAL-ENERGY CT

DECT is a valuable tool for liver imaging that can brighten contrast attenuation, reduce artifacts, and increase lesion detection. DECT exploits the fact that all materials attenuate X rays to a degree unique to that material at low versus high energy. Unlike conventional CT (single-energy CT [SECT]), DECT obtains two separate sets of CT data, one from low-energy and one from high-

energy X-ray photon spectra.[34] In particular, iodine contrast can be delineated from calcium and organic material by DECT, even if they have similar HU values at SECT.

Image Reconstructions

Various vendor-specific implementations of DECT are available, and a detailed discussion on each of these is beyond the scope of this review article. Nevertheless, all clinical DECT systems produce similar image reconstructions. The DECT image reconstructions most relevant to liver imaging are 120-kVp–like images that closely resemble conventional SECT scans, virtual unenhanced (VUE) images, virtual monochromatic (VMC) images, and material-specific images, particularly the iodine image.[34,35]

Table 2
Scan delay techniques for capturing the late arterial phase[19,20,23]

Method	Advantages	Disadvantages
Fixed Scan Delay	Easiest to perform No additional radiation to determine delay	Does not account for variations in cardiac output or IV catheter issues High frequency of poorly timed late arterial phase examinations in patients with nonaverage cardiac output or poor venous catheter placement
Bolus-Tracking	Individualizes scan delay Aims for a good late arterial scan Full contrast dose used for diagnostic imaging	Additional radiation to assess target vessel density
Test-Bolus	Individualizes scan delay Aims for the optimized late arterial scan Tests IV catheter integrity prior to the full bolus	Least time-efficient to perform Additional radiation to assess target vessel density

Table 3
Multiphase liver CT imaging and contrast bolus timing[20,23]

	Scan Delay after Start of Diagnostic IV Contrast Bolus Injection		
Method	Late Hepatic Arterial Phase	Portal Venous Phase	Delayed Phase
Fixed Scan Delay	35–45 s after start of injection	60–80 s after start of injection	3–5 min after start of injection
Bolus-Tracking	Aortic threshold density: 100–150 HU Image acquisition: 10–30 s after aortic threshold density attained	60–80 s delay after start of injection	3–5 min after start of injection
Test-Bolus	Image acquisition: 10–20 s after peaking aortic enhancement Or Scan delay proportional to time to peak aortic enhancement (see **Table 4**)	60–80 s after start of injection Or Scan delay proportional to time to peak aortic enhancement (see **Table 4**)	3–5 min after start of injection

VUE Images

VUE images resemble true noncontrast scans in appearance.[36,37] VUE images can help differentiate calcium and hemorrhage from iodine enhancement in a lesion or liver tissue to aid diagnosis and allow elimination of a separate noncontrast CT, which simplifies multiphase CT and reduces radiation dose exposure.[35] Although early results are encouraging, the attenuation values on VUE images may depend on the dual-energy scanner, the patient's body habitus, and the acquisition phase of the DECT protocol.[38] Incomplete iodine subtraction and inability to measure HU values on some vendor-specific VUE images are other challenges.[35,38] Also, lipiodol chemoembolization material in a treated lesion may be subtracted on VUE images and hence may be mistaken for contrast enhancement.[39] For evaluation of ambiguous high attenuation foci, VNC images should always be viewed alongside iodine and 120-kVp–like images.

VMC Images

VMC images simulate the appearance of a CT scan acquired with a monochromatic X-ray beam at a given X-ray energy (keV).[40] These images resemble 120-kVp SECT images but with increased attenuation of iodine contrast when reconstructed at low keV (<60 keV) and reduced beam hardening artifact at high keV (>80 keV).[40] Low-keV VMC images (<55 keV) can improve conspicuity of hypervascular liver lesions

(**Fig. 4**)[41] and may be helpful to rescue CT scans with poor contrast enhancement such as from a poor bolus.[42] Portal venous phase DECT scans may benefit from low-keV VMC images to better delineate hypovascular lesions such as metastases and infiltrating liver masses.[41,43]

Iodine Images

Iodine images show the distribution of iodine contrast and can be displayed as a gray-scale image or as a color-coded overlay on the 120-kVp–like image.[44] In comparison with the iodine enhancement assessment on SECT, iodine images and low-keV images provide better image contrast and more reliable measurement of tissue enhancement[45] (**Figs. 5** and **6**). When viewed in conjunction with VNC images, tissue enhancement can be determined without the need for true noncontrast images (**Fig. 6**). For example, calcified lesions may be differentiated from enhancing masses, and tumor thrombi may be differentiated from bland thrombi.[46] Early reports suggest that the use of DECT iodine concentration may be better than SECT as an imaging biomarker of HCC response to local therapy[47 48] (**Fig. 6**).

DIFFUSE LIVER DISEASE

Diffuse liver disease is an important public health problem and a major cause of liver-related morbidity and mortality in the United States and worldwide.[49] Steatosis, iron deposition, inflammation, and cholestasis can lead to diffuse liver

Table 4
Timing bolus scan delay lookup table[26,27]

Time to Peak Aortic Enhancement (s)	Late Arterial Phase Scan Delay (s)	Portal Venous Phase Scan Delay (s)
6	28	60
8	30	60
10	33	60
12	36	60
13	37	62
14	39	63
15 (average patient)	40	68
16	42	71
17	43	74
18	44	78
19	46	80
20	47	84
22	50	91
24	53	97
26	56	104
28	58	110
30	61	116
32	64	122
34	67	129
36	70	136
38	72	140
40	75	147
42	78	154
44	81	161
46	84	167
48	86	172
50	89	179

Scan delays are for 5 cc/s injection, 30-mL timing bolus, and 50-mL saline chase. For portal venous phase scans, add 8 seconds for 4 cc/s or 16 seconds for 3 cc/s IV contrast injections. Scan delays are based on time to peak enhancement correlations, with corrections based on IV contrast bolus durations. Timing boluses must be performed with the same injection rate and saline chase volumes as for the subsequent diagnostic contrast bolus.

parenchymal injury, which if untreated may progress to cirrhosis and its complications.[50] Liver biopsy remains the reference standard for diffuse liver disease diagnosis, but it is invasive, its use can be limited by sampling error, and it is not feasible for monitoring treatment and long-term clinical follow-up.[51] Noninvasive imaging by MRI is the most accurate for liver fat and fibrosis quantification, and US is valuable for fat and fibrosis quantification. Nevertheless, CT is commonly obtained, is highly reproducible, and may be obtained in circumstances when patients are unable to undergo MRI.

Liver Steatosis and Iron Deposition

Liver steatosis is associated with metabolic X syndrome and nonalcoholic fatty liver disease, which may progress to steatohepatitis and cirrhosis.[52] Liver iron overload may be primary (idiopathic) or secondary and, if untreated, can lead to cirrhosis and multiorgan failure.[53] A concern for CT assessment of fat and iron deposition is these two materials have opposite effects on CT attenuation such that the presence of one may interfere with the assessment of the other: fat decreases and iron increases liver attenuation. While SECT may not be sensitive for detection of mild steatosis, several noncontrast 120-kVp SECT thresholds (eg, <37 or <48 HU) have shown value for the detection of moderate to severe steatosis (≥30% fat at histology).[54] Conversely, noncontrast SECT thresholds for iron overload (eg, >75 HU) are suggestive but nonspecific because high liver CT attenuation may be seen in other scenarios such as treatment with amiodarone or colloidal gold, Wilson disease, and glycogen storage disease. When IV contrast is given for SECT, the detection of steatosis or iron deposition becomes even less accurate.

To an extent, DECT mitigates some of the limitations of SECT because material decomposition may allow for more specific quantification of either fat or iron. Unlike water and normal liver tissue that show negligible changes in the attenuation at different kVp settings, liver attenuation varies linearly with varying degrees of liver iron overload and steatosis. In cases of steatosis, the CT attenuation increases with higher kVp imaging. Conversely, in cases of iron deposition, the CT attenuation decreases slightly with higher kVp imaging. But clinical study results for DECT quantification of deposition disease have been mixed particularly for low levels of steatosis and iron deposition[55–58] (**Table 5**). Better results are seen with DECT quantification of liver iron in patients with moderate to severe iron overload, which is a population wherein MRI quantification is less accurate.[59–62] Potentially, newer multimaterial decomposition algorithms may allow for differentiation of iron from other materials including fat, and large cohort clinical studies for the validation of DECT are warranted.

Liver Fibrosis

Liver fibrosis results from repeated injury to the liver. Fibrosis staging carries important prognostic implications as the early stage can be treated and

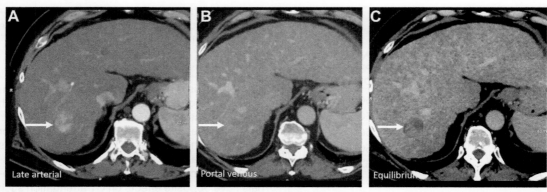

Fig. 3. HCC on multiphase CT. HCC (*arrow*) on the late arterial (*A*), portal venous (*B*), and equilibrium (*C*) phases. Although faint washout is seen in the portal venous phase, the tumor washout and pseudocapsule features are best seen in the equilibrium phase. This case shows the importance of including an equilibrium phase for the evaluation of HCC.

even reversed with antiviral therapy for hepatitis B or C and lifestyle modifications in nonalcoholic steatohepatitis.[63] Among imaging techniques, MRI and US elastography are most commonly used in clinical practice.[64] Nevertheless, several CT methods of staging fibrosis are being studied. Morphologic measures of fibrosis include the liver segmental volume ratio[65] and liver surface nodularity score, which are simple methods but may require specialized software.[66] Contrast-enhanced CT methods include perfusion CT that can show correlation of contrast mean transient time and arterial fractional flow with the fibrosis stage. Such methods require dedicated CT protocols, a high radiation dose, and software. Simpler measurement of the hepatic extracellular volume fraction (fECV) in equilibrium and noncontrast phases, as calculated by the formula—fECV (%) = liver enhancement/aorta enhancement × (100 - Hematocrit [%]), showed good prediction of cirrhosis and modest prediction of fibrosis stage at routine imaging.[64,67] DECT further simplifies fECV calculation from a single equilibrium (delayed) phase scan without need for an additional unenhanced scan.[68] Further studies are needed to validate the role of DECT in quantifying liver fibrosis.

FUTURE DIRECTIONS

Several advances in CT loom on the horizon and promise to be available within the next 5 to 10 y. Artificial intelligence (AI) is already changing radiology practice[69] and will improve many basic aspects of our specialty. Deep learning using convolutional neural networks is used to reduce image noise, reduce the required radiation dose, increase contrast attenuation, and reduce artifacts at CT.[3,70] (**Fig. 7**). Deep learning in image recognition promises to reduce the radiologist's workload and improve diagnostic consistency[69] for detecting and characterizing focal[71,72] and diffuse liver diseases.[73]

Photon-counting CT (PCCT) uses tiny detectors that sort incident photons by energy. Theoretically, these small detectors should provide superior spatial resolution, reduce the required radiation dose, reduce beam hardening artifact, and provide more detailed spectral delineation of the imaged body parts than possible with existing clinical CT

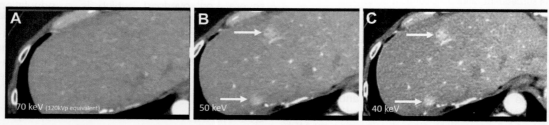

Fig. 4. DECT low-energy VMC images improve lesion conspicuity. Axial contrast-enhanced DECT VMC images at the level of liver obtained during the late arterial phase of contrast enhancement. Two hypervascular liver metastases (*arrows*) are barely seen in the 70-keV VMC image (*A*) and are more conspicuous in the 50-keV (*B*) and 40-keV (*C*) VMC images.

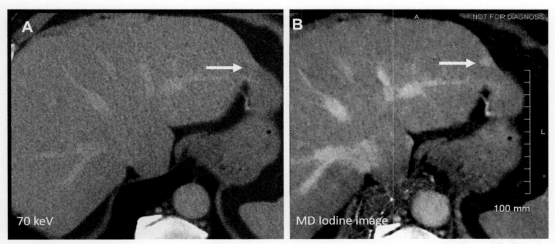

Fig. 5. Improved lesion visibility on material density (MD) iodine image. Axial contrast-enhanced 70-keV (*A*) and iodine (*B*) images of the liver obtained during portal venous of contrast enhancement. An incidental small lesion in the left lobe lateral segment is better seen in the iodine image owing to its inherent superior contrast. Although the lesion eventually turned out to be a hemangioma (in MRI not shown here), this example highlights the benefit of iodine images for detection of small lesions.

scanners, all of which use energy-integrating detectors.[74,75] PCCT should enable reconstruction of more accurate material-specific maps and differentiate more than two materials,[74] as needed for the quantification of hepatic steatosis, iron, and contrast enhancement. In parallel, novel noniodine contrast agents that can be given simultaneously with iodine agents yet appear in different colors in DECT and even more vividly in PCCT are under development.[74,76] These contrast agents generally use high atomic number reporter atoms, such as tantalum, bismuth, gold, ytterbium, or hafnium,

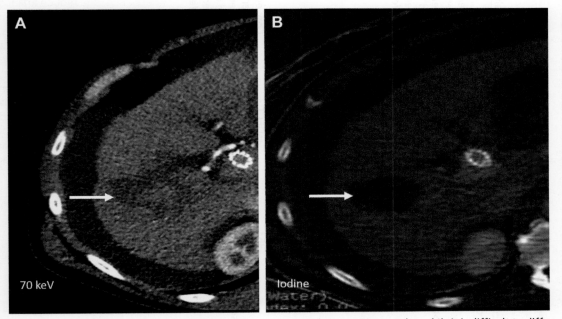

Fig. 6. Therapy monitoring after HCC ablation. Based on the 70-keV VMC image alone (*A*), it is difficult to differentiate between hemorrhage versus residual enhancement in the ablation bed (*arrow*). The iodine image (*B*) confirms lack of enhancement/residual disease in the ablation bed. The example highlights the benefit of iodine images in material differentiation, especially when unenhanced CT is not available for interpretation.

Table 5
Publications on liver fat and iron quantification via DECT

Studies on fat quantification[50–53]

Authors, Year	Cases (n)	DECT Platform and Phases Acquired	Modality Compared	DECT Method for Quantification	Reference Comparison	Liver Biopsy Results	Results
Zheng et al[55] (2013, retrospective)	52	ssDECT (unenhanced SECT and DECT)	Conventional unenhanced SECT (liver attenuation and liver-spleen attenuation difference/ratio)	Analysis of VMC images (1) ΔHU and spectral curve analysis (2) ROI for fat pixel on dual-energy subtraction imaging (DESI) (subtracting VMC at 75 keV from 50 keV)	Unenhanced SECT	None	Distinctive curve patterns at different grades of hepatic steatosis can be created on spectral CT. Subtraction images help in quantitative and qualitative assessment. Overall, DECT has advantages over SECT.
Patel et al[57] (2013, retrospective)	363	ssDECT (unenhanced SECT and contrast-enhanced DECT)	Conventional unenhanced SECT (liver attenuation and liver-spleen attenuation difference)	Two-material decomposition algorithm fat (iodine)	Unenhanced SECT	None	Good correlation between the fat density and fat HU measurements (liver-spleen difference) on water images and SECT. A threshold of 1027 mg/mL can identify 90% of steatotic livers on contrast-enhanced DECT studied. But the study showed poor correlation between fat density measurements

Study	No.	DECT technique	DECT measurement	Other imaging compared	Reference standard	Independent correlation	Findings
							and the degree of steatosis.
Hyodo et al[56] (2017, prospective)	33	ssDECT (contrast-enhanced DECT)	Percentage of fat volume fraction from multimaterial decomposition algorithm		Magnetic resonance spectroscopy	Yes	For hepatic fat quantification on contrast-enhanced study, DECT is accurate and reproducible. This may obviate the need for the unenhanced scan.
Kramer et al[58] (2017, prospective)	50	ssDECT (unenhanced DECT)	VMI (range = 70–140 keV) and material decomposition images	Unenhanced SECT, gray-scale US, US-SWE proton density fat fraction MRI	Magnetic resonance spectroscopy	None	Excellent correlation between MRS and both proton density fat fraction MRI and SECT. DECT-based material decomposition did not add value over conventional SECT in quantifying fat.
Studies on iron quantification[54-57]							
Joe et al[59] (2011, retrospective)	87	dsDECT (unenhanced DECT)	ΔHU between 80 kVp and140 kVp	3T MRI (iron indexes calculated on T1 and T2W sequences. R2 or R2* method not used	Histology	Yes	ΔHU significantly correlated with the degree of iron accumulation. At clinically important levels of LIC, DECT and MRI have similar accuracy. ΔHU of 13.8 provides specific threshold to exclude significant LIC.

(continued on next page)

Table 5
(continued)

Authors, Year	Cases (n)	DECT Platform and Phases Acquired	Modality Compared	DECT Method for Quantification	Reference Comparison	Liver Biopsy Results	Results
Luo et al[60] (2015, prospective)	56 (MRI data from 34 patients)	dsDECT (unenhanced DECT)	1.5 T MRI (spine echo–based R2* technique)	VIC analyzed using three-material decomposition algorithm	MRI R2* technique	No	DECT-based VIC showed significant correlation with MRI-R2* and MRI-measured LIC. Diagnostic performance of DECT was similar to MRI above clinically significant iron levels.
Werner et al[62] (2019, retrospective)	110 (147 scans from 110 patients)	dsDECT (unenhanced DECT)	Serum ferritin and transfused iron (estimated amount)	VIC analyzed using three-material decomposition algorithm	Serum ferritin and estimated amount of transfused iron	No	DECT-based VIC algorithm strongly correlates with serum ferritin levels and estimated amount of transfused iron
Ma et al[61] (2020, retrospective)	31	dlDECT (unenhanced DECT)	MRI (R2* technique)	ΔHU in VMC images – between lower (50 keV) and higher (120 keV) energy levels	MRI R2* technique	No	ΔHU showed a strong linear correlation with liver R2*. The study also calculated R2* and ΔHU of cardiac muscles, but the correlation was wk.

Abbreviations: dlDECT, dual detector layer DECT; dsDECT, dual-source DECT; HU, Hounsfield units; LIC, liver iron content; MRS, MR spectroscopy; ROI, region of interest; SECT, single-energy CT; ssDECT, single-source DECT; SWE, shear wave elastography; US, ultrasound; VIC, virtual iron content.

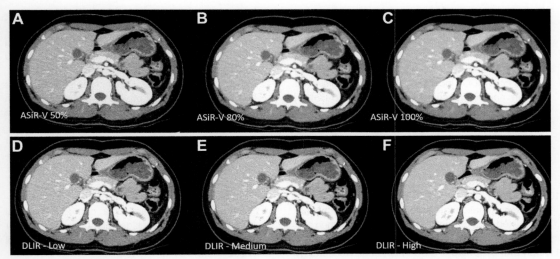

Fig. 7. Deep learning image reconstruction (DLIR) for improved CT image quality. The figure shows a CT image reconstructed at different iterative reconstruction strengths (*A–C*) and DLIR levels (*D–F*). High DLIR strength image (*F*) has the least amount of noise and most optimal image quality. Although iterative reconstruction images may reduce image noise, such images have been associated with unacceptable image texture as in (*C*), which was reconstructed with 100% iterative reconstruction strength. DLIRs allow for reduction in image noise with better preservation of image texture (*F*).

and may provide CT attenuation benefits even with SECT.[77] Multicontrast PCCT examinations, such as with iodine and gadolinium contrast agents in a single acquisition, could provide both the arterial and venous phase examination of the liver with perfect image coregistration.[76,78] Of course, such images would further improve the value of AI for liver CT analysis.

SUMMARY

CT remains a cornerstone of liver disease evaluation. Wide-detector and dual-energy CT technologies allow for improved detection and characterization of focal liver lesions and, to a lesser extent, assessment of liver steatosis, iron deposition, and fibrosis. Attention to CT technique, and in particular accurately capturing the late arterial phase, improves the evaluation for HCC and other hypervascular tumors. Emerging technologies including artificial intelligence, photon-counting CT, and novel contrast agents will further improve the capabilities of liver CT diagnoses.

DISCLOSURE

N.K. is a consultant for General Electric Healthcare. A.R.K. reports research grant from General Electric Healthcare, Philips Healthcare, and Pancreas Cancer Action Network. A.F. has nothing to declare. B.M.Y. reports grants from General Electric Healthcare, Philips Healthcare, Guerbet, and NIH; is a shareholder of Nextrast; is a consultant for General Electric Healthcare; is a speaker for General Electric Healthcare, Philips Healthcare, and Canon Medical Systems; reports book royalties from Oxford University Press; and reports patent royalties from UCSF.

REFERENCES

1. Boll DT, Merkle EM. Diffuse liver disease: strategies for hepatic CT and MR imaging. Radiographics 2009;29(6):1591–614.
2. McCollough CH, Leng S, Yu L, et al. Dual- and multienergy CT: principles, technical approaches, and clinical applications. Radiology 2015;276(3):637–53.
3. Lell MM, Kachelriess M. Recent and upcoming technological developments in computed tomography: high speed, low dose, deep learning, multienergy. Invest Radiol 2020;55(1):8–19.
4. Ginat DT, Gupta R. Advances in computed tomography imaging technology. Annu Rev Biomed Eng 2014;16:431–53.
5. Ramirez-Giraldo JC, Grant K, Primak AN. Thomas Flohr new approaches to reduce radiation while maintaining image quality in multi-detector-computed tomography. Curr Radiol Rep 2015;3.
6. Soloff EV, Desai N, Busey JM, et al. Feasibility of wide detector three-pass arterial phase liver CT in patients with cirrhosis: timing of hyperenhancing lesion peak conspicuity. Abdom Radiol (Ny) 2020; 45(8):2370–7.

7. Fang W, Wang CH, Yu YF, et al. The feasibility of 1-stop examination of coronary CT angiography and abdominal enhanced CT. Medicine (Baltimore) 2018;97(32):e11651.

8. Palorini F, Origgi D, Granata C, et al. Adult exposures from MDCT including multiphase studies: first Italian nationwide survey. Eur Radiol 2014;24(2):469–83.

9. Israel GM, Cicchiello L, Brink J, et al. Patient size and radiation exposure in thoracic, pelvic, and abdominal CT examinations performed with automatic exposure control. AJR Am J Roentgenol 2010;195(6):1342–6.

10. Kalra MK, Maher MM, Toth TL, et al. Comparison of Z-axis automatic tube current modulation technique with fixed tube current CT scanning of abdomen and pelvis. Radiology 2004;232(2):347–53.

11. Yeh BM, Shepherd JA, Wang ZJ, et al. Dual-energy and low-kVp CT in the abdomen. AJR Am J Roentgenol 2009;193(1):47–54.

12. Lee KH, Lee JM, Moon SK, et al. Attenuation-based automatic tube voltage selection and tube current modulation for dose reduction at contrast-enhanced liver CT. Radiology 2012;265(2):437–47.

13. Marin D, Nelson RC, Schindera ST, et al. Low-tube-voltage, high-tube-current multidetector abdominal CT: improved image quality and decreased radiation dose with adaptive statistical iterative reconstruction algorithm–initial clinical experience. Radiology 2010;254(1):145–53.

14. Desai GS, Uppot RN, Yu EW, et al. Impact of iterative reconstruction on image quality and radiation dose in multidetector CT of large body size adults. Eur Radiol 2012;22(8):1631–40.

15. Seyal AR, Arslanoglu A, Abboud SF, et al. CT of the Abdomen with Reduced Tube Voltage in Adults: A Practical Approach. Radiographics 2015;35(7):1922–39.

16. Prakash P, Kalra MK, Kambadakone AK, et al. Reducing abdominal CT radiation dose with adaptive statistical iterative reconstruction technique. Invest Radiol 2010;45(4):202–10.

17. Mileto A, Guimaraes LS, McCollough CH, et al. State of the art in abdominal CT: the limits of iterative reconstruction algorithms. Radiology 2019;293(3):491–503.

18. Chung BM, Park HJ, Park SB, et al. Differentiation of small arterial enhancing hepatocellular carcinoma from non-tumorous arterioportal shunt with an emphasis on the precontrast CT scan. Abdom Imaging 2015;40(7):2200–9.

19. Hennedige T, Yang ZJ, Ong CK, et al. Utility of non-contrast-enhanced CT for improved detection of arterial phase hyperenhancement in hepatocellular carcinoma. Abdom Imaging 2014;39(6):1247–54.

20. Kim HC, Kim AY, Han JK, et al. Hepatic arterial and portal venous phase helical CT in patients treated with transcatheter arterial chemoembolization for hepatocellular carcinoma: added value of unenhanced images. Radiology 2002;225(3):773–80.

21. Brink JA. Use of high concentration contrast media (HCCM): principles and rationale–body CT. Eur J Radiol 2003;45(Suppl 1):S53–8.

22. Heiken JP, Brink JA, McClennan BL, et al. Dynamic incremental CT: effect of volume and concentration of contrast material and patient weight on hepatic enhancement. Radiology 1995;195(2):353–7.

23. Laghi A, Iannaccone R, Rossi P, et al. Hepatocellular carcinoma: detection with triple-phase multi-detector row helical CT in patients with chronic hepatitis. Radiology 2003;226(2):543–9.

24. Ichikawa T, Kitamura T, Nakajima H, et al. Hypervascular hepatocellular carcinoma: can double arterial phase imaging with multidetector CT improve tumor depiction in the cirrhotic liver? AJR Am J Roentgenol 2002;179(3):751–8.

25. Bae KT. Intravenous contrast medium administration and scan timing at CT: considerations and approaches. Radiology 2010;256(1):32–61.

26. Liu YI, Kamaya A, Jeffrey RB, et al. Multidetector computed tomography triphasic evaluation of the liver before transplantation: importance of equilibrium phase washout and morphology for characterizing hypervascular lesions. J Comput Assist Tomogr 2012;36(2):213–9.

27. Lim JH, Choi D, Kim SH, et al. Detection of hepatocellular carcinoma: value of adding delayed phase imaging to dual-phase helical CT. AJR Am J Roentgenol 2002;179(1):67–73.

28. Lam A, Fernando D, Sirlin CC, et al. Value of the portal venous phase in evaluation of treated hepatocellular carcinoma following transcatheter arterial chemoembolisation. Clin Radiol 2017;72(11):994.e9–16.

29. Chu LL, Joe BN, Westphalen AC, et al. Patient-specific time to peak abdominal organ enhancement varies with time to peak aortic enhancement at MR imaging. Radiology 2007;245(3):779–87.

30. Schneider JG, Wang ZJ, Wang W, et al. Patient-tailored scan delay for multiphase liver CT: improved scan quality and lesion conspicuity with a novel timing bolus method. AJR Am J Roentgenol 2014;202(2):318–23.

31. Iannaccone R, Laghi A, Catalano C, et al. Hepatocellular carcinoma: role of unenhanced and delayed phase multi-detector row helical CT in patients with cirrhosis. Radiology 2005;234(2):460–7.

32. Liu YI, Shin LK, Jeffrey RB, et al. Quantitatively defining washout in hepatocellular carcinoma. AJR Am J Roentgenol 2013;200(1):84–9.

33. Monzawa S, Ichikawa T, Nakajima H, et al. Dynamic CT for detecting small hepatocellular carcinoma: usefulness of delayed phase imaging. AJR Am J Roentgenol 2007;188(1):147–53.

34. De Cecco CN, Darnell A, Rengo M, et al. Dual-energy CT: oncologic applications. AJR Am J Roentgenol 2012;199(5 Suppl):S98–105.

35. Morgan DE. Dual-energy CT of the abdomen. Abdom Imaging 2014;39(1):108–34.

36. Zhang LJ, Peng J, Wu SY, et al. Liver virtual non-enhanced CT with dual-source, dual-energy CT: a preliminary study. Eur Radiol 2010;20(9):2257–64.

37. De Cecco CN, Muscogiuri G, Schoepf UJ, et al. Virtual unenhanced imaging of the liver with third-generation dual-source dual-energy CT and advanced modeled iterative reconstruction. Eur J Radiol 2016;85(7):1257–64.

38. De Cecco CN, Darnell A, Macias N, et al. Virtual unenhanced images of the abdomen with second-generation dual-source dual-energy computed tomography: image quality and liver lesion detection. Invest Radiol 2013;48(1):1–9.

39. Lee JM, Yoon JH, Joo I, et al. Recent advances in CT and MR imaging for evaluation of hepatocellular carcinoma. Liver Cancer 2012;1(1):22–40.

40. Yu L, Leng S, McCollough CH. Dual-energy CT-based monochromatic imaging. AJR Am J Roentgenol 2012;199(5 Suppl):S9–15.

41. Yamada Y, Jinzaki M, Tanami Y, et al. Virtual monochromatic spectral imaging for the evaluation of hypovascular hepatic metastases: the optimal monochromatic level with fast kilovoltage switching dual-energy computed tomography. Invest Radiol 2012;47(5):292–8.

42. Lv P, Zhou Z, Liu J, et al. Can virtual monochromatic images from dual-energy CT replace low-kVp images for abdominal contrast-enhanced CT in small- and medium-sized patients? Eur Radiol 2019;29(6):2878–89.

43. Caruso D, De Cecco CN, Schoepf UJ, et al. Can dual-energy computed tomography improve visualization of hypoenhancing liver lesions in portal venous phase? Assessment of advanced image-based virtual monoenergetic images. Clin Imaging 2017;41:118–24.

44. Patino M, Prochowski A, Agrawal MD, et al. Material separation using dual-energy CT: current and emerging applications. Radiographics 2016;36(4):1087–105.

45. Agrawal MD, Pinho DF, Kulkarni NM, et al. Oncologic applications of dual-energy CT in the abdomen. Radiographics 2014;34(3):589–612.

46. Qian LJ, Zhu J, Zhuang ZG, et al. Differentiation of neoplastic from bland macroscopic portal vein thrombi using dual-energy spectral CT imaging: a pilot study. Eur Radiol 2012;22(10):2178–85.

47. Lee JA, Jeong WK, Kim Y, et al. Dual-energy CT to detect recurrent HCC after TACE: initial experience of color-coded iodine CT imaging. Eur J Radiol 2013;82(4):569–76.

48. Lee SH, Lee JM, Kim KW, et al. Dual-energy computed tomography to assess tumor response to hepatic radiofrequency ablation: potential diagnostic value of virtual noncontrast images and iodine maps. Invest Radiol 2011;46(2):77–84.

49. Schuppan D, Afdhal NH. Liver cirrhosis. Lancet 2008;371(9615):838–51.

50. Chalasani N, Younossi Z, Lavine JE, et al. The diagnosis and management of nonalcoholic fatty liver disease: Practice guidance from the American Association for the Study of Liver Diseases. Hepatology 2018;67(1):328–57.

51. Kose S, Ersan G, Tatar B, et al. Evaluation of percutaneous liver biopsy complications in patients with chronic viral hepatitis. Eurasian J Med 2015;47(3):161–4.

52. Fotbolcu H, Zorlu E. Nonalcoholic fatty liver disease as a multi-systemic disease. World J Gastroenterol 2016;22(16):4079–90.

53. Adams P, Brissot P, Powell LW. EASL international consensus conference on haemochromatosis. J Hepatol 2000;33(3):485–504.

54. Pickhardt PJ, Park SH, Hahn L, et al. Specificity of unenhanced CT for non-invasive diagnosis of hepatic steatosis: implications for the investigation of the natural history of incidental steatosis. Eur Radiol 2012;22(5):1075–82.

55. Zheng X, Ren Y, Phillips WT, et al. Assessment of hepatic fatty infiltration using spectral computed tomography imaging: a pilot study. J Comput Assist Tomogr 2013;37(2):134–41.

56. Hyodo T, Hori M, Lamb P, et al. Multimaterial decomposition algorithm for the quantification of liver fat content by using Fast-Kilovolt-Peak switching dual-energy CT: experimental validation. Radiology 2017;282(2):381–9.

57. Patel BN, Kumbla RA, Berland LL, et al. Material density hepatic steatosis quantification on intravenous contrast-enhanced rapid kilovolt (peak)-switching single-source dual-energy computed tomography. J Comput Assist Tomogr 2013;37(6):904–10.

58. Kramer H, Pickhardt PJ, Kliewer MA, et al. Accuracy of Liver fat quantification with advanced CT, MRI, and ultrasound techniques: prospective comparison with MR spectroscopy. AJR Am J Roentgenol 2017;208(1):92–100.

59. Joe E, Kim SH, Lee KB, et al. Feasibility and accuracy of dual-source dual-energy CT for noninvasive determination of hepatic iron accumulation. Radiology 2012;262(1):126–35.

60. Luo XF, Xie XQ, Cheng S, et al. Dual-energy CT for patients suspected of having liver iron overload: can virtual iron content imaging accurately quantify liver iron content? Radiology 2015;277(1):95–103.

61. Ma J, Song ZQ, Yan FH. Separation of hepatic iron and fat by dual-source dual-energy computed tomography based on material decomposition: an animal study. PLoS One 2014;9(10):e110964.

62. Werner S, Krauss B, Haberland U, et al. Dual-energy CT for liver iron quantification in patients with haematological disorders. Eur Radiol 2019;29(6): 2868–77.

63. Lee YA, Wallace MC, Friedman SL. Pathobiology of liver fibrosis: a translational success story. Gut 2015;64(5):830–41.

64. Horowitz JM, Venkatesh SK, Ehman RL, et al. Evaluation of hepatic fibrosis: a review from the society of abdominal radiology disease focus panel. Abdom Radiol (Ny) 2017;42(8):2037–53.

65. Furusato Hunt OM, Lubner MG, Ziemlewicz TJ, et al. The liver segmental volume ratio for noninvasive detection of cirrhosis: comparison with established linear and volumetric measures. J Comput Assist Tomogr 2016;40(3):478–84.

66. Smith AD, Branch CR, Zand K, et al. Liver surface nodularity quantification from routine ct images as a biomarker for detection and evaluation of cirrhosis. Radiology 2016;280(3):771–81.

67. Varenika V, Fu Y, Maher JJ, et al. Hepatic fibrosis: evaluation with semiquantitative contrast-enhanced CT. Radiology 2013;266(1):151–8.

68. Lamb P, Sahani DV, Fuentes-Orrego JM, et al. Stratification of patients with liver fibrosis using dual-energy CT. IEEE Trans Med Imaging 2015;34(3): 807–15.

69. Hosny A, Parmar C, Quackenbush J, et al. Artificial intelligence in radiology. Nat Rev Cancer 2018; 18(8):500–10.

70. Higaki T, Nakamura Y, Tatsugami F, et al. Improvement of image quality at CT and MRI using deep learning. Jpn J Radiol 2019;37(1):73–80.

71. Vivanti R, Szeskin A, Lev-Cohain N, et al. Automatic detection of new tumors and tumor burden evaluation in longitudinal liver CT scan studies. Int J Comput Assist Radiol Surg 2017;12(11):1945–57.

72. Yasaka K, Akai H, Abe O, et al. Deep learning with convolutional neural network for differentiation of liver masses at dynamic contrast-enhanced CT: A preliminary study. Radiology 2018;286(3):887–96.

73. Choi KJ, Jang JK, Lee SS, et al. Development and Validation of a deep learning system for staging liver fibrosis by using contrast agent-enhanced CT images in the liver. Radiology 2018;289(3):688–97.

74. Willemink MJ, Persson M, Pourmorteza A, et al. Photon-counting CT: technical principles and clinical prospects. Radiology 2018;289(2):293–312.

75. Symons R, Reich DS, Bagheri M, et al. Photon-counting computed tomography for vascular imaging of the head and neck: first in vivo human results. Invest Radiol 2018;53(3):135–42.

76. Symons R, Krauss B, Sahbaee P, et al. Photon-counting CT for simultaneous imaging of multiple contrast agents in the abdomen: An in vivo study. Med Phys 2017;44(10):5120–7.

77. Yeh BM, FitzGerald PF, Edic PM, et al. Opportunities for new CT contrast agents to maximize the diagnostic potential of emerging spectral CT technologies. Adv Drug Deliv Rev 2017;113:201–22.

78. Si-Mohamed S, Thivolet A, Bonnot PE, et al. Improved peritoneal cavity and abdominal organ imaging using a biphasic contrast agent protocol and spectral photon counting computed tomography K-edge imaging. Invest Radiol 2018;53(10):629–39.

Abbreviated MR Protocols for Chronic Liver Disease and Liver Cancer

Guillermo Carbonell, MD[a,b,c], Bachir Taouli, MD, MHA[a,b],*

KEYWORDS

• Abbreviated magnetic resonance imaging • Hepatocellular carcinoma • Screening • Fat • Fibrosis

KEY POINTS

- Abbreviated MR imaging (AMRI) protocols represent a cheaper and less time-consuming alternative to full MR imaging protocols in hepatocellular carcinoma (HCC) surveillance/screening and for evaluation of diffuse liver disease.
- There are 3 different AMRI protocols used for HCC screening/surveillance, including noncontrast AMRI, dynamic AMRI, and hepatobiliary AMRI, each with its pros and cons.
- More data on the diagnostic value of AMRI protocols are needed.

INTRODUCTION

MR imaging has become an increasingly important imaging technique for assessment of patients with chronic liver disease and for liver cancer evaluation. The use of multiparametric imaging and recent technologic advances in MR imaging, aligned with the lack of ionizing radiation, has established MR imaging as one of the most powerful imaging tools for assessing liver disease.[1,2] These advances, however, usually entail complex, time-consuming, and costly protocols.

Based on the benefits of diagnostic MR imaging and attempting to minimize the disadvantages, abbreviated MR imaging (AMRI) protocols have been proposed as potential alternatives for liver disease evaluation. The purpose of AMRI protocols is to minimize the length of full MR imaging examinations by using a reduced number of MR imaging sequences in order to decrease acquisition and interpretation times and to reduce costs without losing diagnostic sensitivity and accuracy.[3]

Compared with a complete MR imaging protocol, AMRI approaches have shown important reductions in study acquisitions times,[4,5] enabling the possibility of scheduling and evaluating more patients in a shorter period of time. Furthermore, these abbreviated studies would improve radiologists' workflow with a smaller number of sequences to review and interpret.[6] Moreover, shorter reports could be obtained and delivery times to the clinicians also would be reduced, potentially improving health care quality.

In terms of cost saving and cost-effectiveness, several studies suggest that AMRI protocols may be consider a valid alternative to the current evaluation methods for assessing liver disease. A study carried out by Lima and colleagues[7] demonstrated that AMRI may be a cost-effective strategy for liver cancer surveillance rather than ultrasound (US) examination.

AMRI protocols already have been tested successfully in different organs, including breast,[8] liver,[9] pancreas,[10] and prostate,[11] among others. Specifically, AMRI protocols in liver are focused mainly on hepatocellular carcinoma (HCC) screening and surveillance, and in diffuse liver disease.[3,9]

---

[a] BioMedical Engineering and Imaging Institute, Icahn School of Medicine at Mount Sinai, One Gustave L. Levy Place, New York, NY 10029-6574, USA; [b] Department of Diagnostic, Molecular and Interventional Radiology, Icahn School of Medicine at Mount Sinai, One Gustave L. Levy Place, New York, NY 10029-6574, USA; [c] Department of Radiology, Virgen de la Arrixaca University Clinical Hospital, University of Murcia, Spain
* Corresponding author.
E-mail address: bachir.taouli@mountsinai.org

Magn Reson Imaging Clin N Am 29 (2021) 321–327
https://doi.org/10.1016/j.mric.2021.05.003
1064-9689/21/© 2021 Elsevier Inc. All rights reserved.

CLINICAL APPLICATIONS
Hepatocellular Carcinoma Screening and Surveillance

Current guidelines for hepatocellular carcinoma screening and surveillance

HCC has been the most rapidly rising cause of cancer-related death in the United States over the past 20 years and currently is the third cause of cancer-related mortality worldwide.[12] To improve overall survival of at-risk population (adult patients with cirrhosis and/or chronic hepatitis B virus [HBV]), the American Association for the Study of Liver Diseases (AASLD) and the European Association for the Study of the Liver (EASL) guidelines recommends surveillance using US every 6 months[13,14] with or without alpha fetoprotein (AFP).

Despite the practice guidelines recommending the use of standard US for surveillance of individuals at risk of developing HCC, some caveats should be mentioned. The ability of US examinations to fully image the liver parenchyma may be limited due to several factors, such as obesity, advanced liver cirrhosis, alcoholic, or nonalcoholic fatty liver disease (NAFLD)-related cirrhosis, and other technical factors.[15–18] Moreover, recent studies suggest that US has low sensitivity for early-stage tumors, with only 63% for detecting early HCC and 20% for very-early-stage HCC.[19,20] More sensitive surveillance techniques should be investigated.

Regarding the added value of AFP to US, according to the EASL guidelines, the available data show that tumor biomarkers, including AFP, are suboptimal in terms of cost effectiveness for routine surveillance of early HCC.[14] On the other hand, the AASLD guidelines state that AFP could be optionally combined with US in surveillance strategies.[13] Other emerging blood biomarkers for HCC have been explored with promising results. The GALAD score (a serum biomarker-based model combining gender, age, *Lens culinaris* agglutinin-reactive AFP [AFP-L3], total AFP, and des-γ-carboxyprothrombin)[21] and liquid biopsy/circulating tumor DNA[22,23] have shown promising results and may have a role in surveillance protocols in the future.

Abbreviated MR imaging protocols for hepatocellular carcinoma screening and surveillance

Conventional contrast-enhanced (CE)-MRI has shown superior diagnostic sensitivity for HCC detection compared with US, particularly for early-stage tumors.[16,17,24] MR imaging, however, is more expensive, longer examination times are required, and imaging review and interpretation are more challenging and time consuming for radiologists. These facts question the suitability of conventional MR imaging for HCC surveillance. AMRI protocols represent a potential alternative because they solve some of these disadvantages of full MR imaging protocols.

Several AMRI protocols, combining different sequences with and without contrast agents, have been described for HCC screening (**Fig. 1**). Most of these studies have retrospectively evaluated the performance of simulated/reconstructed AMRI protocols, extracting the relevant sequences from complete MR imaging examinations, while prospective studies using real AMRI protocols are lacking (**Table 1**):

Noncontrast Abbreviated MR Imaging These type of protocols are simpler and cheaper than the CE approaches avoiding the potential risks of using gadolinium-based contrast agents. They consist of diffusion-weighted imaging (DWI) with or without T2-weighted imaging (T2WI).[25–29] Some studies also explored the combination of T2WI and DWI

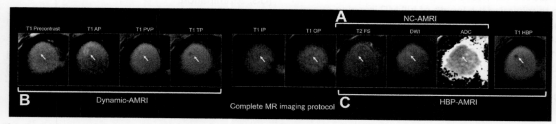

Fig. 1. A 56-year-old man with HCV cirrhosis with hepatocellular carcinoma in segment 8. Complete gadoxetate-enhanced MR imaging study is divided into 3 AMRI protocols: (*A*) NC-AMRI, including T2WI, DWI; (*B*) Dyn-AMRI, including T1WI dynamic (precontrast, arterial phase, portal venous phase, and transitional phase); and (*C*) HBP-AMRI, including T1WI HBP post-gadoxetate, T2WI, and DWI. Axial T2WI FS shows a mildly hyperintense lesion in the hepatic dome, with no fat in T1WI IP/OP, with corresponding mild hyperintensity in DWIs (b800) and hypointensity in ADC map (*arrows*). Axial T1WI precontrast, arterial phase, portal venous phase, transitional phase and HBP demonstrates a 10-mm lesion with arterial hyperenhancement, washout in portal venous phase, and hypointensity in HBP (*arrows*). ADC, apparent diffusion coefficient; AP, arterial phase; DWI, diffusion weighted imaging; FS, fat saturation; HBP, hepatobiliary phase; IP, in phase; OP, out of phase; PVP, portal venous phase; TP, transitional phase.

Table 1
Summary of published abbreviated MR imaging studies for hepatocellular carcinoma detection

Study, Year	Screening Population	Study Design	Sample Size	Hepatocellular Carcinoma Prevalence	Reference Standards	Abbreviated MR Imaging Sequences	Sensitivity	Specificity
NC-AMRI								
Sutherland et al,[25] 2017	Yes	P	192	3.0%	Combined[a]	DWI	83.0%	98.0%
Besa et al,[26] 2017	No	R	174	35.6%	Pathology	DWI	87.1%	93.8%
McNamara et al,[27] 2018	No	R	37	54.1%	Pathology	DWI	78.0%	88.0%
Vietti-Violi et al,[28] 2020	Yes	R	237	5.5%	Combined[a]	T2WI + DWI	61.5%	95.5%
Park et al,[29] 2020	Yes	P	382	11.3%	Combined[a]	T2WI + DWI	79.1%	97.9%
Kim et al,[30] 2014	No	R	157	85.9%	Pathology	T2WI + DWI + T1WI	92.5%	NA
Han et al,[31] 2018	No	R	247	70.8%	Combined[a]	T2WI + DWI + T1WI	84.6%	81.9%
Chan et al,[32] 2019	No	R	188	NA	Radiology	T2WI + DWI + T1WI	84.5%	92.7%
Whang et al,[33] 2020	No	R	263	53.2%	Combined[a]	T2WI + DWI + T1IP/OP	86.1%	92.7%
Dyn-AMRI								
Besa et al,[26] 2017	No	R	174	35.6%	Pathology	CE-T1WI	88.7%	100%
Lee et al,[36] 2018	No	R	156	Unclear	Radiology	CE-T1WI	High LI-RADS concordance with full MR imaging	
Khatri et al,[37] 2020	No	R	86	32.6%	Combined[a]	CE-T1WI + T2WI	92.1%	88.6%
Vietti-Violi et al,[28] 2020	Yes	R	237	5.5%	Combined[a]	CE-T1WI + T2WI + DWI	84.6%	99.8%
HBP-AMRI								
Besa et al,[26] 2017	No	R	174	35.6%	Pathology	HBP HBP + DWI	91.9% 83.9%	91.1% 94.6%
Brunsing et al,[38] 2019	Yes	R	141	8.5%	Combined[a]	HBP	92.0%	91.0%
Marks et al,[39] 2015	No	R	298	16.4%	Combined[a]	HBP + T2WI HBP + T2WI + DWI	82.6% 83.7%	93.2% 93.2%
Tillman et al,[4] 2018	No	R	79	16.5%	Combined[a]	HBP + T2WI	85.2%	NA
Vietti-Violi et al,[28] 2020	Yes	R	237	5.5%	Combined[a]	HBP + T2WI + DWI	80.8%	94.9%
Whang et al,[33] 2020	No	R	263	53.2%	Combined[a]	HBP + T2WI + DWI	89.7%	92.7%

Abbreviations: NA, non applicable; NPV, negative predictive value; P, prospective design; PPV, positive predictive value; R, retrospective design; IP/OP, in-phase/out of phase.
[a] "Combined" refers to pathology and/or imaging assessment.

with T1-weighted imaging (T1WI) sequences.[30–33] According to the current literature, per-patient sensitivity on noncontrast (NC)-AMRI showed a wide range between 61.5% and 92.5%, with high specificity (88.0%–97.9%).[25–33] A retrospective study by Vietti-Violi and colleagues[28] in at-risk patients reported low sensitivity (61.5%) for HCC screening using a combination on T2WI and DWI. However, 2 prospective studies performed in at-risk patients showed that NC-AMRI protocols had similar to better sensitivity than US (AMRI vs US sensitivity: 83% vs 100%, respectively, and 79.1% vs 27.9, respectively).[25,29] In cases of positive findings, a recall study using multiphasic CT or MR imaging is needed in order to characterize the observations applying the Liver Imaging Reporting and Data System (LI-RADS) criteria, devised to standardize imaging analysis for HCC screening and surveillance, diagnosis and treatment response assessment.[34]

Dynamic Abbreviated MR Imaging These protocols are based on dynamic (Dyn) CE-T1WI sequences (unenhanced, arterial, portal venous, and delayed/transitional phases) after the administration of a contrast agent (typically extracellular, but gadoxetate disodium also can be used). The main advantage of Dyn-AMRI protocols is that in cases of positive findings, no further confirmation generally is required because major LI-RADS criteria can be applied to multiphasic imaging. Different studies have used CE-T1WI sequences alone[26,35,36] or in combination with T2WI[35,37] or T2WI and DWI.[28] Dyn-AMRI protocols, based on CE-T1WI sequences, have shown high per-patient sensitivity (84.6.6%–92.1%) and specificity (88.6%–100%).[26,28,37] Furthermore, a study carried out by Lee and colleagues[36] showed high concordance in LI-RADS categorization of liver observations between the complete MR imaging exploration and the Dyn-AMRI.

Gadoxetate-enhanced hepatobiliary phase abbreviated MR imaging Protocols that are based on the T1WI hepatobiliary phase (HBP) obtained approximately 20 minutes after gadoxetate disodium administration. For the HBP-AMRI, the contrast agent is injected outside the MR imaging room with no need for automated injector or Dyn sequences, which reduces study time and simplifies the study. Several investigators have assessed T1WI HBP alone[26,38] and in combination with T2WI,[4,39] DWI,[26] or both.[28,33,39] Reported per-patient diagnostic performance of HBP-AMRI protocols showed higher sensitivity (80.8%–92.0%) and specificity (92.8%–96.1%) compared

with other AMRI approaches, however, not consistently in screening populations.[4,26,28,33,38,39]

Screening and Assessment of Liver Fat and Fibrosis

Current evaluation method

NAFLD is one of the most common causes of chronic liver disease in adults, with a prevalence of up to 20% to 30% in developed countries.[40] This entity represents a wide spectrum of pathologies ranging from simple steatosis to nonalcoholic steatohepatitis (NASH).[41] Moreover, with late diagnosis and lack of treatment, this entity may lead to a progressive liver fibrosis and cirrhosis.[42] Iron overload can be another important cofactor for developing liver fibrosis in patients with NALFD and NASH, so its evaluation also is important.[43] Currently, standard of reference for assessing derived complications of the disease like steatohepatitis, fibrosis, and iron overload is percutaneous biopsy. It does have considerable limitations and complications, however, some of which, although infrequent, potentially are fatal.[44] In recent years, different noninvasive method, such as serum biomarkers and elastography techniques, have been proposed as potential alternatives for evaluation of NAFLD, grading of steatosis, diagnosis of NASH, and staging of liver fibrosis.[45] Furthermore, MR imaging has shown potential in evaluating iron overload within the liver, using specific MR imaging methods, including relaxometry techniques.[46]

Abbreviated MR imaging protocol for assessing liver fat and fibrosis

Multiparametric MR imaging, including MR elastography (MRE) examination, proton-density fat fraction (PDFF), and T2* sequences have emerged as powerful noninvasive methods to assess liver fibrosis, steatosis, and iron overload[2,45] (**Fig. 2**). To the best of the authors' knowledge, only 1 study, carried out by Cunha and colleagues,[47] has evaluated an abbreviated protocol combining different MR imaging sequences to assess different characteristics of NAFLD. They prospectively evaluated an AMRI protocol to assess quantitative imaging features of patients with obesity and NAFLD, and tested its use during treatment. The AMRI protocol consisted of a combination of T2WI single-shot, fast spin-echo, volumetric, 3-dimensional, 3-point Dixon images with water and fat separation for manual visceral adipose tissue measurements, iterative decomposition of water and fat with echo asymmetry and least-squares estimation sequence (IDEAL IQ) for liver fat fraction and iron overload estimations, and liver 2-dimensional gradient-echo MRE sequence for liver stiffness analysis. They concluded that this

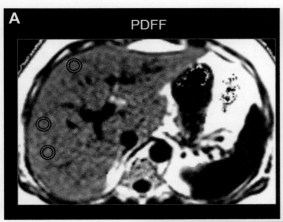
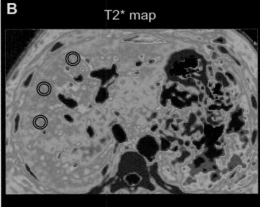
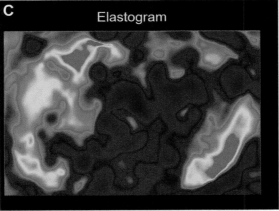

Fig. 2. A 63-year-old man with NASH and stage 3 fibrosis. AMRI protocol performed for liver fat/iron/fibrosis assessment demonstrates liver steatosis on (*A*) PDFF map (TR: 15.6 ms/TE: 2.38 ms, 4.76 ms, 7.14 ms, 9.52 ms, 11.90 ms, and 14.28 ms) with regions of interest measuring PDFF at 24%, (*B*) T2* map (TR: 1.93 ms/TE: 2.38 ms, 4.76 ms, 7.15 ms, 9.53 ms, 11.91 ms, 14.29 ms, 16.67 ms, and 19.06 ms) performed for iron quantification showing no iron overload (T2* 22.1 ms) and (*C*) elastogram obtained with 2-dimensional EPI MRE sequence showing elevated liver stiffness (4.3 kPa). EPI, echo planar imaging; TR, repetition time; TR, echo time.

abbreviated approach was a feasible, cheaper, and accessible option for screening and monitoring patients with obesity and NAFLD.

LIMITATIONS AND FUTURE PERSPECTIVES

There still are few data on diagnostic accuracy of different AMRI approaches and these protocols are not yet supported by professional societies guidelines. In addition, in order to gain clinical adoption, a Current Procedural Terminology code and insurance reimbursement for these studies should be obtained. Prospective and multicenter studies comparing AMRI protocols with the standards of reference for each disease are lacking. Furthermore, cost-effectiveness analysis should be performed.

SUMMARY

AMRI is emerging as a potential alternative for HCC surveillance and for diffuse liver disease

assessment. AMRI protocols are faster and may represent a low-cost alternative to a complete MR imaging protocol. The most accurate, time-effective, and cost-effective protocol, however, as well as the target population in each scenario needs to be defined. Prospective and multicentric studies, exploring different AMRI protocols versus the current standard of reference for each, should be performed.

CLINICS CARE POINTS

- AMRI protocols represent a cheaper and less time-consuming alternative than full MR imaging protocols in HCC surveillance/screening, and evaluation of liver fat, fibrosis, and iron overload.

- There are 3 different AMRI protocols for HCC screening, including NC-AMRI, Dyn-AMRI, and HBP-AMRI, each with its pros and cons.
- There still are few data, and larger studies are necessary.

DISCLOSURE

Grant support: Bayer Healthcare, Takeda, Regeneron.

REFERENCES

1. Taouli B, Ehman RL, Reeder SB. Advanced MRI methods for assessment of chronic liver disease. AJR Am J Roentgenol 2009;193(1):14–27.
2. Yin M, Glaser KJ, Talwalkar JA, et al. Hepatic MR elastography: clinical performance in a series of 1377 consecutive examinations. Radiology 2016; 278(1):114–24.
3. Canellas R, Rosenkrantz AB, Taouli B, et al. Abbreviated MRI protocols for the abdomen. Radiographics 2019;39(3):744–58.
4. Tillman BG, Gorman JD, Hru JM, et al. Diagnostic per-lesion performance of a simulated gadoxetate disodium-enhanced abbreviated MRI protocol for hepatocellular carcinoma screening. Clin Radiol 2018;73(5):485–93.
5. Weiss J, Martirosian P, Notohamiprodjo M, et al. Implementation of a 5-minute magnetic resonance imaging screening protocol for prostate cancer in men with elevated prostate-specific antigen before biopsy. Invest Radiol 2018;53(3):186–90.
6. Oldrini G, Derraz I, Salleron J, et al. Impact of an abbreviated protocol for breast MRI in diagnostic accuracy. Diagn Interv Radiol 2018;24(1):12.
7. Lima PH, Fan B, Bérubé J, et al. Cost-utility analysis of imaging for surveillance and diagnosis of hepatocellular carcinoma. Am J Roentgenol 2019;213(1): 17–25.
8. Mango VL, Morris EA, Dershaw DD, et al. Abbreviated protocol for breast MRI: are multiple sequences needed for cancer detection? Eur J Radiol 2015; 84(1):65–70.
9. Brunsing RL, Fowler KJ, Yokoo T, et al. Alternative approach of hepatocellular carcinoma surveillance: abbreviated MRI. Hepatoma Res 2020;6:59.
10. Macari M, Lee T, Kim S, et al. Is gadolinium necessary for MRI follow-up evaluation of cystic lesions in the pancreas? Preliminary results. Am J Roentgenol 2009;192(1):159–64.
11. Polanec SH, Lazar M, Wengert GJ, et al. 3D T2-weighted imaging to shorten multiparametric prostate MRI protocols. Eur Radiol 2018;28(4):1634–41.
12. Marrero JA, Kulik LM, Sirlin CB, et al. Diagnosis, staging, and management of hepatocellular carcinoma: 2018 practice guidance by the American Association for the Study of Liver Diseases. Hepatology 2018;68(2):723–50.
13. Heimbach JK, Kulik LM, Finn RS, et al. AASLD guidelines for the treatment of hepatocellular carcinoma. Hepatology 2018;67(1):358–80.
14. European Association For The Study Of The Liver. EASL clinical practice guidelines: management of hepatocellular carcinoma. J Hepatol 2018;69(1): 182–236.
15. Simmons O, Fetzer DT, Yokoo T, et al. Predictors of adequate ultrasound quality for hepatocellular carcinoma surveillance in patients with cirrhosis. Aliment Pharmacol Ther 2017;45(1):169–77.
16. Nam CY, Chaudhari V, Raman SS, et al. CT and MRI improve detection of hepatocellular carcinoma, compared with ultrasound alone, in patients with cirrhosis. Clin Gastroenterol Hepatol 2011;9(2): 161–7.
17. Colli A, Fraquelli M, Casazza G, et al. Accuracy of ultrasonography, spiral CT, magnetic resonance, and alpha-fetoprotein in diagnosing hepatocellular carcinoma: a systematic review. Am J Gastroenterol 2006;101(3):513–23.
18. Samoylova ML, Mehta N, Roberts JP, et al. Predictors of ultrasound failure to detect hepatocellular carcinoma. Liver Transpl 2018;24(9):1171–7.
19. Singal A, Volk ML, Waljee A, et al. Meta-analysis: surveillance with ultrasound for early-stage hepatocellular carcinoma in patients with cirrhosis. Aliment Pharmacol Ther 2009;30(1):37–47.
20. Tzartzeva K, Obi J, Rich NE, et al. Surveillance imaging and alpha fetoprotein for early detection of hepatocellular carcinoma in patients with cirrhosis: a meta-analysis. Gastroenterology 2018;154(6): 1706–18.
21. Yang JD, Addissie BD, Mara KC, et al. GALAD score for hepatocellular carcinoma detection in comparison with liver ultrasound and proposal of GALADUS score. Cancer Epidemiol Prev Biomarkers 2019; 28(3):531–8.
22. Cai J, Chen L, Zhang Z, et al. Genome-wide mapping of 5-hydroxymethylcytosines in circulating cell-free DNA as a non-invasive approach for early detection of hepatocellular carcinoma. Gut 2019; 68(12):2195–205.
23. Xu R-h, Wei W, Krawczyk M, et al. Circulating tumour DNA methylation markers for diagnosis and prognosis of hepatocellular carcinoma. Nat Mater 2017; 16(11):1155–61.
24. Hanna RF, Miloushev VZ, Tang A, et al. Comparative 13-year meta-analysis of the sensitivity and positive predictive value of ultrasound, CT, and MRI for detecting hepatocellular carcinoma. Abdom Radiol 2016;41(1):71–90.
25. Sutherland T, Watts J, Ryan M, et al. Diffusion-weighted MRI for hepatocellular carcinoma

screening in chronic liver disease: Direct comparison with ultrasound screening. J Med Imaging Radiat Oncol 2017;61(1):34–9.

26. Besa C, Lewis S, Pandharipande PV, et al. Hepatocellular carcinoma detection: diagnostic performance of a simulated abbreviated MRI protocol combining diffusion-weighted and T1-weighted imaging at the delayed phase post gadoxetic acid. Abdom Radiol 2017;42(1):179–90.

27. McNamara MM, Thomas JV, Alexander LF, et al. Diffusion-weighted MRI as a screening tool for hepatocellular carcinoma in cirrhotic livers: correlation with explant data—a pilot study. Abdom Radiol 2018;43(10):2686–92.

28. Vietti-Violi NV, Lewis S, Liao J, et al. Gadoxetate-enhanced abbreviated MRI is highly accurate for hepatocellular carcinoma screening. Eur Radiol 2020; 30(11):6003–13.

29. Park HJ, Jang HY, Kim SY, et al. Non-enhanced magnetic resonance imaging as a surveillance tool for hepatocellular carcinoma: comparison with ultrasound. J Hepatol 2020;72(4):718–24.

30. Kim YK, Kim YK, Park HJ, et al. Noncontrast MRI with diffusion-weighted imaging as the sole imaging modality for detecting liver malignancy in patients with high risk for hepatocellular carcinoma. Magn Reson Imaging 2014;32(6):610–8.

31. Han S, Choi J-I, Park MY, et al. The diagnostic performance of liver MRI without intravenous contrast for detecting hepatocellular carcinoma: a case-controlled feasibility study. Korean J Radiol 2018; 19(4):568–77.

32. Chan MV, McDonald SJ, Ong Y-Y, et al. HCC screening: assessment of an abbreviated non-contrast MRI protocol. Eur Radiol Exp 2019;3(1):49.

33. Whang S, Choi MH, Choi J-I, et al. Comparison of diagnostic performance of non-contrast MRI and abbreviated MRI using gadoxetic acid in initially diagnosed hepatocellular carcinoma patients: a simulation study of surveillance for hepatocellular carcinomas. Eur Radiol 2020;30(8):4150–63.

34. Chernyak V, Fowler KJ, Kamaya A, et al. Liver Imaging Reporting and Data System (LI-RADS) version 2018: imaging of hepatocellular carcinoma in at-risk patients. Radiology 2018;289(3):816–30.

35. Hecht EM, Holland AE, Israel GM, et al. Hepatocellular carcinoma in the cirrhotic liver: gadolinium-enhanced 3D T1-weighted MR imaging as a stand-alone sequence for diagnosis. Radiology 2006;239(2): 438–47.

36. Lee JY, Huo EJ, Weinstein S, et al. Evaluation of an abbreviated screening MRI protocol for patients at risk for hepatocellular carcinoma. Abdom Radiol 2018;43(7):1627–33.

37. Khatri G, Pedrosa I, Ananthakrishnan L, et al. Abbreviated-protocol screening MRI vs. complete-protocol diagnostic MRI for detection of hepatocellular carcinoma in patients with cirrhosis: An equivalence study using LI-RADS v2018. J Magn Reson Imaging 2020;51(2):415–25.

38. Brunsing RL, Chen DH, Schlein A, et al. Gadoxetate-enhanced Abbreviated MRI for Hepatocellular Carcinoma Surveillance: Preliminary Experience. Radiol Imaging Cancer 2019;1(2):e190010.

39. Marks RM, Ryan A, Heba ER, et al. Diagnostic per-patient accuracy of an abbreviated hepatobiliary phase gadoxetic acid–enhanced MRI for hepatocellular carcinoma surveillance. Am J Roentgenol 2015; 204(3):527–35.

40. Angulo P. Nonalcoholic fatty liver disease. N Engl J Med 2002;346(16):1221–31.

41. Hashimoto E, Taniai M, Tokushige K. Characteristics and diagnosis of NAFLD/NASH. J Gastroenterol Hepatol 2013;28:64–70.

42. Bataller R, Brenner DA. Liver fibrosis. J Clin Invest 2005;115(2):209–18.

43. George DK, Goldwurm S, Macdonald GA, et al. Increased hepatic iron concentration in nonalcoholic steatohepatitis is associated with increased fibrosis. Gastroenterology 1998;114(2):311–8.

44. Rockey DC, Caldwell SH, Goodman ZD, et al. Liver biopsy. Hepatology 2009;49(3):1017–44.

45. Castera L, Vilgrain V, Angulo P. Noninvasive evaluation of NAFLD. Nat Rev Gastroenterol Hepatol 2013; 10(11):666–75.

46. Hernando D, Levin YS, Sirlin CB, et al. Quantification of liver iron with MRI: state of the art and remaining challenges. J Magn Reson Imaging 2014;40(5): 1003–21.

47. Cunha GM, Villela-Nogueira CA, Bergman A, et al. Abbreviated mpMRI protocol for diffuse liver disease: a practical approach for evaluation and follow-up of NAFLD. Abdom Radiol 2018;43(9): 2340–50.

MR Imaging Contrast Agents
Role in Imaging of Chronic Liver Diseases

Silvia D. Chang, MD, FRCPC, FSAR[a], Guilherme Moura Cunha, MD[b],
Victoria Chernyak, MD, MS[c],*

KEYWORDS

• MR imaging • Liver • Hepatocellular carcinoma • Gadolinium

KEY POINTS

• Contrast-enhanced MR imaging is critical in the assessment of complications in patients with chronic liver disease, of which the most concerning is hepatocellular carcinoma (HCC).
• Two types of gadolinium-based MR imaging contrast agents are most beneficial to patients with chronic liver disease: extracellular and hepatobiliary agents.
• The choice of the contrast agent follows institutional preferences and clinical context, emphasizing either sensitivity or specificity.
• Extracellular agents are more specific for HCC diagnosis, whereas hepatobiliary agents offer the highest sensitivity for detection.

INTRODUCTION

Chronic liver disease (CLD) causes significant health-care burden, with more than 1.5 billion individuals affected worldwide.[1] This population is at high risk of complications, such as hepatic failure and development of primary liver cancer. Historically, the clinical standard for assessing CLD has been histology analysis through tissue sampling. However, liver biopsy has risks and limitations that make it unsuitable for longitudinal assessment, as well as for cancer screening, diagnosis, and staging.[2] Contrast-enhanced MR imaging allows for noninvasive assessment of liver disease and diagnosis and staging of its complications, mainly, hepatocellular carcinoma (HCC).[3–6] Different categories of gadolinium-based MR imaging contrast agents can be used for liver imaging: extracellular agents (ECAs), hepatobiliary agents (HBAs), reticuloendothelial agents, and blood pool agents.[7] In patients with CLD, both ECAs and HBAs offer numerous advantages, and therefore, both are used in clinical practice.[8] This review focuses on these two classes of contrast agents and their utility in patients with CLD. The review first discusses these agents individually, highlighting their advantages and limitations, and then addresses their clinical use and future directions.

EXTRACELLULAR AGENTS
Background

Gadolinium is a metal with paramagnetic properties and high relaxivity (ie, ability to reduce T1 and/or T2 at low doses), resulting in signal enhancement in T1-weighted images and signal loss in T2-weight images. Gadolinium-based contrast agents (GBCAs) are produced by the chelation of gadolinium to organic ligands to increase its stability while reducing the toxicity of the free metal ion.[9] Different types of gadolinium-based

[a] Department of Radiology, University of British Columbia, Vancouver General Hospital, 899 West 12th Avenue, Vancouver, British Columbia V5Z 1M9, Canada; [b] Department of Radiology, University of Washington, 1959 NE Pacific Street 2nd Floor, Seattle, WA 98195, USA; [c] Department of Radiology, Beth Israel Deaconess Medical Center, 330 Brookline Avenue, Boston, MA 02215, USA
* Corresponding author.
E-mail address: vichka17@hotmail.com
Twitter: @SilviaChangMD (S.D.C.); @VChernyakMD (V.C.)

Magn Reson Imaging Clin N Am 29 (2021) 329–345
https://doi.org/10.1016/j.mric.2021.05.014
1064-9689/21/© 2021 Elsevier Inc. All rights reserved.

chelate ECAs are available for clinical use (**Table 1**).

The dose of gadolinium-based ECAs is usually 0.1 mmol/kg or 0.2 mL/kg of body weight administrated intravenously.[10] The rate of injection is 2 to 3 mL/s, usually followed by a 15- to 20-mL saline flush to clear the contrast from the intravenous line. ECAs enter the liver via the portal vein and the hepatic artery and rapidly distribute into the extracellular space. An equilibrium distribution into the extracellular interstitial space is usually reached around 5 minutes after the injection. ECAs are primarily excreted by the kidneys with an elimination half-life of 80 minutes.[9] MR imaging of the liver is performed before and after the injection of ECAs, often with fat saturation that improves liver contrast/noise ratio, as well as the sensitivity for extrahepatic findings.[11] After contrast administration, dynamic imaging (ie, arterial phase [AP], portal venous phase [PVP], and delayed phase) is required for liver lesion characterization.[12] In patients with CLD, dynamic imaging with acquisition of adequate AP is crucial because most HCCs and some HCC precursors will present with AP hyperenhancement (APHE).[13] For detection and characterization of these AP hyperenhancing observations, the late AP is preferred, the subtype of AP when the hepatic artery and branches are fully enhanced, the portal vein is enhanced more than the liver parenchyma, and the hepatic veins are not enhanced.[12] Radiologists should be mindful about the timing of the AP because the absence of portal vein enhancement indicates an early AP acquisition, when hypervascular observation may not yet be enhanced, and therefore not yet be visualized (**Fig. 1**). Following the AP, PVP occurs 60 to 80 seconds after contrast injection, and delayed phase (DP) occurs 2 to 5 minutes after contrast injection. In both PVP and DP, the portal vein and the hepatic vein enhancement is more than the background liver. An ECA full diagnostic protocol includes precontrast and postcontrast images, with additional sequences to help in lesion characterization (**Table 2**). Abbreviated MR imaging protocols using ECAs for HCC screening and surveillance have also been proposed[14] and are discussed in detail in another chapter of the current issue.

Advantages of Extracellular Agents in Patients with Chronic Liver Disease

Hepatocellular carcinoma diagnosis

In patients with CLD, the main advantage of ECA-enhanced MR imaging is its ability to accurately characterize focal liver observations. Patients with CLD are at increased risk of developing HCC, as well as other primary liver malignancies, and therefore, characterization of any observation detected during screening or surveillance is imperative. In patients at risk, the high specificity and positive predictive value of contrast-enhanced MR imaging for HCC diagnosis obviates the need for pathologic confirmation.[6] The Liver Imaging Reporting And Data System (LI-RADS) was introduced in 2011 to promote standardization of liver imaging in patients at risk of or with HCC.[15] In the LI-RADS, focal observations found on imaging in patients at risk are assigned ordinal categories (LR-1 to LR-5) to reflect the probability of HCC based on the combination of imaging features, namely, nonrim APHE, nonperipheral washout, enhancing capsule, and threshold growth (**Fig. 2**). An additional category (LR-M) communicates the probability of non-HCC malignancies.[15]

Nonrim APHE is defined as nonrim-like enhancement in the AP, unequivocally greater in whole or in part than the background liver, with the enhancing component having higher intensity than the liver in the AP.[12] The presence of APHE yields high sensitivity and high overall accuracy for HCC diagnosis, especially for progressed tumors.[16,17] Further, the presence of APHE in association with other postcontrast imaging features

Table 1
Gadolinium-based extracellular contrast agents

Trade Name	Generic Name	Short Name	Structure
Dotarem	Gadoterate meglumine	Gd-DOTA	Ionic, macrocyclic
Gadavist	Gadobutrol	Gd-DO3A-butrol	Ionic, macrocyclic
Magnevist	Gadopentetate dimeglumine	GD-DTPA	Ionic, linear
Omniscan	Gadodiamide	Gd-DTPA-BMA	Nonionic, linear
OptiMARK	Gadoversetamide	Gd-DTPA-BMEA	Nonionic, linear
ProHance	Gadoteridol	Gd-HP-DO3A	Nonionic, macrocyclic

From: fda.gov/drugs/postmarket-drug-safety-information-patients-and-providers/information-gadolinium-based-contrast-agents, last accessed October 5, 2020.

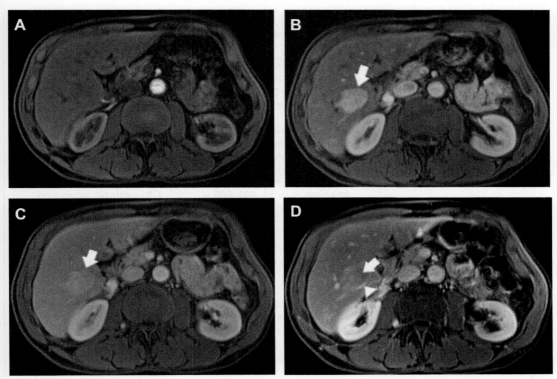

Fig. 1. MR imaging scans with an extracellular contrast agent in a 59-year-old man with hepatitis C and an AFP of 730 demonstrating an HCC (LI-RADS 5 observation). The early arterial phase (*A*) is too early to detect the hepatocellular carcinoma, which is well seen on the late arterial phase (*B*) as a hypervascular enhancing observation (*arrow*) in the right lobe of the liver in segments V and VI. The HCC demonstrates slight washout (*arrow*) on the portal venous phase (*C*). The washout (*arrow*) and enhancing capsule (*arrowhead*) is more obvious on the 3-minute delayed phase (*D*). AFP, alpha fetoprotein.

(eg, nonperipheral washout, enhancing capsule) maximizes the specificity for HCC diagnosis.[16] Therefore, AP images are arguably the most important contrast phase in patients with CLD. APHE has been shown to be more frequently depicted with ECAs than with HBAs, with at least two factors responsible for this finding.[18] First, ECAs are administered in higher volume, which results in a larger intravenous bolus, facilitating its tracking and the acquisition of the optimally timed late AP.[10] Second, transient severe motion (TSM) artifacts, that is, respiratory motion artifacts mostly associated with AP acquisitions and resulting in image degradation, have been shown to happen less frequently in patients administered with ECAs than with HBAs.[19] In addition, ECAs provide higher image contrast in the vascular phases than HBAs in patients with and without cirrhosis, which is likely to result in a clearer depiction of observations with APHE.[20,21]

In addition to APHE, two additional imaging features are important for the diagnosis of HCC with high confidence: nonperipheral washout and

enhancing capsule. The LI-RADS defines nonperipheral washout as visually assessed reduction in enhancement from the earlier to later phase, resulting in hypoenhancement relative to the liver that is not more pronounced in the periphery of the observation.[12] With ECAs, the appraisal of washout can be done on either the portal venous or delayed phase; because in some HCCs, washout is more clearly depicted on delayed phases, use of ECAs results in improved diagnostic accuracy.[22] As a standalone feature, nonperipheral washout on ECA-enhanced MR imaging results in 62% to 95% specificity for HCC diagnosis.[16] Conversely, the progressive liver parenchymal enhancement observed with HBAs can be a cofounder for the assessment of washout, negatively affecting the specificity for HCC diagnosis, as discussed further in this article. Enhancing capsule is similarly more frequently depicted with ECAs because the surrounding parenchymal enhancement observed with HBAs may make the enhancing capsule less conspicuous.[23] On ECA-enhanced MR imaging, the

Table 2
Suggested extracellular agents and gadoxetate disodium–enhanced liver MR imaging protocols

Phases	Extracellular Agent	Hepatobiliary Agent
Precontrast acquisitions	Coronal 2D T2-weighted SSFSE Axial 2D or 3D T1-weighted GRE (in-phase and out-of-phase) Axial 2D T2-weighted SSFSE Axial 2D T2-weighted SSFSE with fat saturation (Optional) Axial diffusion-weighted imaging, b = 50, 400, 800 s/mm^2 Axial 2D or 3D T1-weighted GRE with fat saturation	Coronal 2D T2-weighted SSFSE Axial 2D or 3D T1-weighted GRE (in-phase and out-of-phase) Axial 2D or 3D T1-weighted GRE with fat saturation
GBCA Injection →	*Gadolinium-based ECA (0.1 mmol/kg of body weight)*	*Gadoxetate disodium (0.025 mmol/kg of body weight)*
≈20 s after contrast injection	Axial 2D or 3D T1-weighted GRE with fat saturation—arterial phase	Axial 2D or 3D T1-weighted GRE with fat saturation—arterial phase
≈60–80 s after contrast injection	Axial 2D or 3D T1-weighted GRE with fat saturation—portal venous phase	Axial 2D or 3D T1-weighted GRE with fat saturation—portal venous phase
		Axial 2D T2-weighted SSFSE Axial 2D T2-weighted SSFSE with fat saturation (optional)
≈2–5 min after contrast injection	Axial 2D or 3D T1-weighted GRE with fat saturation—delayed phase Coronal 2D or 3D T1-weighted GRE with fat saturation—delayed phase (optional)	Axial 2D or 3D T1-weighted GRE with fat saturation—transitional phase
		Axial diffusion-weighted imaging, b = 50, 400, 800 s/mm^2
≈20 min after contrast injection		Axial 2D or 3D T1-weighted GRE with fat saturation—hepatobiliary phase Coronal 2D or 3D T1-weighted GRE with fat saturation—hepatobiliary phase (optional)

Abbreviations: GBCA, gadolinium-based contrast agent; GRE, gradient echo; SSFSE, single-shot fast spin echo.

detection of an enhancing capsule yields higher than 95% per-lesion specificity and positive predictive value for HCC diagnosis in patients at risk.[24]

In light of the aforementioned considerations, ECAs have been shown to provide the highest specificity, as well as high sensitivity, positive predictive value, and overall accuracy for HCC diagnosis in populations at risk. In two recent meta-analyses, ECA-enhanced MR imaging was reported to have 92% to 96% specificity and 72% to 76% sensitivity for HCC diagnosis.[5,25]

The ability to accumulate in the extracellular space offers an additional advantage to ECAs for lesion characterization. Lesions with expanded extracellular space, such as intrahepatic cholangiocarcinomas and some metastases, will show progressive enhancement on delayed phases, as

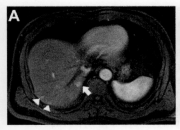
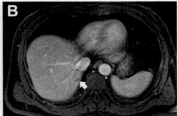

Fig. 2. MR imaging with an extracellular contrast agent in a 48-year-old man with hepatitis B. The late arterial phase (A) demonstrates 3 nonrim hyperenhancing observations (arrows), the largest one centrally near the right hepatic vein, and inferior vena cava measures 12 mm. On the portal venous phase (B), the largest lesion shows washout, in keeping with an LI-RADS 5 observation. The other two hypervascular observations did not show washout, in keeping with LI-RADS 3 observations.

opposed to the characteristic washout of HCCs, supporting the imaging-based differentiation[26] (Fig. 3). The differential between HCC and non-HCC malignancies in patients at risk is of utmost importance because management and treatment options significantly differ.[27]

Other advantages

Once thought to be associated only with HCCs, vascular invasion (ie, tumor in vein; LR-TIV), is a relatively complication of all primary malignancies arising in patients with CLD. In a recent meta-analysis, 71% of LR-TIVs were due to HCC and 29% were secondary to other malignancies.[28] But probably, more important than its etiology, the detection of tumor in the vein in patients with CLD has significant management implications. The presence of TIV is a contraindication to liver transplantation and to most locoregional therapies.[29] Although no studies have directly compared MR imaging agents for the assessment of LR-TIV, ECAs yield higher signal/noise ratios

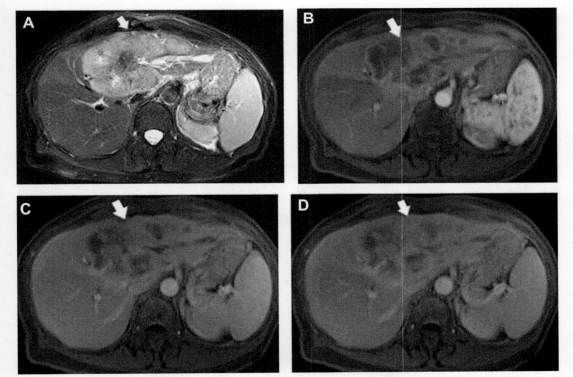

Fig. 3. MR imaging with an ECA in a 74-year-old woman with hepatitis B and cholangiocarcinoma. The T2-weighted image (A) shows a large heterogenous hyperintense mass (arrow) that demonstrates (C) rim hyperenhancement on the arterial phase (B) with delayed central enhancement on the portal venous phase (C) and delayed images (D). Imaging features meet criteria for LR-M category (Probably or definitely malignant, not HCC specific) and are commonly seen in intrahepatic cholangiocarcinoma, which was surgically proven.

(SNRs) and overall enhancement of vascular structures[20,30] and are likely to improve the visualization of tumor in the vein (**Fig. 4**). ECAs are also the preferred agents for the evaluation of extrahepatic tumor spread.[11] Altogether, ECA-enhanced MR imaging permits simultaneous diagnosis and staging of HCCs, potentially better informing treatment planning and prognosis than other contrast agents.

Limitations of Extracellular Agents in Patients with Chronic Liver Disease

Although APHE confers high sensitivity for HCC greater than 2 cm, in the absence of additional imaging features, it may have limited diagnostic performance.[16] Arteriovenous shunts commonly occur in patients with CLD, presenting on imaging as AP hyperenhancing observations. Although rare, other benign entities may also present with APHE in patients with CLD.[15] These AP hyperenhancing observations on ECA-enhanced studies in the context of CLD increase the risk of false-positive HCC diagnosis.[31] Another potential pitfall associated with ECAs in patients with CLD refers

to the enhancement of fibrous tissue surrounding cirrhotic nodules, which can be mistakenly perceived as an enhancing capsule and also potentially increase the risk of false positives.[11] In these situations, the lack of an additional contrast mechanism as enabled by other agents (eg, HBAs) limits the ability of further differentiation, negatively affecting specificity. The sensitivity of ECAs for HCC precursors and hypovascular or infiltrative HCCs is also relatively limited and needs to be acknowledged when using these contrast agents.[11,32]

HEPATOBILIARY CONTRAST AGENTS
Background

HBAs are gadolinium-based intravenous MR imaging contrast agents with dual properties. These agents diffuse into the extracellular space in a similar fashion as ECAs but are also actively transported by membrane proteins into functioning hepatocytes, subsequently excreted through the bile ducts.[33] The hepatocyte uptake results in intense hepatic parenchymal enhancement, adding another contrast mechanism to liver imaging that

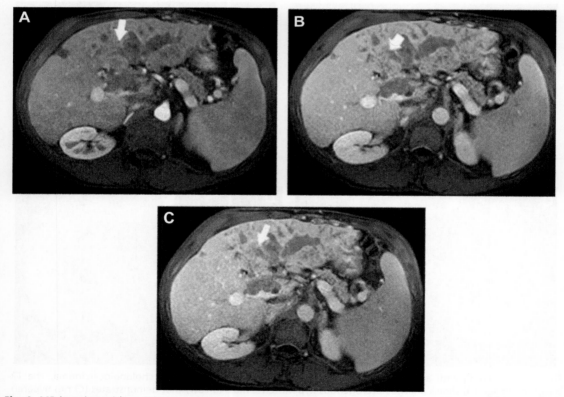

Fig. 4. MR imaging with an ECA in a 53-year-old man with hepatis C cirrhosis demonstrating an infiltrative HCC with TIV. Arterial (*A*), portal venous (*B*), and delayed (*C*) phase images showing a large infiltrative mass in segments I, II, and III with areas of mild hypervascularity and washout invading into the portal vein (*arrow*).

expands the opportunities for lesion detection, characterization, and functional assessment. To maximize this contrast mechanism, hepatobiliary phase (HBP) images are acquired at 20 minutes after injection, when most livers reach marked cellular uptake. For focal lesions, the appearance on HBP is determined by the presence or absence of functional hepatocytes and the expression of functional transporters responsible for HBA uptake in relation to the background liver parenchyma. For full diagnostic examinations, the HBP is acquired in addition to conventional dynamic postcontrast phases (ie, AP and PVP). The nomenclature of the postcontrast phase is slightly different than with ECAs, reflecting its contrast mechanism and distribution (see **Table 2**). The higher relaxivity of gadoxetate allows for lower dosage than ECAs, at 0.025 mmol/kg,[33] with most centers often using a standard dose of 10 mL. Abbreviated MR imaging protocols that include HBP for HCC screening have been investigated[14] and are also discussed in another chapter of the current issue.

Currently, two contrast agents are recognized as HBAs: gadobenate dimeglumine (MultiHance; Bracco) and gadoxetate disodium (Eovist or Primovist; Bayer Healthcare), herein referred as gadoxetate. Approximately 5% of the administered dose of gadobenate dimeglumine is excreted via hepatocytes, and the HBP occurs 1 to 3 hours after contrast injection.[33] With gadoxetate, approximately 50% of the administered dose is excreted by the hepatocytes, and the HBP occurs 15 to 20 min after injection in patients with no significant liver dysfunction.[34] In practice, gadoxetate is the most commonly used HBA. The use of gadobenate dimeglumine is less practical, given the relatively long delay between contrast administration and the onset of the HBP, relatively low hepatobiliary excretion, and a comparative paucity of the literature assessing its use in the setting of background liver dysfunction.[35]

Advantages of Gadoxetate in Patients with Chronic Liver Disease

Improved sensitivity for hepatocellular carcinoma

In patients at risk of liver malignancy, the main advantage of gadoxetate is offered by the acquisition of the HBP and the resulting high liver-to-lesion contrast. Owing to its high SNR and contrast/noise ratio, the HBP may depict HCCs with higher conspicuity than other sequences or contrast agents.[36,37] In some cases, lesions are detected in the HBP and are only retrospectively

identified and characterized on other sequences.[38]

Compared with other imaging modalities used for HCC diagnosis (eg, contrast-enhanced ultrasound, computed tomography [CT], and MR imaging with ECAs), gadoxetate-enhanced MR imaging has the highest overall per-lesion sensitivity (86%) and positive predictive value (94%).[39] Furthermore, MR imaging with gadoxetate is the most sensitive modality for detection of small HCCs ($\leq$2 cm), with a sensitivity of 84% to 96%.[39,40] It is important to note, however, that the aforementioned performance is established in patients without cirrhosis or with well-compensated cirrhosis. Because severe liver dysfunction reduces the visualization of HCCs in the HBP, the sensitivity of gadoxetate-enhanced MR imaging in patients with severe liver dysfunction may be reduced, but the exact impact of liver dysfunction on gadoxetate-enhanced MR imaging sensitivity is not known.

Given its high sensitivity for HCC in patients with well-compensated cirrhosis, gadoxetate-enhanced MR imaging is the imaging modality of choice in clinical scenarios wherein locoregional treatment and resection are the preferred treatment options for small HCCs, for example, in Asian countries.[41] In these scenarios, gadoxetate-enhanced MR imaging is more cost-effective than CT or MR imaging with ECAs, associated with an increased number of quality-adjusted life years, lower direct costs, and an incremental cost-effectiveness ratio of $12,000.[42,43]

As previously described in this article, APHE is a hallmark of HCC. However, it develops relatively late during hepatocarcinogenesis, as the lesion progresses from early HCC to progressed HCC.[13] In contradistinction, the expression of organic anion transporting polypeptide 8 (OATP-8), a transporter responsible for gadoxetate cellular uptake of gadoxetate, begins to decline at the earlier stages, as early as a low-grade dysplastic nodule.[44] As a result, relatively reduced gadoxetate uptake occurs in the early stages of hepatocarcinogenesis, before the development of APHE.[44] Eighty-two percent of high-grade dysplastic nodules and 76% of early HCCs are hypointense on the HBP.[45] Furthermore, up to 38% of early HCCs may be seen only on the HBP and not be discernible on any other sequence.[46]

HBP hypointense nodules without APHE are unique to HBA-enhanced MR imaging. On pathology, 74% of HBP hypointense nodules without APHE are HCCs, and 10% are dysplastic nodules.[47] Of HCCs with APHE, 29% to 44% are visible as HBP hypointense nodules without

APHE on prior imaging.[48,49] The rate of progression to hypervascular HCC of HBP hypointense nodules without APHE is 16% to 43% within 24 months (**Fig. 5**).[50,51] In such nodules, the pooled rate of hypervascular transformation is 28% overall, with the pooled 1-, 2-, and 3-year cumulative incidence rates of 18%, 25%, and 30%, respectively.[52] On the other hand, only a small fraction (1%–4%) of the nodules that lack APHE and are hyperintense on the HBP progress to HCC, with a 1-year hypervascularization rate of less than 2%.[53,54] HBP hypointense nodules without APHE are also markers of increased HCC development elsewhere, with the cumulative 3-year rate of HCC elsewhere in the liver being 22%, compared with 6% in patients with no nodules.[55]

Other advantages

In addition to providing improved sensitivity, gadoxetate-enhanced MR imaging may offer some advantages for improved specificity of HCC diagnosis. Arterioportal shunts, common in cirrhotic livers, may contribute to false-positive diagnosis because differentiation from small HCCs may be difficult in cases wherein the shape is round or oval or when the shunt is centrally located.[31] Because the shunts do not represent true space-occupying lesions, they commonly appear similar to background liver parenchyma on the HBP. Eighty-five percent to 94% of nodular vascular pseudolesions are isointense to the background on the HBP, which helps to distinguish them from small HCCs.[56]

Limitations of Hepatobiliary Agents in Patients with Chronic Liver Disease

Mistiming of the AP with gadoxetate is more frequent with gadoxetate than with ECA and can be explained by the smaller bolus of contrast than other gadolinium chelates, resulting in a narrow imaging window for AP acquisition. Because a test bolus is not used to prevent undesirable liver parenchymal enhancement before the full dose, options for bolus timing are limited. Advanced techniques such as multiple AP acquisitions with fluoroscopic triggering may help to ensure correct timing of the late AP.[57] The incidence of TSM is the highest with gadoxetate, ranging from 5% to

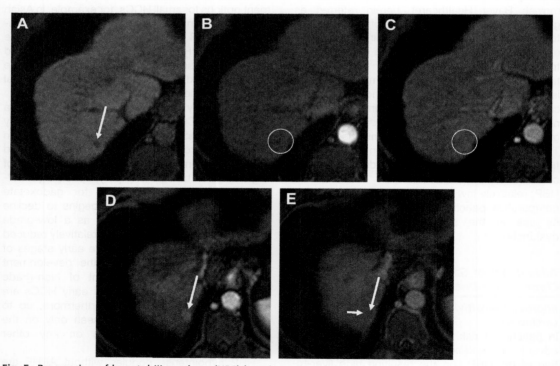

Fig. 5. Progression of hepatobiliary phase (HBP) hypointense nodule without arterial phase hyperenhancement (APHE) in a 59-year-old man with alcoholic cirrhosis. Initial MR imaging in HBP (*A*) demonstrates a 6-mm HBP hypointense nodule (*arrow*). No associated signal abnormality is seen in this region (*circle*) on the arterial phase (*B*) or portal venous phase (*C*). MR imaging 6 months later demonstrates new arterial phase hyperenhancement (*arrow*, *D*), new portal venous phase washout (*long arrow*, *E*), and new enhancing capsule (*short arrow*, e) and threshold growth to 11 mm, resulting in LR-5 (definite HCC) categorization.

22%[19] **(Fig. 6)**. Although TSM is now a well-established phenomenon, the underlying mechanisms causing it remain unknown.[58] Despite that, several technical strategies may help decrease TSM frequency. These include one-to-one dilution of gadoxetate with normal saline, injection at a slower rate, multiple AP acquisition, advanced motion-resistant or free-breathing techniques, modified breathing commands, and patient coaching.[59–61]

Gadoxetate use affects the assessment of washout. With gadoxetate, the progressive parenchymal enhancement may result in a perceived relative hypointensity of focal observations with lower OATP expression, rather than the washout as seen with ECAs.[23] As a result, hypointensity in an observation during the transitional phase (TP) or HBP does not equal washout seen in the portal venous or delayed phases with ECAs. For example, the combination of APHE and TP hypointensity is 86% to 95% specific for HCC, compared with 98% to 100% specificity when the assessment of washout is restricted to the PVP.[62,63] As a result, the LI-RADS restricts assessment of washout with gadoxetate to the PVP in order to maintain the specificity of the LR-5 category as close to 100% as possible.[15] Furthermore, the early parenchymal enhancement with gadoxetate also can obscure visualization of an enhancing capsule.[64] Unlike washout, however, the presence of an enhancing capsule can be assessed on either the PVP or TP on gadoxetate-enhanced MR imaging.[15,23]

While in patients with early or well-compensated cirrhosis, the pharmacokinetics of gadoxetate is similar to that seen in noncirrhotic livers, the hepatocellular uptake may be diminished in patients with decompensated cirrhosis, leading to decreased parenchymal enhancement during the TP and the HBP and/or delayed peak enhancement.[65] Recognition of adequacy of the HBP is crucial for accurate interpretation. If an observation is isointense to the parenchyma on the HBP owing to suboptimal parenchymal enhancement, HBP isointensity should not be interpreted as an ancillary feature favoring benignity. The HBP is

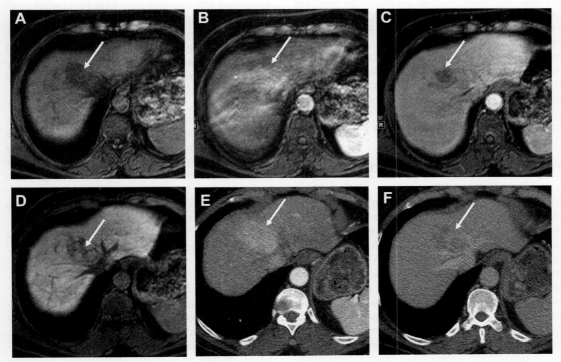

Fig. 6. Transient severe motion in a 54-year-old man with hepatitis C cirrhosis. Precontrast T1-weighted (A), arterial phase (AP) (B), portal venous phase (PVP) (C), and hepatobiliary phase (HBP) (D) demonstrate a 55-mm observation (arrow) with nonperipheral washout (C) and mosaic appearance on HBP (D). The AP is the only phase that is degraded by respiratory motion, confirming transient severe motion. Note that the severe motion artifact precludes assessment for the presence or absence of arterial phase hyperenhancement. CT in the arterial phase (E) and portal venous phase (F) performed 2 weeks later demonstrates nonrim APHE (arrow, E) and nonperipheral washout (arrow, F), allowing for LR-5 (definite HCC) categorization.

considered adequate if the signal intensity of the liver parenchyma is unequivocally hyperintense relative to the intrahepatic blood vessels; otherwise, the HBP is considered suboptimal.[66] Advanced cirrhosis with severe hepatic dysfunction is the most common cause of a suboptimal HBP. Other causes include diffuse iron overload, steatosis, and cholestasis. In patients with a suboptimal HBP, the use of ECAs is preferred.

EXTRACELLULAR VERSUS HEPATOBILIARY CONTRAST AGENTS

The choice of using ECAs versus HBAs is mostly determined by institutional preferences, as it can be by the clinical setting. In North America, multiple institutions use ECAs routinely, reserving the use of HBAs as a problem-solving tool when further evaluation in needed. However, neither North American nor European current guidelines favor one type of contrast agent over another.[6,27] Guidelines in Asia use HBAs as the frontline contrast agent because the emphasis is on improved sensitivity, especially for small ≤2-cm HCC.[41,67] Although depending on the clinical context, one contrast may be preferred over the other, no exceptional differences in overall diagnostic performance between ECAs and HBAs have been reported. In a recent meta-analysis including 31 studies, sensitivities and specificities for HCC were not significantly different between ECAs and HBAs, even in subgroup analyses accounting for the study design, underlying liver disease, lesion size, or reference standard.[25] A comparison of the two agents is presented in **Table 3**.

Emerging Data and Future Directions

Screening and surveillance
In patients at higher risk of HCC, imaging surveillance is recommended for early tumor detection.[27] Although biannual ultrasound is the clinical standard, the sensitivity of ultrasound for small HCCs is suboptimal and may be less than 50% depending on the lesion size and patient characteristics.[27,68] To address this gap and relying on the high sensitivity of contrast-enhanced MR imaging for liver lesions, abbreviated MR imaging protocols have been proposed with the aim of improving early HCC detection in patients at risk.[14] The two types of contrast agents have been investigated. Abbreviated MR imaging protocols using ECAs rely on the high sensitivity of these agents for detection of hypervascular observations, whereas abbreviated protocols using gadoxetate exploit the high liver-to-lesion contrast in the HBP for lesion detection. Although large prospective clinical trials are still needed to support the wide adoption of abbreviated MR imaging protocols in the setting of HCC screening and surveillance, both contrast agents seem comparably promising, with encouraging results being reported with each of these AMRI protocols.[4,69,70]

Patient outcomes and prognosis
Several studies assessed the clinical implication of the presence of HBP hypointense nodules without APHE in patients with early HCCs.[71–75] These nodules have been found to be potential predictors of HCC development in the background liver. The presence of such nodules on pretreatment MR imaging is associated with 68% increase in risk of HCC recurrence and significantly lower overall survival rates.[71] An addition of gadoxetate-enhanced MR imaging to CT prior to definitive surgical or locoregional treatment is associated with 28% to 33% decreased risk of HCC recurrence and 35% decreased risk of overall mortality.[72,73] In addition, treatment of HBP hypointense nodules without APHE at the same time as early HCC resection was shown to improve the 1-, 3-, and 5-year recurrence-free survival rates.[46] Gadoxetate-enhanced MR imaging may also be predictive of postsurgical outcomes after liver transplantation. HBP hypointense satellite nodules and peritumoural hypointensity on the HBP of the pretransplant MR imaging were shown to be independently associated with tumor recurrence after transplantation.[76]

For decades, imaging detection and diagnostic criteria for primary liver cancers in patients with CLD have been addressed monotonically. HCCs have been mostly described as a single entity despite their known variability in the molecular profile and biology. More recently, physicians and researchers have been more interested in individual tumor biology and biologic behavior, with a few investigating their relation to imaging features. Two studies have reported worse biologic behavior, assessed by the rate of postsurgical recurrence, in both HCC and non-HCC malignancies when these present with LR-M features.[77,78] Another study has found LI-RADS imaging features (eg, enhancing capsule) as potential predictors of high-grade HCCs.[79] Rhee and colleagues[80] reported irregular rim APHE to be more frequent in macrotrabecular HCC subtypes, as well as in HCCs expressing cytokeratin 19 (CK19), both associated with more aggressive behavior. Although these features can be confidently assessed with ECAs, MR imaging with gadoxetate provides additional information and seems particularly promising. Different levels of molecular transporter expression and activity in

Table 3
Comparison of extracellular and hepatobiliary contrast agents

Feature	Extracellular	Hepatobiliary
Uptake	Nonspecific extracellular space	Hepatobiliary and extracellular space
Excretion	Renal	Half biliary, half renal
Cost	Most economical	More expensive
Arterial Phase	Easier to optimize Less motion artifact	More challenging to optimize owing to smaller bolus Prone to motion artifact owing to transient tachypnea
Washout	Can use portal venous and delayed phases	Use the portal venous phase
Enhancing Capsule	See on portal venous and delayed phases	May not be well seen on the transitional phase owing to the enhancing adjacent parenchyma
Hepatic Dysfunction	Not affected	May have a suboptimal hepatobiliary phase
Sensitivity and Specificity for Detecting HCC	More specific	More sensitive

tumors of variable differentiation result in different levels of gadoxetate uptake and, therefore, may offer an insight into tumor differentiation.[81] The tumor/liver signal intensity ratio of ≤ 0.522 on the HBP has been shown to be predictive of CK19-positive HCC.[82] Up to 15% of HCCs are isointensity or hyperintensity on the HBP owing to the preserved expression of OATP-8.[44] HCCs demonstrating HBP hyperintensity express molecular features of mature hepatocytes, with weak expression of stem cell markers, and are commonly associated with more favorable outcomes, such as decreased likelihood of microvascular invasion (MVI) and increased rates of peliosis.[83,84] HCCs with isointensity or hyperintensity on the HBP have been shown to have longer recurrence-free and overall survival than HBP hypointense HCCs.[83–86]

Additional prognostic information offered by gadoxetate-enhanced MR imaging is the peritumoral hypointensity on the HBP as a predictor of MVI (**Fig. 7**). In two studies, MVI was significantly more frequent in HCCs with peritumoral HBP hypointensity than in HCCs without this feature (46%–64% vs 12%–26%, $P<.005$).[87,88] The odds of MVI are 5 to 20 times higher in HCCs with peritumoral HBP hypointensity, with a reported hazard ratio of 4.5 for prediction of postresection recurrence.[88,89] As evidence-based data emerge and knowledge accrues, the role of contrast-enhanced MR imaging in patients with CLD and at risk of primary liver tumors is likely to expand beyond detection and diagnosis to provide a more comprehensive assessment that includes tumor biology and prognostic information.

New-generation contrast agents
Newer agents use macrocyclic chelates to decrease the risk of dissociation that can result in gadolinium retention. Other agents that continue to be investigated use endogenous components, such as iron and manganese, so that retention is less of an issue. Protein-based targeted agents are also being investigated to determine their efficacy in assessing early fibrosis.[90] New agents are also being investigated for noninvasive assessment of fibrotic or inflammatory tissue at the molecular level, which may impact treatment with various drugs.[91] Perfusion imaging and quantitative contrast uptake analysis have also been investigated to assess the degree of fibrosis and hepatic dysfunction in patients with CLD.[3,91]

Safety Considerations

Adverse reactions to gadolinium-based MR imaging contrast agents are infrequent.[10] Most reactions are mild and transient, such as headache, nausea, and vomiting, occurring in less than 1% of patients.[92] The incidence of allergic reactions is also low. In a large series report of 141,623 doses, 0.079% presented with immediate hypersensitivity reactions.[93] The most common reported reaction was urticaria, with anaphylaxis representing less than 10% of all reaction cases. Other studies have also reported very low rates

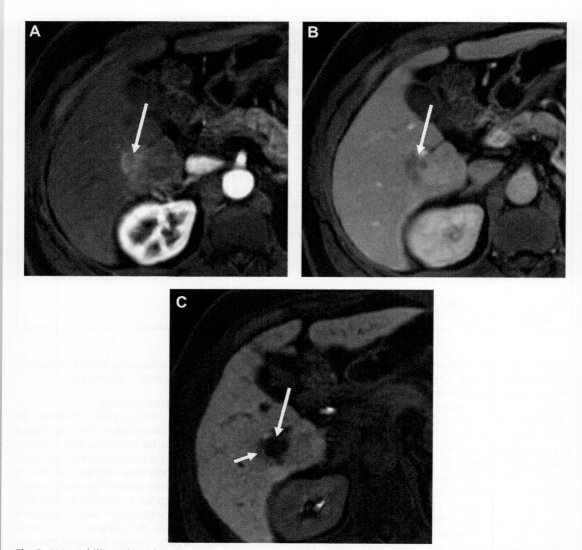

Fig. 7. Hepatobiliary phase (HBP) halo in a 55-year-old man with hepatitis C cirrhosis. MR imaging in the arterial phase (*A*) and portal venous phase (*B*) demonstrates a 19-mm observation with nonrim arterial phase hyperenhancement (*arrow, A*) and nonperipheral washout (*arrow, B*), categorized LR-5 (definite HCC). The observation is hypointense on the HBP (*long arrow, C*). Note the ill-defined area of decreased signal intensity around the observation (*short arrow*), consistent with the HBP hypointense halo. Resection confirmed HCC with microvascular invasion.

of anaphylaxis to gadolinium, in the range of 0.001% to 0.01%.[92,94–96]

Other serious and equally rare complications of GBCA administration are nephrogenic systemic fibrosis (NSF) and gadolinium deposition within the brain tissue. The former is a complication of gadolinium use in patients with end-stage renal disease,[97] and the latter is a dose-dependent retention in patients who have undergone repeated use of galodinium.[98] NSF is a late complication characterized by progressive thickening of the skin, believed to be related to the dissociation of gadolinium from the chelate, lending to gadolinium ion accumulation in the soft tissues. The overall risk of NSF associated with MR imaging contrast agents is extremely low, particularly at standard doses of macrocyclic agents and newer linear agents (group II agents), when the risk is considered virtually inexistent.[99] In patients with kidney disease and a potential risk of NSF, these group II agents can be administered with caution, at the lowest dose possible to obtain the required information to make the diagnosis.[99] Gadolinium deposition in the brain has been only recently described, and its effects are still unknown. It has been associated with linear agents rather than macrocyclic agents because the latter are more thermodynamically stable.[100–102] Owing to the unknown significance of this process, it is recommended that GBCAs are administered at the approved standard doses only, avoiding frequent use, if possible.[99]

Gadolinium can pass into the placenta or be excreted in very low amounts in the breast milk,[103,104] but there has been no known evidence of mutagenic or teratogenic effects from maternal administration[105] or of harmful effects to infants who have ingested breast milk from a lactating patient who received GBCAs.[103] The current recommendation is that these agents are administered with caution to pregnant or lactating women, considering the risks and benefits of their use.[99]

SUMMARY

Contrast-enhanced MR imaging is essential in the evaluation of patients with CLD, particularly in the assessment of associated complications, such as detection and characterization of liver lesions. The two classes of contrast agents discussed in this article (ie, ECAs and HBAs) are equally suitable for patients with CLD. The choice of using one over another should follow institutional preferences as well as emphasis on specificity or sensitivity as per the clinical context. The recent expansions in the clinical applications of contrast-enhanced MR imaging in patients with CLD lay out a promising landscape to improve further the medical care of this population.

CLINICS CARE POINTS

- Contrast-enhanced MR imaging is critical in the assessment of complication in patients with chronic liver disease, of which the most concerning is hepatocellular carcinoma (HCC).

- Two types of gadolinium-based MR imaging contrast agents are most beneficial to patients with chronic liver disease: extracellular and hepatobiliary agents.

- The choice of the agent often follows institutional preferences and clinical context. Extracellular agents are more often more specific for HCC diagnosis, whereas hepatobiliary agents offer the highest sensitivity for detection.

DISCLOSURE

S.D. Chang has nothing to disclose. G.M. Cunha has nothing to disclose. V. Chernyak is a consultant at Bayer.

REFERENCES

1. Moon AM, Singal AG, Tapper EB. Contemporary epidemiology of chronic liver disease and cirrhosis. Clin Gastroenterol Hepatol 2020;18(12): 2650–66.
2. Moura Cunha G, Navin PJ, Fowler KJ, et al. Quantitative magnetic resonance imaging for chronic liver disease. Br J Radiol 2021;94(1121):20201377.
3. Lee HJ, Hong SB, Lee NK, et al. Validation of functional liver imaging scores (FLIS) derived from gadoxetic acid-enhanced MRI in patients with chronic liver disease and liver cirrhosis: the relationship between Child-Pugh score and FLIS. Eur Radiol 2021. https://doi.org/10.1007/s00330-021-07955-1.
4. Brunsing RL, Chen DH, Schlein A, et al. Gadoxetate-enhanced Abbreviated MRI for Hepatocellular Carcinoma Surveillance: Preliminary Experience. Radiol Imaging Cancer 2019;1(2):e190010.
5. Feng Z, Zhao H, Guan S, et al. Diagnostic performance of MRI using extracellular contrast agents versus gadoxetic acid for hepatocellular carcinoma: A systematic review and meta-analysis. Liver Int 2021;41(5):1117–28.
6. Ayuso C, Rimola J, Vilana R, et al. Diagnosis and staging of hepatocellular carcinoma (HCC): current guidelines. Eur J Radiol 2018;101:72–81.
7. Schuhmann-Giampieri G. Liver contrast media for magnetic resonance imaging: interrelations between pharmacokinetics and imaging. Invest Radiol 1993;28(8):753–61.
8. Tang A, Abukasm K, Moura Cunha G, et al. Imaging of hepatocellular carcinoma: a pilot international survey. Abdom Radiol (NY) 2021;46(1): 205–15.
9. Hao D, Ai T, Goerner F, et al. MRI contrast agents: basic chemistry and safety. J Magn Reson Imaging 2012;36(5):1060–71.
10. Gandhi SN, Brown MA, Wong JG, et al. MR contrast agents for liver imaging: what, when. How Radiographics 2006;26(6):1621–36.
11. Choi JY, Lee JM, Sirlin CB. CT and MR imaging diagnosis and staging of hepatocellular carcinoma: part II. Extracellular agents, hepatobiliary agents, and ancillary imaging features. Radiology 2014;273(1):30–50.
12. Available at: https://www.acr.org/Clinical-Resources/Reporting-and-Data-Systems/LI-RADS/CT-MRI-LI-RADS-v2018, Accessed April 29, 2021.
13. Kim CK, Lim JH, Park CK, et al. Neoangiogenesis and sinusoidal capillarization in hepatocellular

carcinoma: correlation between dynamic CT and density of tumor microvessels. Radiology 2005; 237(2):529–34.

14. An JY, Peña MA, Cunha GM, et al. Abbreviated MRI for Hepatocellular Carcinoma Screening and Surveillance. Radiographics 2020;40(7):1916–31.

15. Chernyak V, Fowler KJ, Kamaya A, et al. Liver Imaging Reporting and Data System (LI-RADS) Version 2018: Imaging of Hepatocellular Carcinoma in At-Risk Patients. Radiology 2018;289(3):816–30.

16. Tang A, Bashir MR, Corwin MT, et al. LI-RADS Evidence Working Group. Evidence Supporting LI-RADS Major Features for CT- and MR Imaging-based Diagnosis of Hepatocellular Carcinoma: A Systematic Review. Radiology 2018;286(1):29–48.

17. Yim JH, Kim YK, Min JH, et al. Diagnosis of recurrent HCC: intraindividual comparison of gadoxetic acid MRI and extracellular contrast-enhanced MRI. Abdom Radiol (NY) 2019;44(7):2366–76.

18. Min JH, Kim JM, Kim YK, et al. Prospective intraindividual comparison of magnetic resonance imaging with gadoxetic acid and extracellular contrast for diagnosis of hepatocellular carcinomas using the liver imaging reporting and data system. Hepatology 2018;68(6):2254–66.

19. Shah MR, Flusberg M, Paroder V, et al. Transient arterial phase respiratory motion-related artifact in MR imaging of the liver: an analysis of four different gadolinium-based contrast agents. Clin Imaging 2017;41:23–7.

20. Schalkx HJ, van Stralen M, Coenegrachts K, et al. Liver perfusion in dynamic contrast-enhanced magnetic resonance imaging (DCE-MRI): comparison of enhancement in Gd-BT-DO3A and Gd-EOB-DTPA in normal liver parenchyma. Eur Radiol 2014;24(9):2146–56.

21. Vernuccio F, Cannella R, Gozzo C, et al. Hepatic enhancement in cirrhosis in the portal venous phase: what are the differences between gadoxetate disodium and gadobenate dimeglumine? Abdom Radiol (NY) 2020;45(8):2409–17.

22. Lee SE, An C, Hwang SH, et al. Extracellular contrast agent-enhanced MRI: 15-min delayed phase may improve the diagnostic performance for hepatocellular carcinoma in patients with chronic liver disease. Eur Radiol 2018;28(4):1551–9.

23. Santillan C, Fowler K, Kono Y, et al. LI-RADS major features: CT, MRI with extracellular agents, and MRI with hepatobiliary agents. Abdom Radiol (NY) 2018;43(1):75–81.

24. Cerny M, Bergeron C, Billiard JS, et al. LI-RADS for MR imaging diagnosis of hepatocellular carcinoma: performance of major and ancillary features. Radiology 2018;288(1):118–28.

25. Kim DW, Choi SH, Kim SY, et al. Diagnostic performance of MRI for HCC according to contrast agent type: a systematic review and meta-analysis. Hepatol Int 2020;14(6):1009–22.

26. Welle CL, Guglielmo FF, Venkatesh SK. MRI of the liver: choosing the right contrast agent. Abdom Radiol (NY) 2020;45(2):384–92.

27. Marrero JA, Kulik LM, Sirlin CB, et al. Diagnosis, Staging, and Management of Hepatocellular Carcinoma: 2018 Practice Guidance by the American Association for the Study of Liver Diseases. Hepatology 2018;68(2):723–50.

28. Kim DH, Choi SH, Park SH, et al. The Liver Imaging Reporting and Data System tumor-in-vein category: a systematic review and meta-analysis. Eur Radiol 2021;31(4):2497–506.

29. Baheti AD, Dunham GM, Ingraham CR, et al. Clinical implications for imaging of vascular invasion in hepatocellular carcinoma. Abdom Radiol (NY) 2016;41(9):1800–10.

30. Feuerlein S, Gupta RT, Boll DT, et al. Hepatocellular MR contrast agents: enhancement characteristics of liver parenchyma and portal vein after administration of gadoxetic acid in comparison to gadobenate dimeglumine. Eur J Radiol 2012;81(9):2037–41.

31. Parente DB, Perez RM, Eiras-Araujo A, et al. MR imaging of hypervascular lesions in the cirrhotic liver: a diagnostic dilemma. Radiographics 2012;32(3):767–87.

32. Rosenkrantz AB, Lee L, Matza BW, et al. Infiltrative hepatocellular carcinoma: comparison of MRI sequences for lesion conspicuity. Clin Radiol 2012;67(12):e105–11.

33. Frydrychowicz A, Lubner MG, Brown JJ, et al. Hepatobiliary MR imaging with gadolinium-based contrast agents. J Magn Reson Imaging 2012;35(3):492–511.

34. Ringe KI, Husarik DB, Sirlin CB, et al. Gadoxetate disodium-enhanced MRI of the liver: part 1, protocol optimization and lesion appearance in the non-cirrhotic liver. AJR Am J Roentgenol 2010;195(1):13–28.

35. Filippone A, Blakeborough A, Breuer J, et al. Enhancement of liver parenchyma after injection of hepatocyte-specific MRI contrast media: a comparison of gadoxetic acid and gadobenate dimeglumine. J Magn Reson Imaging 2010;31(2):356–64.

36. Frericks BB, Loddenkemper C, Huppertz A, et al. Qualitative and quantitative evaluation of hepatocellular carcinoma and cirrhotic liver enhancement using Gd-EOB-DTPA. AJR Am J Roentgenol 2009;193(4):1053–60.

37. Tirkes T, Mehta P, Aisen AM, et al. Comparison of dynamic phase enhancement of hepatocellular carcinoma using gadoxetate disodium vs

gadobenate dimeglumine. J Comput Assist To-mogr 2015;39(4):479–82.

38. Park MJ, Kim YK, Lee MW, et al. Small hepatocel-lular carcinomas: improved sensitivity by combining gadoxetic acid-enhanced and diffusion-weighted MR imaging patterns. Radi-ology 2012;264(3):761–70.

39. Hanna RF, Miloushev VZ, Tang A, et al. Compara-tive 13-year meta-analysis of the sensitivity and positive predictive value of ultrasound, CT, and MRI for detecting hepatocellular carcinoma. Ab-dom Radiol (NY) 2016;41(1):71–90.

40. Liu X, Jiang H, Chen J, et al. Gadoxetic acid disodium-enhanced magnetic resonance imaging outperformed multidetector computed tomography in diagnosing small hepatocellular carcinoma: A meta-analysis. Liver Transpl 2017;23(12):1505–18.

41. Omata M, Cheng AL, Kokudo N, et al. Asia–Pacific clinical practice guidelines on the management of hepatocellular carcinoma: a 2017 update. Hepatol Int 2017;11(4):317–70.

42. Nishie A, Goshima S, Haradome H, et al. Cost-effectiveness of EOB-MRI for Hepatocellular Carci-noma in Japan. Clin Ther 2017;39(4):738–750 e4.

43. Suh CH, Kim KW, Park SH, et al. Performing Ga-doxetic acid-enhanced MRI After CT for guiding curative treatment of early-stage hepatocellular carcinoma: a cost-effectiveness analysis. Am J Roentgenol 2018;210(2):W63–9.

44. Kitao A, Matsui O, Yoneda N, et al. The uptake transporter OATP8 expression decreases during multistep hepatocarcinogenesis: correlation with gadoxetic acid enhanced MR imaging. Eur Radiol 2011;21(10):2056–66.

45. Kim BR, Lee JM, Lee DH, et al. Diagnostic Perfor-mance of Gadoxetic Acid-enhanced Liver MR Im-aging versus Multidetector CT in the Detection of Dysplastic Nodules and Early Hepatocellular Car-cinoma. Radiology 2017;285(1):134–46.

46. Matsuda M, Ichikawa T, Amemiya H, et al. Preoper-ative gadoxetic Acid-enhanced MRI and simulta-neous treatment of early hepatocellular carcinoma prolonged recurrence-free survival of progressed hepatocellular carcinoma patients after hepatic resection. HPB Surg 2014;2014:641685.

47. Nakamura S, Nouso K, Kobayashi Y, et al. The diagnosis of hypovascular hepatic lesions showing hypo-intensity in the hepatobiliary phase of Gd-EOB- DTPA-enhanced MR imaging in high-risk pa-tients for hepatocellular carcinoma. Acta Med Okayama 2013;67(4):239–44.

48. Yamamoto A, Ito K, Tamada T, et al. Newly devel-oped hypervascular hepatocellular carcinoma dur-ing follow-up periods in patients with chronic liver disease: observation in serial gadoxetic acid-enhanced MRI. Am J Roentgenol 2013;200(6): 1254–60.

49. Ichikawa S, Ichikawa T, Motosugi U, et al. Was hy-pervascular hepatocellular carcinoma visible on previous gadoxetic acid-enhanced magnetic reso-nance images? Liver Cancer 2015;4(3):154–62.

50. Kim YS, Song JS, Lee HK, et al. Hypovascular hy-pointense nodules on hepatobiliary phase without T2 hyperintensity on gadoxetic acid-enhanced MR images in patients with chronic liver disease: long-term outcomes and risk factors for hypervas-cular transformation. Eur Radiol 2016;26(10): 3728–36.

51. Yang HJ, Song JS, Choi EJ, et al. Hypovascular hy-pointense nodules in hepatobiliary phase without T2 hyperintensity: long-term outcomes and added value of DWI in predicting hypervascular transfor-mation. Clin Imaging 2018;50:123–9.

52. Suh CH, Kim KW, Pyo J, et al. Hypervascular trans-formation of hypovascular hypointense nodules in the hepatobiliary phase of gadoxetic acid-enhanced MRI: a systematic review and meta-anal-ysis. Am J Roentgenol 2017;209(4):781–9.

53. Sano K, Ichikawa T, Motosugi U, et al. Outcome of hypovascular hepatic nodules with positive uptake of gadoxetic acid in patients with cirrhosis. Eur Ra-diol 2017;27(2):518–25.

54. Matsuda M, Tsuda T, Yoshioka S, et al. Incidence for progression of hypervascular HCC in hypovas-cular hepatic nodules showing hyperintensity on gadoxetic acid-enhanced hepatobiliary phase in patients with chronic liver diseases. Jpn J Radiol 2014;32(7):405–13.

55. Komatsu N, Motosugi U, Maekawa S, et al. Hepato-cellular carcinoma risk assessment using gadox-etic acid-enhanced hepatocyte phase magnetic resonance imaging. Hepatol Res 2014;44(13): 1339–46.

56. Sun HY, Lee JM, Shin CI, et al. Gadoxetic acid-enhanced magnetic resonance imaging for differ-entiating small hepatocellular carcinomas (< or =2 cm in diameter) from arterial enhancing pseudolesions: special emphasis on hepatobiliary phase imaging. Invest Radiol 2010;45(2):96–103.

57. Min JH, Kim YK, Kang TW, et al. Artifacts during the arterial phase of gadoxetate disodium-enhanced MRI: Multiple arterial phases using view-sharing from two different vendors versus single arterial phase imaging. Eur Radiol 2018; 28(8):3335–46.

58. Well L, Weinrich JM, Adam G, et al. Transient se-vere respiratory motion artifacts after application of gadoxetate disodium: what we currently know. RoFo 2018;190(1):20–30.

59. Xiao YD, Ma C, Liu J, et al. Transient severe motion during arterial phase in patients with Gadoxetic acid administration: Can a five hepatic arterial sub-phases technique mitigate the artifact? Exp Ther Med 2018;15(3):3133–9.

60. Kim YK, Lin WC, Sung K, et al. Reducing Artifacts during Arterial Phase of Gadoxetate Disodium-enhanced MR Imaging: Dilution Method versus Reduced Injection Rate. Radiology 2017;283(2):429–37.

61. Polanec SH, Bickel H, Baltzer PAT, et al. Respiratory motion artifacts during arterial phase imaging with gadoxetic acid: Can the injection protocol minimize this drawback? J Magn Reson Imaging 2017;46(4):1107–14.

62. Choi SH, Lee SS, Kim SY, et al. Intrahepatic cholangiocarcinoma in patients with cirrhosis: differentiation from hepatocellular carcinoma by using gadoxetic acid-enhanced MR Imaging and Dynamic CT. Radiology 2017;282(3):771–81.

63. Joo I, Lee JM, Lee DH, et al. Noninvasive diagnosis of hepatocellular carcinoma on gadoxetic acid-enhanced MRI: can hypointensity on the hepatobiliary phase be used as an alternative to washout? Eur Radiol 2015;25(10):2859–68.

64. Dioguardi Burgio M, Picone D, Cabibbo G, et al. MR-imaging features of hepatocellular carcinoma capsule appearance in cirrhotic liver: comparison of gadoxetic acid and gadobenate dimeglumine. Abdom Radiol (NY) 2016;41(8):1546–54.

65. Kim AY, Kim YK, Lee MW, et al. Detection of hepatocellular carcinoma in gadoxetic acid-enhanced MRI and diffusion-weighted MRI with respect to the severity of liver cirrhosis. Acta Radiol 2012;53(8):830–8.

66. Hope TA, Fowler KJ, Sirlin CB, et al. Hepatobiliary agents and their role in LI-RADS. Abdom Imaging 2015;40(3):613–25.

67. Xie DY, Ren ZG, Zhou J, et al. Critical appraisal of Chinese 2017 guideline on the management of hepatocellular carcinoma. Hepatobiliary Surg Nutr 2017;6(6):387–96.

68. Brunsing RL, Fowler KJ, Yokoo T, et al. Alternative approach of hepatocellular carcinoma surveillance: abbreviated MRI. Hepatoma Res 2020;6:59.

69. Vietti Violi N, Lewis S, Liao J, et al. Gadoxetate-enhanced abbreviated MRI is highly accurate for hepatocellular carcinoma screening. Eur Radiol 2020;30(11):6003–13.

70. Khatri G, Pedrosa I, Ananthakrishnan L, et al. Abbreviated-protocol screening MRI vs. complete-protocol diagnostic MRI for detection of hepatocellular carcinoma in patients with cirrhosis: An equivalence study using LI-RADS v2018. J Magn Reson Imaging 2020;51(2):415–25.

71. Toyoda H, Kumada T, Tada T, et al. Non-hypervascular hypointense nodules on Gd-EOB-DTPA-enhanced MRI as a predictor of outcomes for early-stage HCC. Hepatol Int 2015;9(1):84–92.

72. Kim HD, Lim YS, Han S, et al. Evaluation of early-stage hepatocellular carcinoma by magnetic resonance imaging with gadoxetic acid detects additional lesions and increases overall survival. Gastroenterology 2015;148(7):1371–82.

73. Shim JH, Han S, Shin YM, et al. Prognostic performance of preoperative gadoxetic acid-enhanced MRI in resectable hepatocellular carcinoma. J Magn Reson Imaging 2015;41(4):1115–23.

74. Lee DH, Lee JM, Lee JY, et al. Non-hypervascular hepatobiliary phase hypointense nodules on gadoxetic acid-enhanced MRI: risk of HCC recurrence after radiofrequency ablation. J Hepatol 2015;62(5):1122–30.

75. Inoue M, Ogasawara S, Chiba T, et al. Presence of non-hypervascular hypointense nodules on Gadolinium-ethoxybenzyl-diethylenetriamine pentaacetic acid-enhanced magnetic resonance imaging in patients with hepatocellular carcinoma. J Gastroenterol Hepatol 2017;32(4):908–15.

76. Kim AY, Sinn DH, Jeong WK, et al. Hepatobiliary MRI as novel selection criteria in liver transplantation for hepatocellular carcinoma. J Hepatol 2018;68(6):1144–52.

77. Jeon SK, Joo I, Lee DH, et al. Combined hepatocellular cholangiocarcinoma: LI-RADS v2017 categorisation for differential diagnosis and prognostication on gadoxetic acid-enhanced MR imaging. Eur Radiol 2019;29(1):373–82.

78. Choi SH, Lee SS, Park SH, et al. LI-RADS Classification and Prognosis of Primary Liver Cancers at Gadoxetic Acid-enhanced MRI. Radiology 2019;290(2):388–97.

79. Wei H, Jiang H, Liu X, et al. Can LI-RADS imaging features at gadoxetic acid-enhanced MRI predict aggressive features on pathology of single hepatocellular carcinoma? Eur J Radiol 2020;132:109312.

80. Rhee H, An C, Kim HY, et al. Hepatocellular carcinoma with irregular rim-like arterial phase hyperenhancement: more aggressive pathologic features. Liver Cancer 2019;8(1):24–40.

81. Erra P, Puglia M, Ragozzino A, et al. Appearance of hepatocellular carcinoma on gadoxetic acid-enhanced hepato-biliary phase MR imaging: a systematic review. Radiol Med 2015;120(11):1002–11.

82. Choi SY, Kim SH, Park CK, et al. Imaging Features of Gadoxetic Acid-enhanced and Diffusion-weighted MR Imaging for Identifying Cytokeratin 19-positive Hepatocellular Carcinoma: A Retrospective Observational Study. Radiology 2018;286(3):897–908.

83. Yamashita T, Kitao A, Matsui O, et al. Gd-EOB-DTPA-enhanced magnetic resonance imaging and alpha-fetoprotein predict prognosis of early-stage hepatocellular carcinoma. Hepatology 2014;60(5):1674–85.

84. Kitao A, Matsui O, Yoneda N, et al. Hypervascular hepatocellular carcinoma: correlation between biologic features and signal intensity on gadoxetic

acid-enhanced MR images. Radiology 2012; 265(3):780–9.

85. Choi JW, Lee JM, Kim SJ, et al. Hepatocellular carcinoma: imaging patterns on gadoxetic acid-enhanced MR Images and their value as an imaging biomarker. Radiology 2013;267(3):776–86.

86. Fujita N, Nishie A, Asayama Y, et al. Significance of the signal intensity of gadoxetic acid-enhanced MR imaging for predicting the efficacy of hepatic arterial infusion chemotherapy in hepatocellular carcinoma. Magn Reson Med Sci 2016;15(1):111–20.

87. Huang M, Liao B, Xu P, et al. Prediction of Microvascular Invasion in Hepatocellular Carcinoma: Preoperative Gd-EOB-DTPA-Dynamic Enhanced MRI and Histopathological Correlation. Contrast Media Mol Imaging 2018;2018:9674565.

88. Lee S, Kim SH, Lee JE, et al. Preoperative gadoxetic acid-enhanced MRI for predicting microvascular invasion in patients with single hepatocellular carcinoma. J Hepatol 2017;67(3): 526–34.

89. Shin SK, Kim YS, Shim YS, et al. Peritumoral decreased uptake area of gadoxetic acid enhanced magnetic resonance imaging and tumor recurrence after surgical resection in hepatocellular carcinoma: A STROBE-compliant article. Medicine 2017;96(33):e7761.

90. Salarian M, Turaga RC, Xue S, et al. Early detection and staging of chronic liver diseases with a protein MRI contrast agent. Nat Commun 2019;10(1):4777.

91. Zhou IY, Catalano OA, Caravan P. Advances in functional and molecular MRI technologies in chronic liver diseases. J Hepatol 2020;73(5): 1241–54.

92. Bleicher AG, Kanal E. Assessment of adverse reaction rates to newly approved MRI contrast agent: Review of 23,553 administrations of gadobenate dimeglumine. Am J Roentgenol 2008;191: W307–11.

93. Jung JW, Kang HR, Kim MH, et al. Immediate hypersensitivity reaction to gadolinium-based MR contrast media. Radiology 2012;264:414–22.

94. Murphy KJBJ, Cohan RH. Adverse reactions to gadolinium contrast media: a review of 36 cases. AJR Am J Roentgenol 1996;167:847–9.

95. Runge VM. Safety of approved MR contrast media for intravenous injection. J Magn Reson Imaging 2000;12(2):205–13.

96. Runge VM. Safety of magnetic resonance contrast media. Top Magn Reson Imaging 2001;12(4):309–14.

97. Ersoy H, Rybicki FJ. Biochemical safety profiles of gadolinium based extracellular contrast agents and nephrogenic systemic fibrosis. J Magn Reson Imaging 2007;26:1190–7.

98. Kanda T, Ishii K, Kawaguchi H, et al. High signal intensity in the dentate nucleus and globus pallidus on unenhanced T1-weighted MR images: relationship with increasing cumulative dose of a gadolinium-based contrast material. Radiology 2014;270:834–41.

99. Available at: www.ACR.org/-/media/ACR/Files/Clinical-Resource/Contrast_Media.pdf. Accessed April 29, 2021.

100. Errante Y, Cirimele V, Mallio CA, et al. Progressive increase of T1 signal intensity of the dentate nucleus on unenhanced magnetic resonance images is associated with cumulative doses of intravenously administered gadodiamide in patients with normal renal function, suggesting dechelation. Invest Radiol 2014;49:685–90.

101. Radbruch A, Weberling LD, Kieslich PJ, et al. Gadolinium retention in the dentate nucleus and globus pallidus is dependent on the class of contrast agent. Radiology 2015;275:783–91.

102. Kromrey ML, Liedtke KR, Ittermann T, et al. Intravenous injection of gadobutrol in an epidemiological study group did not lead to a difference in relative signal intensities of certain brain structures after 5 years. Eur Radiol 2017;27:772–7.

103. Rofsky NM, Weinreb JC, Litt AW. Quantitative analysis of gadopentate diglumine excreted in breast milk. J Magn Resson Imaging 1993;3:131–2.

104. Webb JA, Thomsen HS, Morcos SK. The use of iodinated and gadolinium contrast media during pregnancy and lactation. Eur Radiol 2005;15(6): 1234–40.

105. De Santis M, Straface G, Cavaliere AF, et al. Gadolinium periconceptional exposure: pregnancy and neonatal outcome. Acta Obstet Gynecol Scand 2007;86(1):99–101.

MR Imaging of Diffuse Liver Disease

Robert M. Marks, MD[a,b],*, Kathryn J. Fowler, MD[c], Mustafa R. Bashir, MD[d]

KEYWORDS

• Liver • Diffuse • MR imaging • Fat • Iron

KEY POINTS

- Chemical shift imaging, proton density fat fraction, and T2*/R2* maps can aid in detection and quantification of liver fat and iron.
- MR elastography can quantify liver fibrosis.
- MR cholangiopancreatography aids in detection of biliary anomalies and diseases.
- Multiphasic MR imaging with or without postcontrast phases can identify and monitor diffuse liver diseases.

INTRODUCTION

The liver performs many vital functions for the human body. It stores essential vitamins and minerals, such as iron and vitamins A, D, K, and B$_{12}$. It synthesizes proteins, such as blood clotting factors, albumin, and glycogen, as well as cholesterol, carbohydrates, and triglycerides. Additionally, it acts as a detoxifier, metabolizing and helping to clear alcohol, drugs, and ammonia. Diffuse liver disease typically occurs when one of these processes breaks down. Typical MR imaging protocols for liver imaging include T2-weighted (T2w), chemical shift imaging, and precontrast and postcontrast T1-weighted (T1w) sequences. This article discusses MR imaging of diffuse liver diseases and their typical imaging findings.

IMAGING TECHNIQUE FOR LIVER DISEASE
Typical Liver MR Imaging Protocol

The technical parameters for the typical liver MR imaging protocol are shown in **Table 1**. T2w imaging is a mainstay in liver imaging because it serves for lesion detection and characterization.[1] Most focal liver lesions are hyperintense on T2w imaging compared with the relatively dark liver. Many benign entities, such as cysts and hemangiomas, are markedly hyperintense on T2w images, whereas malignant neoplasms, such as hepatocellular carcinoma (HCC), intrahepatic cholangiocarcinoma (iCCA), and metastases, typically are mild to moderately hyperintense compared with liver parenchyma but less so than benign lesions (**Fig. 1**). Fat suppression may help make lesions more conspicuous on T2w imaging.

Fat-suppressed, noncontrast, T1w gradient-echo imaging serves primarily as a baseline for postcontrast imaging. The timing recommendations for postcontrast imaging are described in **Table 2**. Because liver signal intensity is brighter than most tissues due to its glycogen content, T1w imaging can be used to characterize focal nodular hyperplasia and some hepatic adenomas, which typically are isointense to the liver, unlike nonhepatocellular lesions. Dynamic contrast-enhanced T1w imaging allows for definitive characterization of multiple benign and malignant liver lesions, such as hemangiomas, focal nodular

[a] Department of Radiology, Naval Medical Center San Diego, 34800 Bob Wilson Drive, Suite 204, San Diego, CA 92134, USA; [b] Department of Radiology, Uniformed Services University of the Health Sciences, 4301 Jones Bridge Road, Bethesda, MD 20814, USA; [c] Department of Radiology, University of California San Diego, 200 West Arbor Drive, San Diego, CA 92103, USA; [d] Department of Radiology, Duke University, Box 3808, Durham, NC 27710, USA
* Corresponding author. Department of Radiology, Naval Medical Center San Diego, 34800 Bob Wilson Drive, Suite 204, San Diego, CA 92134.
E-mail address: robert.m.marks.mil@mail.mil

Magn Reson Imaging Clin N Am 29 (2021) 347–358
https://doi.org/10.1016/j.mric.2021.05.004
1064-9689/21/Published by Elsevier Inc.

Table 1
Technical considerations for typical liver MR imaging protocol

Sequence	Acquisition Type	Slice Thickness	Fat Saturation	Other
T2w imaging	2-D single shot or 2-D fast spin echo	$\leq$8 mm; slice gap, $\leq$2 mm	Optional	Axial and coronal planes are recommended.
T1w IP and OP imaging	Dual-phase acquisition is recommended, IP and OP can be generated as part of Dixon acquisition	If 2-D: $\leq$8 mm; slice gap $\leq$2 mm If 3-D: $\leq$6 mm	None	OP should be acquired before IP.
DWI	Single-shot echo-planar imaging with $\geq$2 b values (including b value = 0 s/mm^2–50 s/mm^2 and b value = 400 s/mm^2–1000 s/mm^2	$\leq$8 mm; slice gap, $\leq$2 mm	N/A	Parallel imaging is recommended to reduce artifacts. Higher b values can improve specificity for malignant lesions but have lower SNR.
T1w imaging	3-D is strongly recommended	$\leq$5 mm	Strongly recommended	Postcontrast acquisition parameters should match precontrast parameters to facilitate subtraction.

Abbreviations: 2-D, 2-dimensional; 3-D, 3-dimensional; IP, in phase; OP, opposed phase; SNR, signal-to-noise ratio.
Data from The LI-RADS v2018 Manual.[39]

hyperplasia, HCC, iCCA, and both hypervascular and hypovascular metastatic liver lesions based on distinct patterns of perfusion.

Chemical shift imaging is composed of in-phase/opposed-phase pulse sequences that exploit the differences in fat and water proton frequency when exposed to the same magnetic field.[2] In the context of diffuse liver disease, chemical shift imaging is used most frequently to detect hepatic steatosis. When fat and water occupy the same voxel, signal loss occurs in the opposed-phase images compared with the in-phase images, as in the setting of hepatic steatosis (**Fig. 2**).[3] Typically, the opposed-phase images are acquired at a shorter echo time than the in-phase images, so that any loss of signal within the liver on opposed-phase images, compared with in-phase images, can be attributed to some degree of hepatic steatosis. Due to a lack of corrections for signal decay, however, T1 weighting, and other confounding factors, in-phase/opposed-phase imaging provides at best a subjective measure of hepatic steatosis and is not highly accurate for liver fat quantification. Subjective assessment of steatosis remains useful for characterizing the presence or absence of fat within a mass and, because the in-phase/opposed-phase images may be generated (at no expense of time) as part of a Dixon-based T1w

precontrast series, they remain a valuable component of a complete diagnostic liver protocol.

Additionally, chemical shift imaging can be used to evaluate for the presence of abnormal iron deposition in the liver. As iron accumulates in the liver, the iron induces inhomogeneities in the local magnetic field that cause more rapid T2* relaxation, which manifests in loss of signal in the liver on images acquired at a longer echo time compared with those acquired with a shorter echo time.[4] Thus, in dual-echo imaging, when the in-phase images are obtained at a later echo time than the opposed-phase images, excessive signal loss in the liver on the in-phase images compared with the opposed-phase images is the typical manifestation of the presence of abnormal amounts of iron in the liver (**Fig. 3**).

Optional Protocol Additions

Diffusion-weighted imaging

Diffusion-weighted imaging (DWI) exploits the random motion of unrestricted water molecules. Water that is held in a hollow viscus, such as the gallbladder, or cerebral spinal fluid, is able to move relatively freely in its microenvironment, whereas water in solid organ and tumor interstitium is more restricted in its movement because of interactions with cell membranes and macromolecules.[5] In a diffusion-weighted sequence,

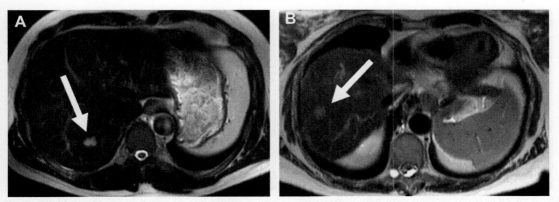

Fig. 1. (*A*) A 32-year-old man with a T2 markedly bright hemangioma in segment VII. This is compared with (*B*) the mildly bright HCC in segment VIII in this 72-year-old woman with hepatitis C cirrhosis.

Table 2
Technical considerations of postcontrast liver MR imaging protocols

Sequence	Timing	Other
Arterial phase	15–30 s after the start of injection	Late arterial phase is recommended. Bolus tracking is recommended.
Portal venous phase	60–80 s after the start of injection	Typical rate of injection is 3–5 mL/s
Delayed phase	2–5 min after injection	With extracellular contrast agent
Transitional phase	2–5 min after injection	With gadoxetate
Hepatobiliary Phase	~20 min with gadoxetate 1–3 h with gadobenate	Only with hepatobiliary agents

Data from The LI-RADS v2018 Manual.[39]

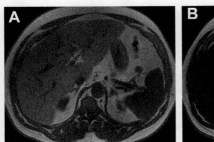 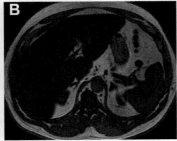

Fig. 2. A 49-year old man with hepatic steatosis. There is drop in signal from (*A*) the in-phase image compared with (*B*) the opposed-phase image, indicating fat deposition in the liver.

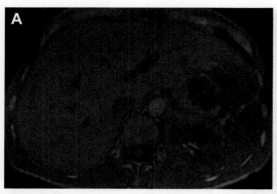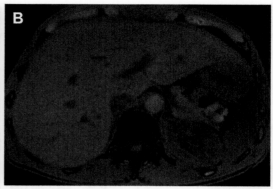

Fig. 3. A 49-year-old woman with hemochromatosis. There is subtle loss of signal in (A) the in-phase image compared with (B) the opposed-phase image, indicating T2* effect.

motion-probing gradients are applied to equally dephase and rephase stationary protons that experience both gradients at the same strength. Protons in water molecules that move between the application of those gradients are not completely rephased, resulting in signal loss proportional to the distance they have traveled. As a result, the signal from freely moving water, for example, in the cerebral spinal fluid or gallbladder, is strongly attenuated with increasing diffusion gradients, whereas the signal from water in a high-cellularity environment, such as the spleen, a lymph node, or a highly cellular tumor, is much less attenuated and appears relatively hyperintense on DWI.[6] In the liver, DWI is used to evaluate for highly cellular tumors like HCC and iCCA as well as complex fluid collections like liver abscesses (**Fig. 4**). Likewise, diffuse processes like cirrhosis or inflammation that increase the extracellular matrix macromolecular structure or cellularity, respectively, also result in a pattern of diffusely restricted diffusion within the liver.

Proton density fat fraction

Standard (dual-echo) chemical shift imaging provides a subjective quantification of liver fat content. By collecting additional data and correcting for a variety of confounding factors, however, the signal contribution from liver fat (in the form of triglycerides) can be quantified relative to signal from water in the form of proton density fat fraction (PDFF). This has been validated against histology and spectroscopy as a highly accurate noninvasive method of fat quantification in the liver. PDFF estimation techniques typically incorporate at least 6 echoes in order to collect enough data to estimate and remove the effects of T2* decay and multifrequency signal interference effects caused by protons in fat.[7] These sequences may be proton density–weighted in order to remove the effect of T1 relaxation or may incorporate explicit T1 corrections. The reconstruction of

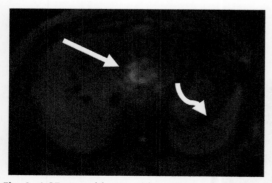

Fig. 4. A 25-year-old man with an abscess (*straight arrow*) in the left lobe of the liver. The high b-value DWI shows that the abscess is brighter than the visualized spleen (*curved arrow*) indicating restricted diffusion.

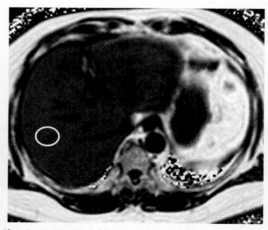

Fig. 5. A 63-year-old man with a history of NAFLD. This PDFF image shows bright signal in the liver with an ROI over the right lobe, which showed 18% fat within the ROI.

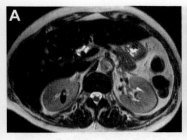
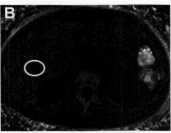

Fig. 6. A 61-year-old woman with hemochromatosis. (*A*) T2w image shows markedly low signal throughout the liver. (*B*) R2* map shows high signal. The ROI shows an average of 230 Hz, which is consistent with a moderate abnormal iron deposition in the liver.

PDFF maps allows for regional interrogation of the liver by placement of a region of interest (ROI) on the images so that the estimated amount of fat can be reported with high accuracy (**Fig. 5**).

Iron quantification
A subjective evaluation of the presence of abnormal iron deposition can be obtained using chemical shift imaging. MR imaging also can be used to quantify iron concentration and assess the severity of iron overload. Empirically, the R2* rate (inverse of T2* time) has been found to be directly proportional to liver iron concentration (LIC) across a range of biologically relevant iron levels, whereas the R2 rate has a more complex but predictable relationship with LIC. Using a multiecho acquisition with progressively increasing echo times, the T2* or T2 signal decay rates can be calculated, inverted to yield R2* or R2, and then used to calculate the LIC using empiric calibration curves that are specific to field strength. T2, T2*, R2, and/or R2* mapping sequences are available options on all current MR vendors (**Fig. 6**).[8]

MR elastography
MR elastography is a noninvasive MR technique for estimating liver stiffness, which is related primarily to liver fibrosis. MR elastography uses mechanical shear waves produced by an external source of vibration, typically at 60 Hz, to evaluate the stiffness of the liver.[9] In normal liver tissue, the wavelengths produced by the shear waves of the liver are short, compared with fibrotic liver tissue with long wavelengths.[10] In the MR imaging scanner, a drumlike acoustic driver, attached to a preprogrammed speaker system to produce vibrations, is placed on the body wall in a region over the liver.[11] A modified phase-contrast sequence, typically a gradient-recalled-echo or spin echo–echo-planar imaging sequence, is used to capture phase shifts induced by tissue displacement from the propagating shear waves.[9] After postprocessing, stiffness maps of the liver can be created to show estimates of liver stiffness

in a given region of the liver (**Fig. 7**). MR elastography has been validated with liver tissue biopsies and also is widely available with all MR imaging vendors. MR elastography also has been investigated for differentiating uncomplicated nonalcoholic fatty liver disease (NAFLD) from nonalcoholic steatohepatitis (NASH) with fibrosis, the presence and response of fibrosis related to chronic hepatitis C viral infection, assessment of treatment response of liver tumors, and to evaluate the stiffness of tumors, which can help in estimating their malignant potential.[9]

MR cholangiopancreatography
MR cholangiopancreatography (MRCP) is an excellent noninvasive alternative to endoscopic retrograde cholangiopancreatography for evaluating the gallbladder and pancreaticobiliary ductal system. By using high-resolution, heavily T2w imaging with very long echo times, MRCP takes advantage of the extremely long T2 time of the fluid in the biliary tree. As a result, signal in that fluid is preserved whereas signal from solid organs is suppressed, allowing for clear visualization of the pancreaticobiliary structures (**Fig. 8**). MRCP can be used to evaluate for entities, such as choledocholithiasis, biliary strictures, congenital anomalies of the cystic and hepatic ducts, postsurgical biliary complications, pancreatic divisum, and cystic pancreatic tumors.[12]

TYPES AND IMAGING DIAGNOSIS OF DIFFUSE LIVER DISEASE
Storage Diseases

Fatty liver disease
Obesity is significantly rising problem in the United States and worldwide. Since 1975, the worldwide overweight and obesity rates have nearly tripled, making NAFLD a significant global threat, affecting 25% of the global adult population.[13,14] Imaging for hepatic steatosis can be helpful because discovery may lead to lifestyle changes for the patient, and in clinical trials of drug candidates for NASH, early improvements in hepatic steatosis may predict downstream therapeutic benefit.[15]

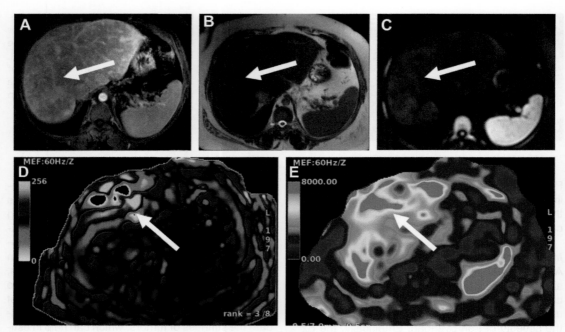

Fig. 7. A 38-year-old woman with Fontan liver disease. (*A*) Delayed postcontrast image of the liver demonstrates delayed enhancing fibrous bands that are mildly bright on (*B*) T2w imaging and (*C*) DWI. (*D*) Wave image and (*E*) elastogram demonstrate significant fibrosis of 4.8 kPa.

Compared with computed tomography (CT) and ultrasound, MR imaging is more accurate for detecting and quantifying hepatic steatosis. Using chemical shift imaging, as discussed previously, areas of fatty liver lose signal in the opposed-phase images compared with the in-phase images. Although typically diffuse, hepatic steatosis can be focal or heterogeneous. Focal fat commonly is seen adjacent to the falciform ligament, periportal regions, and adjacent to the gallbladder fossa. When fat is focal in less common areas of the liver, it can be confused with focal hepatic lesions, such as hypoenhancing metastatic lesions or fat-containing HCC or hepatic adenoma. Compared with a mass, however, focal steatosis typically has no mass effect on surrounding structures and does not displace or compress blood vessels or biliary structures (**Fig. 9**).[3,16]

Iron overload

Abnormal iron overload in the liver can be either primary (genetic hemochromatosis) or secondary (hemosiderosis). Hemochromatosis is an autosomal recessive disease, with a higher incidence in patients from European ancestry, caused by a mutation in the HFE gene. The mutation leads to an increased iron absorption rate from the intestine and progressive deposition of excess iron in tissues.[17] Iron deposition begins in the liver and can progress in severity, with concomitant tissue damage, and eventually lead to cirrhosis. Over time, iron deposition can involve other organs, including the pancreas, leading to diabetes mellitus; the heart, leading to restrictive cardiomyopathy; and the skin, causing dark pigmentation.[18] Hemochromatosis primarily involves the non-reticuloendothelial tissues, resulting in excessive iron deposition in the liver and pancreas with little to no deposition in the spleen and bone marrow. Using chemical shift imaging, primary hemochromatosis is characterized by decreased signal in

Fig. 8. A 34-year-old woman with a clinical concern for a choledocolith. This MRCP shows normal anatomy and normal caliber of the common bile duct (*arrow*) without a filling defect.

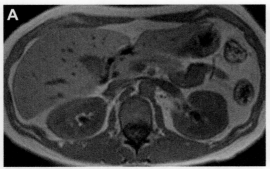
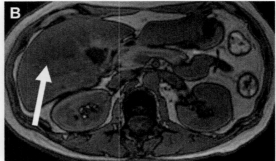

Fig. 9. A 48-year-old woman with the concern on a prior CT for a mass in segment V. (*A*) In-phase and (*B*) opposed-phase images demonstrate focal fat (*arrow*) in segment V, which does not distort blood vessels or liver architecture.

the liver, and occasionally the pancreas, on chemical shift sequences with longer echo times due to the T2* effects (**Fig. 10**). Additionally, the liver frequently is lower in signal intensity than skeletal muscle on T2w images due to iron deposition.

Hemosiderosis occurs in the setting of repeated blood transfusions for treatment of certain anemias as well as iron replacement therapy for diseases, such as end-stage renal disease.[4] The pattern of iron deposition in hemosiderosis is different than in primary hemochromatosis in that the iron deposits in the reticuloendothelial system (RES), leading to decreased signal intensity of liver, bone marrow, and spleen on chemical shift sequences with long echo times and on T2w imaging (**Fig. 11**).[19] As discussed previously, MR imaging also can be used to quantify iron deposition using measurements on T2* or R2* maps.

Excess iron deposition ultimately may lead to cirrhosis and HCC. Cirrhosis is more common in patients with primary hemochromatosis and is rare in patients with secondary hemosiderosis. HCC typically does not contain iron in patients with hemochromatosis, making it more conspicuous on T2w and T1w imaging, where the mass is hyperintense compared with the darker background of the liver.[20]

Coexisting fat and iron deposition

Fat and iron deposition may occur simultaneously in the liver, making the interpretation of chemical shift imaging a challenge. The presence of fat reduces signal intensity on opposed-phase images whereas the presence of iron reduces signal intensity on in-phase images (which typically are obtained with longer echo times than opposed-phase images). Signal intensity losses are detected by comparing the intensity of the liver on in-phase and opposed-phase images, and, when both are reduced, differences between the 2 may be less apparent or undetectable, masking the presence and severity of underlying deposition disease. Using PDFF and T2*/R2* maps to quantify iron fat and iron, respectively, the liver can be evaluated accurately for coexistent fat and iron deposition (**Fig. 12**).

Inflammatory Liver Diseases

Liver inflammation has many causes, including viral hepatitis, alcoholic liver disease, drug-induced liver injury, metabolic fatty liver disease, other deposition diseases such as hemochromatosis, and autoimmune diseases.[21] At the current time, direct or indirect imaging methods for estimation of liver inflammation on MR imaging are

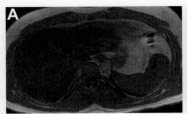
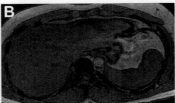
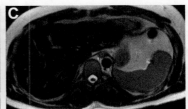

Fig. 10. A 23-year-old man with hemochromatosis. (*A*) In-phase demonstrates lower signal in the liver compared with (*B*) the opposed-phase image obtained at an earlier TE. (*C*) T2w image shows markedly decreased signal in the liver due to T2* effect from the iron accumulation.

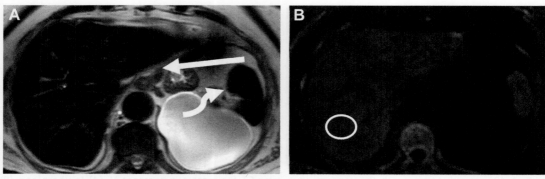

Fig. 11. A 75-year-old woman on iron replacement therapy. (*A*) T2w image shows decreased signal in the liver (*straight arrow*) and spleen (*curved arrow*) consistent with iron deposition in the RES. This pattern is consistent with hemosiderosis. (*B*) R2*map with an ROI in the liver shows an average of 250 Hz consistent with moderate abnormal iron deposition in the liver.

lacking; however, the downstream effects of liver inflammation, such as liver fibrosis, can be detected with imaging techniques like MR elastography, which currently is the most accurate imaging-based test. Ongoing studies are evaluating the possibility of indirectly assessing liver inflammation using advanced MR elastography methods on animal models.[22]

Viral hepatitis

Primary viral hepatitis is caused by 1 of 3 viruses—hepatitis A, hepatitis B, and hepatitis C. Other viruses, such as cytomegalovirus and Epstein-Barr virus, also can affect the liver as part of systemic infection. In the acute setting, MR imaging has no role in diagnosis unless an atypical presentation is present or alternative diagnoses are questioned.

Hepatitis A is highly contagious and is found in the stool and blood of infected individuals. Although the typical course of the disease is short lived, hepatitis A is vaccine preventable and typically cause does not chronic liver disease.

Hepatitis B is the most common cause of viral hepatitis worldwide, infecting more than 30% of the world population.[23] Like hepatitis A, it also is vaccine preventable; however, barriers throughout the world have prevented the vaccine from reaching areas of greatest need. It is estimated that chronic hepatitis B affects more than 290 million people worldwide.[23] Hepatitis B is an oncogenic virus that increases the risk of developing HCC independent of the presence of cirrhosis. In the United States, chronic hepatitis B causes more than 5000 deaths per year due to HCC as well as complications of cirrhosis.[24]

Hepatitis C is less common worldwide than hepatitis B, but it is currently the leading indication for orthotopic liver transplantation in the United States.[25] This is due to hepatitis C causing

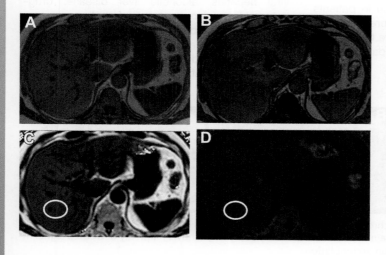

Fig. 12. A 64-year-old man with chronic hepatitis B. (*A*) In-phase and (*B*) opposed-phase images demonstrate drop in signal in the opposed-phase image consistent with hepatic steatosis. (*C*) PDFF with an ROI in the right hepatic lobe demonstrates 22% fat. (*D*) R2* map with an ROI in the right hepatic lobe demonstrates an average of 175 Hz, consistent with mild abnormal iron deposition in the liver. In this case, the amount of fat in the liver and drop of signal in (*B*) the opposed-phase image caused underestimation of the amount of iron in the liver on (*A*) the in-phase image that normally would be lower in signal compared with the in-phase image if there was not fat in the liver.

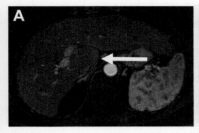
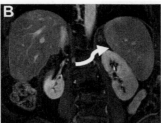

Fig. 13. A 78-year-old woman with primary biliary cirrhosis. (*A*) Axial postcontrast arterial phase image demonstrates hypertrophy of the caudate (*straight arrow*) and lateral left lobe of the liver consistent with cirrhosis. (*B*) Coronal postcontrast delayed image demonstrates splenomegaly (*curved arrow*).

persistent infection and chronic hepatitis leading to cirrhosis in many patients. Although hepatitis C is not vaccine preventable, 2 treatments have become available since 2014, which have been shown to cure most patients with hepatitis C without decompensated cirrhosis or those who have already undergone liver transplantation.[26] Patients with both chronic hepatitis B as well as hepatitis C with advanced fibrosis undergo routine surveillance to detect the presence of cirrhosis and HCC.

Nonalcoholic steatohepatitis

NAFLD is a major problem in the United States. In a minority of patients, NAFLD may progress to NASH, which is characterized by liver inflammation and fibrosis and ultimately can lead to cirrhosis.[27] In the near future, due to the unflagging rise in obesity in the United States and the availability of effective treatments for hepatitis C, cirrhosis caused by NASH is projected to become the leading indication for orthotopic liver transplant in the United States.[28] MR imaging of hepatic steatosis is discussed previously and typically consists of chemical shift imaging for estimation of PDFF. MR elastography also has been investigated for the differentiation of uncomplicated hepatic steatosis from NASH.

MR imaging findings of acute hepatitis

Validated techniques for detection and severity assessment of liver inflammation currently are not available. As such, imaging is not a primary diagnostic test for hepatitis and the imaging features of hepatitis are nonspecific and may include hepatomegaly and increased T2 signal intensity, abnormal enhancement, restricted diffusion, periportal edema, and lymphadenopathy in periportal region.[29,30] Often imaging is performed to rule out other entities that may lead to abnormal liver enzymes, such as portal vein thrombosis, masses, or biliary obstruction. The downstream effects of chronic inflammation include fibrosis, cirrhosis, and portal hypertension.

Cirrhosis

Cirrhosis is defined as liver fibrosis with the formation of regenerative nodules and is a primary risk factor for HCC. Cirrhosis is a growing national problem and is the twelfth overall leading cause of death and the fifth leading cause of death for patients ages 45 years to 54 years in the United States.[31] Causes of cirrhosis include chronic hepatitis B and hepatitis C viral infection, alcoholic liver disease, NASH, hemochromatosis, autoimmune hepatitis, primary and secondary biliary cirrhosis, and primary sclerosing cholangitis

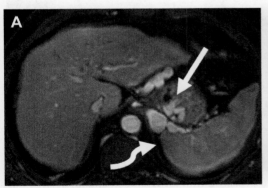
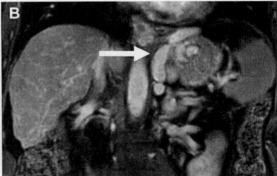

Fig. 14. A 70-year-old man with hepatitis C cirrhosis. (*A*) Axial and (*B*) coronal postcontrast images of the liver demonstrate large gastroesophageal varices (*straight arrows*) and splenomegaly (*curved arrow*) in this cirrhotic patient consistent with portal hypertension.

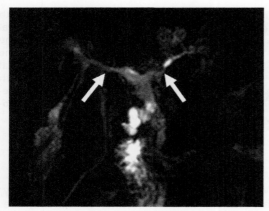

Fig. 15. A 35-year-old man with ulcerative colitis. MRCP image demonstrates mixed narrowing (*arrows*) and prestenotic dilatation of the intrahepatic bile ducts consistent with PSC.

(PSC).[32] Although the prevalence of most major causes of cirrhosis, including hepatitis B and hepatitis C infection and alcoholic liver disease, have remained stable or have decreased over time, the prevalence of NAFLD has increased by more than 10% from 1994 to 2016.[14] Furthermore, NASH-related cirrhosis has shown the most rapid increase as an indication for orthotropic liver transplantation over the past few decades in the United States.[14]

Although early cirrhosis can be associated with a normal morphologic appearance of the liver on cross-sectional imaging, more advanced cirrhosis can manifest as atrophy of the right lobe and segment IV; hypertrophy of the caudate and lateral left lobes; surface nodularity; expansion of spaces between the atrophied liver and the anterior

abdominal wall, hilum, and ligamentum teres; and the findings of portal hypertension, including enlargement of the portal veins, splenomegaly, varices, and ascites (**Figs. 13** and **14**).[33] MR imaging is superior in detecting parenchymal alterations, such as early heterogeneous enhancement, delayed enhancing fibrotic bands, nodules, and hyperintense signal on T2w imaging due to fibrosis.[34] MR elastography, as discussed previously, is the most accurate noninvasive technique for detection and staging of liver fibrosis, including staging of advanced fibrosis related to cirrhosis.

Autoimmune Diseases

Primary sclerosing cholangitis

The most common autoimmune disease affecting the liver is PSC. Although the etiology of PSC is unknown, various factors could be responsible for recurrent biliary duct injury. PSC can overlap clinically with other autoimmune diseases, such as autoimmune hepatitis, pancreatitis, and immunoglobulin G4 disease.[35,36] PSC is more common in men compared with women and has a high association with ulcerative colitis. Due to chronic biliary inflammation and bile duct stasis, patients with PSC have a higher risk for developing cholangiocarcinoma compared with the general population.[37] The classic imaging findings of PSC on MRCP include short segment strictures of the intrahepatic and extrahepatic bile ducts alternating with normal to dilated bile duct segments, causing a beaded appearance (**Fig. 15**). Additional MR imaging findings include peripheral wedge-shaped areas of atrophy with delayed enhancement on postcontrast imaging and periportal edema, which is bright on T2w imaging.[35] A

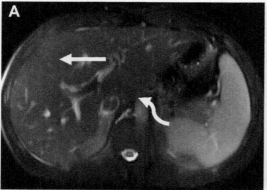
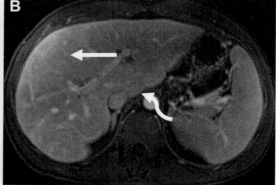

Fig. 16. A 20-year-old man with congestive hepatopathy. (*A*) Axial T2 with fat saturation and (*B*) delayed postcontrast *T1w* image demonstrate abnormal high signal in the peripheral liver on the T2w image with corresponding delayed and reticulated peripheral enhancement (*straight arrows*). The caudate lobe (*curved arrows*) is enlarged and is normal in signal on T2w imaging and has normal enhancement.

primary indication for imaging in patients with PSC is to evaluate for the development of cholangiocarcinoma, which may manifest as a new dominant stricture, eccentric ductal thickening, and/or an intrahepatic mass. Currently, there are no grading or staging systems for assessing PSC disease severity, progression, or regression.

Vascular Diseases

Congestive hepatopathy

Congestive hepatopathy typically presents with elevations of hepatic enzymes and hepatomegaly. The suprahepatic inferior vena cava (IVC) and hepatic veins typically are dilated secondary right to heart dysfunction. On early dynamic contrast-enhanced MR images, there may be reflux of contrast from the suprahepatic IVC into the hepatic veins. In the portal-venous phase, there is slow enhancement near the hepatic veins secondary to the congested hepatic parenchyma, causing patchy, irregular regions of hypoenhancement and a nutmeg appearance (**Fig. 16**).[38] Persistent hepatic congestion can lead to fibrosis and eventually cirrhosis; however, the risk for HCC development in this group of patients is much lower than for patients with cirrhosis of other causes.

SUMMARY

Diffuse liver disease encompasses a large group of heterogeneous disease processes, some of which may have overlapping imaging features. Utilizing MR imaging and optional liver MR imaging techniques, such as DWI, PDFF quantification, T2*/R2* mapping, MR elastography, and MRCP, allows for the diagnosis and monitoring of these disease processes.

CLINICS CARE POINTS

- Chemical shift imaging can aid in detection of liver fat and iron.
- PDFF can quantify liver fat accurately.
- T2*/R2* maps can quantify liver iron deposition.
- MR elastography can quantify liver fibrosis.
- MRCP aids in detection of biliary anomalies and diseases.
- Multiphasic MR imaging with or without postcontrast phases can identify and monitor diffuse liver diseases.

DISCLOSURE

R.M. Marks: no relevant disclosures. The views expressed in this presentation are those of the authors and do not necessarily reflect the official policy or position of the Department of the Navy, Department of Defense, or the US Government. R.M. Marks is a military service member or federal/contracted employee of the United States government. This work was prepared as part of his official duties. Title 17 U.S C. 105 provides that "copyright protection under this title is not available for any work of the United States Government." Title 17 U.S C. 101 defines a U.S. Government work as work prepared by a military service member or employee of the U.S. Government as part of that person's official duties. K.J. Fowler and M.R. Bashir: no relevant disclosures.

REFERENCES

1. Wile GE, Leyendecker JR. Magnetic resonance imaging of the liver: sequence optimization and artifacts. Magn Reson Imaging Clin N Am 2010;18(3): 525–47, xi.
2. Mitchell DG. Focal manifestations of diffuse liver disease at MR imaging. Radiology 1992;185(1):1–11.
3. Venkataraman S, Braga L, Semelka RC. Imaging the fatty liver. Magn Reson Imaging Clin N Am 2002; 10(1):93–103.
4. Labranche R, Gilbert G, Cerny M, et al. Liver iron quantification with MR imaging: a primer for radiologists. Radiographics 2018;38(2):392–412.
5. Koh DM, Collins DJ. Diffusion-weighted MRI in the body: applications and challenges in oncology. AJR Am J Roentgenol 2007;188(6):1622–35.
6. Bammer R, Holdsworth SJ, Veldhuis WB, et al. New methods in diffusion-weighted and diffusion tensor imaging. Magn Reson Imaging Clin N Am 2009; 17(2):175–204.
7. Tang A, Tan J, Sun M, et al. Nonalcoholic fatty liver disease: MR imaging of liver proton density fat fraction to assess hepatic steatosis. Radiology 2013; 267(2):422–31.
8. Henninger B, Alustiza J, Garbowski M, et al. Practical guide to quantification of hepatic iron with MRI. Eur Radiol 2020;30(1):383–93.
9. Hoodeshenas S, Yin M, Venkatesh SK. Magnetic resonance elastography of liver: current update. Top Magn Reson Imaging 2018;27(5):319–33.
10. Venkatesh SK, Yin M, Ehman RL. Magnetic resonance elastography of liver: technique, analysis, and clinical applications. J Magn Reson Imaging 2013;37(3):544–55.
11. Chen J, Yin M, Glaser KJ, et al. MR elastography of liver disease: state of the art. Appl Radiol 2013; 42(4):5–12.

12. Griffin N, Charles-Edwards G, Grant LA. Magnetic resonance cholangiopancreatography: the ABC of MRCP. Insights Imaging 2012;3(1):11–21.

13. Paik JM, Henry L, De Avila L, et al. Mortality related to nonalcoholic fatty liver disease is increasing in the United States. Hepatol Commun 2019;3(11): 1459–71.

14. Younossi ZM, Stepanova M, Younossi Y, et al. Epidemiology of chronic liver diseases in the USA in the past three decades. Gut 2020;69(3):564–8.

15. Harrison SA, Bashir MR, Guy CD, et al. Resmetirom (MGL-3196) for the treatment of non-alcoholic steatohepatitis: a multicentre, randomised, double-blind, placebo-controlled, phase 2 trial. Lancet 2019;394(10213):2012–24.

16. Matsui O, Kadoya M, Takahashi S, et al. Focal sparing of segment IV in fatty livers shown by sonography and CT: correlation with aberrant gastric venous drainage. AJR Am J Roentgenol 1995; 164(5):1137–40.

17. Fleming RE, Britton RS, Waheed A, et al. Pathophysiology of hereditary hemochromatosis. Semin Liver Dis 2005;25(4):411–9.

18. Bacon BR, Adams PC, Kowdley KV, et al, Diseases AAftSoL. Diagnosis and management of hemochromatosis: 2011 practice guideline by the American Association for the Study of Liver Diseases. Hepatology 2011;54(1):328–43.

19. Queiroz-Andrade M, Blasbalg R, Ortega CD, et al. MR imaging findings of iron overload. Radiographics 2009;29(6):1575–89.

20. Guyader D, Gandon Y, Sapey T, et al. Magnetic resonance iron-free nodules in genetic hemochromatosis. Am J Gastroenterol 1999;94(4):1083–6.

21. Koyama Y, Brenner DA. Liver inflammation and fibrosis. J Clin Invest 2017;127(1):55–64.

22. Yin M, Glaser KJ, Manduca A, et al. Distinguishing between hepatic inflammation and fibrosis with MR elastography. Radiology 2017;284(3): 694–705.

23. Foundation THB. Hepatitis B Facts and Figures. The Hepatitis B Foundation. Available at: https://www.hepb.org/what-is-hepatitis-b/what-is-hepb/facts-and-figures/. Accessed January 31, 2020.

24. Murphy SL, Xu J, Kochanek KD, et al. Mortality in the United States, 2017. NCHS Data Brief 2018;(328): 1–8.

25. Hussain SM, Reinhold C, Mitchell DG. Cirrhosis and lesion characterization at MR imaging. Radiographics 2009;29(6):1637–52.

26. Gritsenko D, Hughes G. Ledipasvir/Sofosbuvir (harvoni): improving options for hepatitis C virus infection. P T 2015;40(4):256–76.

27. Shetty A, Syn WK. Health and economic burden of nonalcoholic fatty liver disease in the United States and its impact on veterans. Fed Pract 2019;36(1): 14–9.

28. Parikh ND, Marrero WJ, Wang J, et al. Projected increase in obesity and non-alcoholic-steatohepatitis-related liver transplantation waitlist additions in the United States. Hepatology 2019;70(2):487–95.

29. Chundru S, Kalb B, Arif-Tiwari H, et al. MRI of diffuse liver disease: characteristics of acute and chronic diseases. Diagn Interv Radiol 2014;20(3): 200–8.

30. Alter MJ, Kruszon-Moran D, Nainan OV, et al. The prevalence of hepatitis C virus infection in the United States, 1988 through 1994. N Engl J Med 1999; 341(8):556–62.

31. Scaglione S, Kliethermes S, Cao G, et al. The epidemiology of cirrhosis in the United States: a population-based study. J Clin Gastroenterol 2015; 49(8):690–6.

32. Heidelbaugh JJ, Bruderly M. Cirrhosis and chronic liver failure: part I. Diagnosis and evaluation. Am Fam Physician 2006;74(5):756–62.

33. Horowitz JM, Venkatesh SK, Ehman RL, et al. Evaluation of hepatic fibrosis: a review from the society of abdominal radiology disease focus panel. Abdom Radiol (NY) 2017;42(8):2037–53.

34. Papadatos D, Fowler KJ, Kielar AZ, et al. Cirrhosis and LI-RADS. Abdom Radiol (NY) 2018;43(1):26–40.

35. Khoshpouri P, Habibabadi RR, Hazhirkarzar B, et al. Imaging features of primary sclerosing cholangitis: from diagnosis to liver transplant follow-up. Radiographics 2019;39(7):1938–64.

36. Tanaka A. Immunoglobulin G4-related sclerosing cholangitis. J Dig Dis 2019;20(7):357–62.

37. Palmela C, Peerani F, Castaneda D, et al. Inflammatory bowel disease and primary sclerosing cholangitis: a review of the phenotype and associated specific features. Gut Liver 2018;12(1):17–29.

38. Wells ML, Fenstad ER, Poterucha JT, et al. Imaging findings of congestive hepatopathy. Radiographics 2016;36(4):1024–37.

39. American College of Radiology. The LI-RADS v2018 Manual. 2018. Available at: https://www.acr.org/-/media/ACR/Files/Clinical-Resources/LIRADS/LI-RADS-2018-Manual-5Dec18.pdf?la=en. Accessed June 6, 2020.

Hepatocarcinogenesis
Radiology-Pathology Correlation

Alice Fung, MD[a],*, Krishna P. Shanbhogue, MD[b], Myles T. Taffel, MD[b],
Brian T. Brinkerhoff, MD[c], Neil D. Theise, MD[d]

KEYWORDS

- Liver • Hepatocarcinogenesis • Hepatocellular carcinoma • Dysplastic nodule
- Liver reporting & data system (LI-RADS)

KEY POINTS

- Although cirrhosis is the liver's response to repeated wound healing, hepatocellular carcinoma (HCC) is the result of accumulated genetic and epigenetic changes acquired from chronic inflammation.
- Imaging guidelines used to diagnose HCC reflect the radiologist's suspicion for HCC, are influenced by various priorities in treatment practices, and do not correlate categories with pathologic diagnosis.
- Combined hepatocellular-cholangiocarcinomas (cHCC-CCAs) share imaging characteristics with pure HCC and pure cholangiocarcinoma, including mosaic architecture, but have different treatment and prognosis from either of these types of malignancies. Radiologists should be aware and target different areas of the mosaic to increase the chance of confirming cHCC-CCA by pathology.

INTRODUCTION

Hepatocarcinogenesis is the multistep process by which hepatocellular nodules evolve into precancerous lesions to early cancerous lesions and then to progressed hepatocellular carcinoma (HCC). This complex process is predominantly due to chronic hepatic inflammation and leads to important predictable pathologic changes. Many of these changes are reflected by characteristic imaging findings, allowing for the noninvasive diagnosis of progressed HCC. Understanding the biologic processes, the pathologic changes, and the imaging findings seen throughout hepatocarcinogenesis allows the radiologist to better noninvasively diagnose HCC and recognize its precursor lesions.

CAUSATIVE AGENTS AND MOLECULAR CHANGES OF HEPATOCARCINOGENESIS
Causative Agents

Multiple systemic factors known to cause cirrhosis are also risk factors for HCC with the most common including hepatitis infection, nonalcoholic fatty liver disease (NAFLD), and alcohol consumption.[1] These factors contribute to hepatocarcinogenesis in distinct ways, resulting in additive risk for HCC when more than 1 risk factor is present.[2,3]

Hepatitis viral infection is a major risk factor for the development of HCC. Hepatitis B (HBV) and hepatitis C (HCV) viruses are directly involved in hepatocarcinogenesis given the presence of HCC in noncirrhotic livers.[2] As a DNA virus, HBV directly inserts itself into the host's genome,

a Department of Diagnostic Radiology, Oregon Health & Science University, 3181 SW Sam Jackson Park Road, L-340, Portland, OR 97239, USA; b Department of Radiology, New York University Grossman School of Medicine, 660 First Avenue, 3rd Floor, New York, NY 10016, USA; c Department of Pathology, Oregon Health & Science University, 3181 SW Sam Jackson Park Road, L-113, Portland, OR 97239, USA; d Department of Pathology, MSB 504A, New York University Grossman School of Medicine, 560 First Avenue, New York, NY 10016, USA
* Corresponding author.
E-mail address: funga@ohsu.edu

Magn Reson Imaging Clin N Am 29 (2021) 359–374
https://doi.org/10.1016/j.mric.2021.05.007

causing DNA microdeletions, translocations, and mutations.[3] The virus's HBx gene also affects growth-control genes and suppresses p53-regulated DNA repair, promoting persistent infection and genome instability.[2,3] These processes contribute to the ability of HBV to cause HCC before the liver becomes cirrhotic. HCV promotes hepatocarcinogenesis through its proteins that cause downstream effects on cell proliferation, cell-cycle progression, cellular survival, cell response to stress, and tumor angiogenesis.[3]

NAFLD, a spectrum of progressive liver diseases that includes steatosis, nonalcoholic steatohepatitis, and cirrhosis, is the most common liver disease in Western countries and is projected to become the most common indication for liver transplantation.[4,5] The pathologic mechanisms for the development of HCC in NAFLD have not been clearly established, but are likely related to insulin resistance, hepatic steatosis, high fat and carbohydrate diets, and genetic inheritance.[5]

Molecular Changes

Chronic inflammation is essential in hepatocarcinogenesis and is a major mechanism by which HBV, HCV, and alcohol-related damage occurs.[2,3] With persistent inflammation, repeated cycles of cell injury, death, inflammation, and regeneration can result in aberrant cell signaling and genetic and epigenetic mutations.[3,6,7] Although cirrhosis is the liver's response to this repeated wound healing, HCC is the result of accumulated genetic and epigenetic changes acquired from chronic inflammation. Thus, cirrhosis and HCC evolve in parallel with one another, both developing as a result of the same processes.[6,7]

Key point

Although cirrhosis is the liver's response to repeated wound healing, HCC is the result of accumulated genetic and epigenetic changes acquired from chronic inflammation.

As hepatocytes necrose or become apoptotic, inflammatory cells infiltrate the liver and release free radicals, cytokines, and chemokines.[2] Free radicals promote the formation of genetic mutations, and both cytokines and oxidative stress activate stellate cells to produce increased extracellular matrix as the first step in hepatic fibrosis.[3,8,9] Multiple cytokines, including

interleukin-6 (IL-6) a cytokine associated with increased HCC risk, activate transcription factors with downstream effects on tumorigenesis, metastasis, and angiogenesis.[2]

Chronic inflammation can cause epigenetic changes early in hepatocarcinogenesis with few, if any, genetic or chromosomal structural changes.[7] Epigenetic mechanisms help regulate gene expression, including tumor suppressor genes, and are passed to daughter cells.[3,10] As carcinogenesis progresses, ongoing epigenetic and genetic changes caused by chronic inflammation affect cell survival, proliferation, differentiation, and apoptosis, culminating in genome instability with mutations, telomere erosion, chromosome segregation defects, and oxidative DNA damage.[2,3] These changes escalate during the neoplastic phase, and clonal populations of abnormal cells replace more differentiated cell populations through repetitive growth and expansion.[7] The various combinations of affected genes and regulatory pathways ultimately result in differing clinical courses between patients, between tumors in the same patient, and within different regions of the same tumor. As these changes accumulate, hepatocellular nodules exhibit worsening tumor grades, larger sizes, and worse prognoses.[10]

PREMALIGNANCY THROUGH THE MICROSCOPE

It is difficult, as yet, to correlate well the pathologic lesions identified in clinical human liver specimens with the molecular and experimental data presented previously, given the limited molecular studies of early lesions and the lack of real correlation between animal models of hepatocarcinogenesis and human pathways. The primary premalignant or malignancy-associated hepatocellular lesions in patients with chronic liver disease include small cell change, large cell change, and low-grade and high-grade dysplastic nodules. Although some hepatocellular adenomas are well established as premalignant pathways, the independent complexity of this topic precludes it from being covered in this review.

Large Cell Change

Large cell change (LCC; originally called "large cell dysplasia") is defined as hepatocytes with cellular enlargement, nuclear pleomorphism and hyperchromasia, and multinucleation (**Fig. 1**). They were first identified as a possible premalignant change by Dr Peter Anthony in 1973. In the years since this landmark paper, accumulated data suggest that most LCC is a senescent change seen in

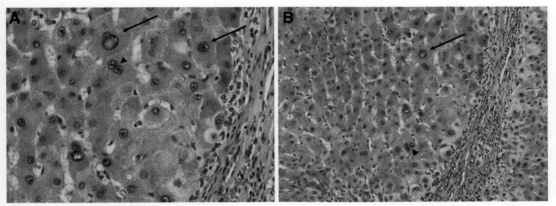

Fig. 1. LCC from an explanted liver. (A) High-power (×20) and (B) low-power (×10) original magnification. Enlarged hepatocytes with nuclear pleomorphism (*long arrows*) and multinucleation (*arrowheads*) are present. LCC is generally considered a malignancy-associated change rather than a directly premalignant lesion.

any chronic liver disease, more a marker of injury that increases risk for HCC development elsewhere in the liver, rather than directly premalignant. However, LCC in hepatitis B may yet be directly premalignant.[11–13] LCC cannot be assessed radiographically because it is a non–mass-forming entity, without specific vascular changes, and occurring within the level of scale of the single hepatic lobule.

Small Cell Change

Small cell change (SCC; originally small cell dysplasia) was originally identified through morphometric studies of LCC and other hepatocytes in chronic liver diseases.[14] SCC, as the name suggests, has smaller than normal cell size, is modestly pleomorphic, with hyperchromatic nuclei, and an increased nuclear:cytoplasmic ratio approaching that of HCC (**Fig. 2**). They also have a tendency to grow in minute, but expansive nodules (<0.1 cm). These are felt to be directly premalignant by morphologic, genetic, and molecular analysis.[12,13,15] SCC cannot be assessed radiographically because, even if showing nodular expansile growth, it is still below the scale of a single hepatic lobule and has no distinctive associated vascular changes.

Dysplastic Nodules

The dysplastic nodule (DN) story began as a radiology story, not as a story written by pathologists. Because of endemic liver disease in Japan and other East Asian nations, ultrasonographic screening for small HCCs was implemented in the early 1980s. For lesions that underwent resection, many could readily be diagnosed as HCC, but some were benign or contained foci of atypia

suggestive of emerging HCC, or, in fact, contained a subnodule of overt HCC. They are recognized as a premalignant lesion in advanced stage (cirrhotic) chronic liver diseases and a significant, if not predominant, multistep pathway of human hepatocarcinogenesis.[16] In general, this pathway has only been considered to occur in the setting of chronic liver disease, although the possibility that it is a pathway in sporadic HCC cannot be excluded.

DNs are defined pathologically as *nodules that are distinct from the surrounding liver parenchyma* in terms of pathologic features such as size, color, texture or the degree to which they bulge from the cut surface of a resection/autopsy specimen but do not have diagnostic features sufficient to diagnosis established HCC.[17] Low-grade dysplastic nodules (LGDN) have no cytologic atypia or only LCC. They contain intact portal tracts and, thus, maintain intact portal and hepatic arterial supply, although low levels of angiogenesis (recognized as arteries that are unpaired, ie, not accompanied by bile ducts in a portal tract) may be recognized[18] (**Fig. 3**). They sometimes have features suggestive of their monoclonality, such as increased iron in an otherwise relatively nonsiderotic liver or copper accumulation in the absence of Wilson disease.

High-grade dysplastic nodules (HGDN) are like LGDN, except they demonstrate features suggestive of progression toward HCC. These may include SCC or "nodule-in-nodule" growth patterns. The latter include nodular growth of SCC, iron resistance in an otherwise siderotic nodule, steatotic foci sometimes with clustering of Mallory-Denk bodies. They may also have atypical architecture suggestive of HCC, such as pseudoacini or thickened trabeculae, but insufficient to confidently diagnose established malignancy. Sometimes these features may be randomly

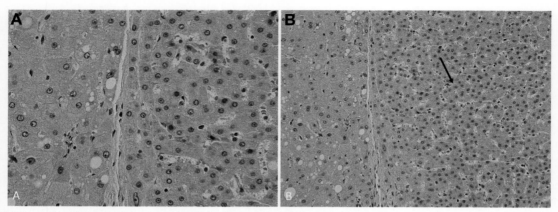

Fig. 2. SCC; HGDN. (*A*) High-power (×20) original magnification shows normal regenerative hepatocytes, but SCC with nuclear crowding with increased nuclear:cytoplasmic ratio, mild pleomorphism, and nuclear hyperchromasia. (*B*) Low-power (×10) original magnification highlights the vaguely nodular growth of the SCC. SCC is generally considered a true, premalignant (dysplastic) change.

scattered in the background nodule, but sometimes they, themselves, are the "nodule-in-nodule." Portal tracts are also always present, but in reduced numbers and there is increasing angiogenesis identified by increasing numbers of unpaired arteries, that is, arteries unaccompanied by bile ducts.[18]

Subnodules of HCC may arise within DNs, although it is not always possible to recognize whether the preexisting lesion was LGDN versus HGDN, depending on how much has been displaced by the emerging HCC. These HCCs have all the classic histologic features of HCC and may be considered truly "in situ" carcinomas if fully contained within the background DN. However, invasion can be subtle, comprising often well-differentiated hepatocytes invading into the stroma of surrounding portal tracts/fibrous septa, the so-called "vaguely nodular" form of early HCC (eHCC).[19,20] The subsequent progression from vaguely nodular to "progressed HCC" is recognized as the growing lesion, rather than spreading subtly by replacing hepatocyte parenchyma or through stromal invasion, becomes a pushing front of highly proliferative tissue. As proliferation speeds up, the pressure on surrounding, nonlesional hepatic tissue leads to atrophy and loss of hepatocytes (see "Pseudocapsule," later in this article).[20]

In brief, accumulating knowledge of DNs allowed for the formation of a theory of human hepatocarcinogenesis.[21] The working hypothesis indicates an early epigenetic or genetic change in a single, now neoplastic hepatocyte. The cell has low proliferation, but is resistant to apoptosis, the relative difference between them allowing the

cell to spread slowly by replacing neighboring hepatocytes, gradually surrounding and incorporating adjacent portal structures as it does so. Over the course of years to decades, diminished stellate cell activation leads to an absence of scar even as the surrounding liver becomes cirrhotic. Thus, in a background of cirrhosis, DNs look like large regenerative nodules, but are relatively preserved islands of hepatic parenchyma made of clonal, neoplastic hepatocytes. Having already taken several steps down the line of neoplasia, they are fertile ground for the final steps

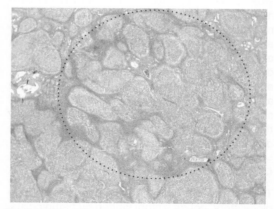

Fig. 3. LGDN. Advanced stage primary sclerosing cholangitis (PSC) with a distinctive nodule corresponding to a distinctive nodule identified radiologically. This nodule (*dotted line*) is composed of normal hepatocytes with increased scar compared with the surrounding parenchyma. In the absence of cytologic and architectural atypia, it is a large-grade DN.

to become HCC. It is these latter steps in which the molecular origins of HCC described previously are likely to be found. The earlier stages remain largely unelucidated.

RADIOLOGY-PATHOLOGY CHANGES OF HEPATOCARCINOGENESIS

Up until collaborations at NYU School of Medicine between pathologists and radiologists directly correlating assessments of the same liver lesions, lesion by lesion, in explant and resection specimens, the understanding of imaging features and how they related to pathologic progression through stages to HCC were poorly recognized.

But just as the early radiologic literature shifted to pathologic studies of DNs and early HCCs, the pendulum swung: research into the basic pathobiology of DNs at the tissue and cellular level receded and an extensive radiographic literature took over the field focused on the clinical implications for diagnosis and treatment of radiographic findings.[20] Multiple radiologic features specific to HCC were recognized, improving the ability to noninvasively diagnose progressed HCC and allowing the creation of imaging guidelines for this purpose. Imaging features suggestive of malignancy although not specific to HCC were also found to improve sensitivity for HCC (**Table 1**).

Table 1
Imaging features suggestive of malignancy, but not specific for HCC; these features are considered ancillary features by LI-RADS

Ancillary Finding	Description	Proposed Pathologic Correlate/ Reasoning
Ultrasound visibility as a discrete nodule	Discrete nodule or mass seen by ultrasound unequivocally corresponding with an observation seen by CT or MRI	• Benign cirrhotic lesions are typically indistinguishable from background liver on grayscale ultrasound. • Ultrasound visibility increases the pretest probability for HCC on diagnostic imaging.[38]
Subthreshold growth	• Unequivocal growth, but by <50% within 6 mo • New mass in any time interval	• The growth rate of a lesion reflects its biological potential of being a tumor. Premalignant and malignant lesions tend to grow more rapidly than benign lesions, which remain stable in size or exhibit slow growth.[38]
Corona enhancement	• Peri-observational enhancement in late arterial phase or early portal venous phase due to venous drainage of tumor • Of various thickness and uniformity	• Corona enhancement occurs when contrast from a progressed HCC drains into surrounding sinusoids and portal venules rather than into the hepatic veins, possibly due to compression or invasion of the hepatic veins by malignant cells.[7,47,56]
Fat-sparing in solid mass	• Relative paucity of fat in a solid mass compared with surrounding steatotic liver • Less steatotic subnodule within a more steatotic outer nodule	• Fat-sparing in solid mass suggests clonal expansion given the decreased fat accumulation compared with surrounding parenchyma. • Fatty change regresses as early HCC evolves into progressed HCC.[7,47]
Restricted diffusion	• Intensity on DWI that is unequivocally higher than liver and/or	• Increased restricted diffusion reflects a malignant lesion's tendency to possess a higher density

(continued on next page)

Table 1
(continued)

Ancillary Finding	Description	Proposed Pathologic Correlate/Reasoning
	ADC unequivocally lower than liver • Not attributable solely to T2 shine-through	of smaller cells and minimal extracellular volume when compared with background liver.[57] These characteristics result in decreased random motion of water molecules when compared with nonneoplastic tissue.
Mild-moderate T2 hyperintensity	• Mildly or moderately higher signal on T2W images than liver. • Nodule's T2 signal is similar to or less than the spleen's without iron deposition.	• Poorly understood. • T2 hyperintensity may reflect increased arterial flow and decreased portal venous flow within the nodule. • Dilated sinusoids and edema within the lesion may also contribute to this feature.[38]
Iron-sparing in solid mass	• Relative paucity of iron in a solid mass compared with surrounding liver	• Regenerative nodules, LGDN, and some HGDNs can have an upregulated iron-transporter system causing increased iron uptake. • Most HGDNs and HCCs exhibit decreased iron content.[7,58]
Transitional phase (TP) hypointensity	• Observation with signal intensity that is, unequivocally lower than surrounding liver in the TP, 3–5 min after gadoxetate disodium injection	• TP hypointensity may be a function of both washout appearance and underexpression of OATP, the membrane transporter responsible for uptake of gadoxetate disodium in normal hepatocytes. • OATP expression decreases during hepatocarcinogenesis resulting in TP hypointensity.[38]
Hepatobiliary phase (HPB) hypointensity	• Observation with signal intensity that is, unequivocally lower than surrounding liver in the HPB, 20 min after gadoxetate disodium injection of 1–3 h after gadobenate dimeglumine injection	• HBP hypointensity has been observed with early and progressed HCC whose cells exhibit decreased OATP expression.[38]

Abbreviations: ADC, apparent diffusion coefficient; CT, computed tomography; DWI, diffusion-weighted imaging; HCC, hepatocellular carcinoma; HGDN, high-grade dysplastic nodules; LGDN, low-grade dysplastic nodules; LI-RADS, Liver Imaging Reporting and Data System; OATP, organic anion-transporting polypeptide.

Diagnostic Imaging Guidelines and Hepatocarcinogenesis

The Liver Imaging Reporting and Data System (LI-RADS) and other imaging guidelines used to diagnose HCC do not attempt to correlate categories with pathologic diagnosis of the various types of hepatocellular nodules (**Fig. 4**).[7] Instead, categories tend to reflect the radiologist's suspicion of HCC, and the diagnostic guidelines are influenced by various priorities in treatment practices.[22] Because liver transplantation is used as a curative treatment in Europe and North America, specificity for HCC is prioritized over sensitivity to avoid false positive diagnoses in Western society guidelines, such as LI-RADS. To contrast, diagnostic guidelines used in Asia, such as the Asian Pacific Association for the Study of the Liver (APASL) and Korean Liver Cancer Association-National Cancer Center favor sensitivity over specificity to maximize early treatment options, including locoregional therapies.[22]

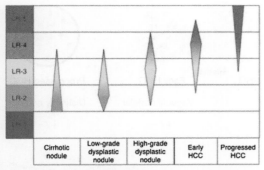

	Cirrhotic nodule	Low-grade dysplastic nodule	High-grade dysplastic nodule	Early HCC	Progressed HCC

Fig. 4. Each LI-RADS category does not correspond to one histologic grade. LI-RADS categories reflect the radiologist's degree of diagnostic suspicion based on observed imaging features, but those categories do not correspond exactly to the histologic categorization described by pathologists. For example, all LI-RADS 5 observations meet imaging criteria for HCC and are very likely to also meet histologic criteria for HCC. However, not all HCCs are LI-RADS 5, some can be categorized as LI-RADS 3 or 4 based on their imaging features. (*From* Narsinh KH, Cui J, Papadatos D, Sirlin CB, Santillan CS. Hepatocarcinogenesis and LI-RADS. *Abdom Radiol (NY).* 2018;43(1):158–168; with permission).

Key point

Imaging guidelines used to diagnose HCC reflect the radiologist's suspicion for HCC, are influenced by various priorities in treatment practices and do not correlate categories with pathologic diagnosis.

Vascular Changes

Radiology view

The unique enhancement pattern of HCC allows differentiation of progressed HCC from other hepatocellular nodules. Regenerative nodules and LGDNs, perfused by intact portal triads, cannot be distinguished from background liver by imaging.[23,24] As hepatocarcinogenesis continues, portal triads diminish and unpaired arteries begin to develop, resulting in the overall hypoenhancing appearance of HGDNs. Progressed HCCs are characterized by nonrim arterial phase hyperenhancement (APHE) due to increased number and size of intranodular abnormal arteries.[24–26] A caveat to this feature is when advanced, infiltrative HCC no longer exhibits APHE, possibly due to tumor cells converting from aerobic metabolism to glycolytic anaerobic metabolism.[27] The lack of

portal venous blood flow in progressed HCC is manifest by nonperipheral washout appearance when the nodule is less enhancing compared with surrounding liver in the portal venous phase, delayed phase, or both on multiphase computed tomography (CT) or MRI enhanced by extracellular gadolinium contrast agents or gadobenate.[24–26] With gadoxetate multiphase MRI, washout appearance is assessed on the portal venous phase, only.

Pathology view

As described previously, LGDN has few unpaired arteries indicative of tumor angiogenesis, but they increase steadily with developing atypia in HGDN, showing highest levels when overt HCC emerges. These arteries and gradual loss of portal tracts are the correlates to changes seen by imaging.

There is also increasing "capillarization" of sinusoids with progression in which sinusoidal endothelial cells lose their morphologic/functional distinctions from normal capillary endothelial cells; however, although capillarization takes place, in part, to high pressure states it is uncertain if it is also reflected in changes recognizable by imaging modalities. As portal tracts decline from LGDN to HGDN to HCC (in which they are completely absent), portal venous supply also diminishes dramatically.[25,26] Thus, early hepatocarcinogenesis is characterized by slowly increasing intranodular arterial flow with preserved portal venous flow. On the other hand, later stages of hepatocarcinogenesis are notable for even higher arterial flow with little to no portal venous flow. Imaging enhancement patterns reflect these vascular changes (**Fig. 5**).

Size

Radiology view

Currently, APASL is the only diagnostic algorithm without a size threshold for the imaging diagnosis of HCC, whereas the 4 other widely used algorithms require a size of 1 cm.[22] Although HCC may range from subcentimeter to many centimeters in size, the greater the size, the better it may be characterized by imaging and accurately differentiated from other lesions, such as hemangiomas, intrahepatic cholangiocarcinomas, metastases, and other hepatocellular nodules.[28,29] In addition, subcentimeter nodules are often difficult to correlate pathologically without the question of sampling error.[30]

Pathology view

The original definitions of dysplastic nodules included size as a primary feature, with cutoffs variably as 1.0 cm or 0.8 cm. This carries over into

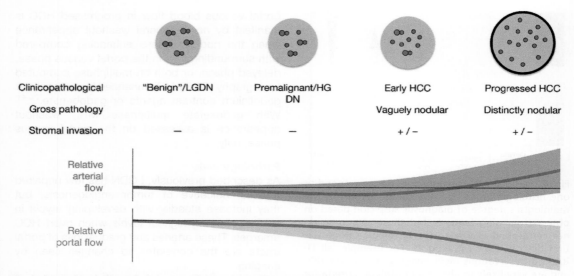

Clinicopathological	"Benign"/LGDN	Premalignant/HG DN	Early HCC	Progressed HCC
Gross pathology			Vaguely nodular	Distinctly nodular
Stromal invasion	–	–	+ / –	+ / –

Relative arterial flow

Relative portal flow

Fig. 5. Vascular changes as hepatocellular nodules progress to HCC. LGDNs possess normal portal triads. As hepatocarcinogenesis progresses, the portal venous flow to the nodule decreases while the arterial flow increases due to the development of unpaired arteries and "capillarization" of sinusoids. Overall, this process results in hypoenhancing HGDNs before the nodule evolves into early or progressed HCC, which tends to be arterially hyperenhancing. (Theise N, Sirlin CB. Hepatocarcinogenesis: Path/LI-RADS Correlation. Liver Imaging Online Course webinar. May 29, 2020. Accessed October 20, 2020. https://www.youtube.com/watch?v=ghWvnBS-N6o&t=66s.)

pathologic examination of tissues, in that the definition of DNs as "distinctive from surrounding parenchyma" particularly relates to size. Thus, their distinctiveness on imaging also often relates to size. Note that some cirrhotic livers have diffusely large nodules (younger patients with autoimmune hepatitis or hepatitis B[31] or patients with regressing fibrosis after treatment of viral hepatitis[32]); these are likely almost entirely large regenerative nodules rather than a multitude of DNs. As noted previously, LCC and SCC are never large enough, even if displaying expansile growth, to achieve resolution by any current imaging modality.

Threshold Growth

Radiology view
Threshold growth as defined by LI-RADS and Organ Procurement and Transplantation Network (OPTN) is increase in size by 50% or more in 6 months or less. This feature is not based on high-level scientific evidence, but rather on biological plausibility and expert opinion.[33] Although not specific for HCC, rapid growth suggests a certain degree of dedifferentiation with well-differentiated HCC generally exhibiting slower growth than moderately or poorly differentiated HCC.[28]

Pathology view
Indeed, as noted previously, DNs are low proliferative lesions compared with regenerating cirrhotic

nodules. Proliferation increases steadily with emergence of HCC and progression from better to more poorly differentiated tumors as demonstrated histologically by increased nuclear:cytoplasmic ratios and cellular crowding within tumors and confirmed by immunostaining for proliferation markers such as Ki-67, which may, in fact, be predicted by CT radiomics.[34]

Fibrous Capsule/Pseudocapsule

Radiology view
Although imaging often suggests the presence of a capsule surrounding a nodule, this appearance does not always correspond to a true histologic capsule. Thus, the radiology term of "capsule" is placed in quotation marks or called capsule appearance.[35] Regardless of whether the nodule possesses a true capsule or a pseudocapsule, the "capsule" appears as a peripheral hyperenhancing rim around a hepatocellular nodule. This rim may be incomplete and is typically thicker and more conspicuous than the finer fibrotic bands surrounding other hepatocellular nodules. The "capsule" should be well-defined, uniform, and smooth along its inner and outer borders without obvious nodularity.[36] This feature is best seen on the portal venous, delayed, and transitional phases of both liver CTs and MRIs and should progressively enhance from the portal venous phase to the delayed or transitional phase.[37] Capsule appearance may also be

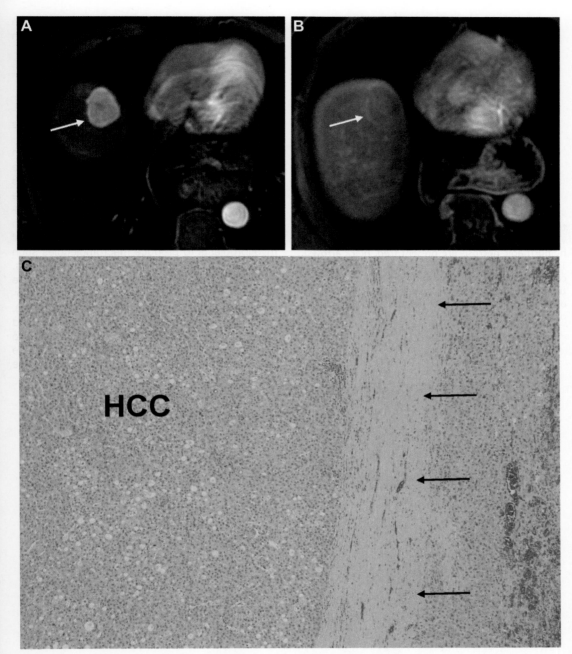

Fig. 6. HCC with true fibrous capsule. (*A*) Axial arterial and (*B*) delayed phase T1-weighted fat-saturated postcontrast images show a segment 8 observation with arterial phase hyperenhancement with washout and capsule appearance (*white arrows*). (*C*) Histology indicates HCC with a relatively uncommon "true" tumor capsule (*dark arrows*), that is dense, hyalinized stroma probably induced by the tumor rather than through compression of surrounding nontumoral liver (note the absence of portal tract remnants in the capsule).

nonenhancing with the same histologic correlations and imaging features as the enhancing "capsule," with the exception of hypoattenuation on all phases of a multiphasic liver CT and hypointensity on all precontrast and postcontrast T1-weighted (T1W) images of a multiphasic liver MR. Variable signal is detected on T2-weighted (T2W) and diffusion-weighted images (DWI).[38] Although the enhancing "capsule" is a major feature for the imaging diagnosis of HCC under LI-RADS

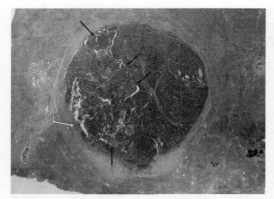

Fig. 7. HCC with thin "pseudocapsule." Following attempted ablation therapy, the tumor has largely survived (*dark blue*), although some foci of hemorrhagic necrosis are present (*red, black arrows*). The thin fibrous capsule surrounding the HCC is cellular and contains remnants of compressed portal tract structures owing to compression of the septa of surrounding liver (*white arrow*). Low-power (×4) original magnification.

and OPTN, the nonenhancing "capsule" is an ancillary feature of LI-RADS favoring HCC in particular.[39]

Pathology view

Two types of tumor capsule are seen histologically. The first is a true tumor capsule usually consisting of relatively dense, but fairly acellular fibrous tissue, usually devoid of elements of the surrounding, nontumoral organ. These are most common in benign tumors (eg, thyroid adenoma), but can be characteristically seen around some malignancies (eg, renal cell carcinoma). These capsules are probably produced by altered signaling by the tumor itself or by tissue neighboring the tumor, with upregulation of TGF-beta, upregulation of local myofibroblasts to produce macromolecules such as collagens, fibronectin, glycosaminoglycans. True capsules like this are unusual in large HCCs, but they are more common around subnodules of HCC within a larger DN or HCC (**Fig. 6**).

On the other hand, pseudocapsules around HCCs, particularly in advanced stage livers to which LI-RADS assessments can be applied, are nearly universal. These are arrived at by the

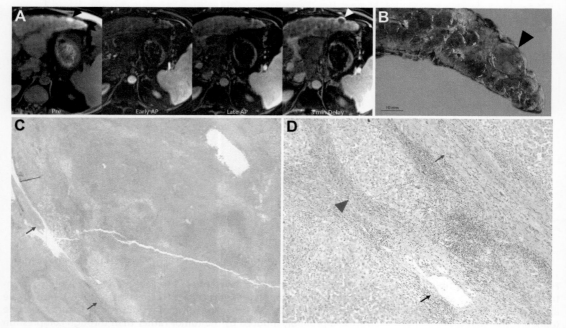

Fig. 8. Well-differentiated HCC with "pseudocapsule." (*A*) T1-weighted fat-saturated images before and after contrast administration denotes a 1.5-cm segment 3 observation with intrinsic T1 hyperintensity (*black arrowhead*), hypoenhancement relative to the background liver and "capsule" (*white arrowhead*). (*B*) Gross pathologic specimen provides correlation of the nodule, which was a well-differentiated hepatocellular carcinoma on pathologic analysis (*black arrowhead*). (*C*) Hematoxylin and eosin stain at ×2 original magnification of the nodule reveals a capsule along the periphery (*white arrows*). (*D*) Hematoxylin and eosin stain of the nodule reveals a pseudocapsule (*red arrow*) that appears similar to adjacent cirrhotic septa (*red arrowhead*). The portal tract remnant (*black arrow*) serves as a histologic hallmark that the pseudocapsule is a secondary process related to the compressive effect of nearby hepatic parenchyma by the tumor. Original magnification ×10.

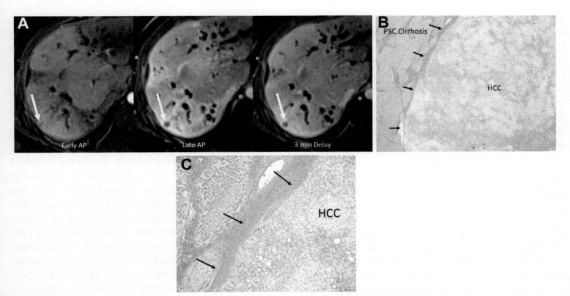

Fig. 9. Well-differentiated HCC with "pseudocapsule." (*A*) T1-weighted fat-saturated images after contrast administration exhibits a segment 7 observation with arterial phase hyperenhancement, washout appearance, and "capsule" (*arrows*). (*B*) A rim of background advanced stage (cirrhotic) primary sclerosing cholangitis (PSC) around a nodule of HCC (defined by *arrows*). Original magnification ×2. (*C*) Well-differentiated HCC with a pseudocapsule (*arrows*) due to compression of surrounding cirrhotic liver. Original magnification ×20.

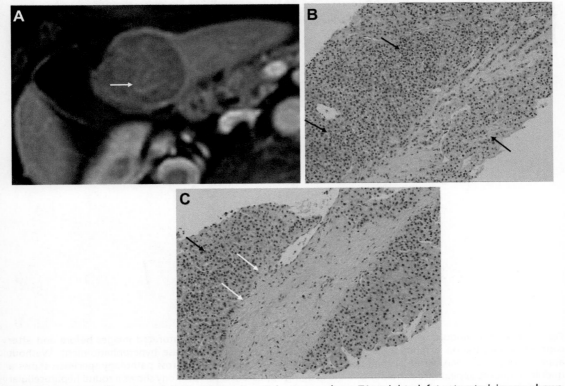

Fig. 10. Mosaic architecture of HCC. (*A*) Axial portal venous phase T1-weighted fat-saturated image shows enhancing fibrous bands (*white arrow*) with washout appearance throughout the rest of the 4.5-cm segment 3 observation. (*B, C*) Percutaneous biopsy specimen shows a moderately differentiated HCC (*black arrows*) intersected by thin and thick fibrous bands (*white arrows*). Low-power (×10) original magnification.

second process of compression of nearby, nontumoral parenchyma (**Fig. 7**). The compressive effects of the enlarging mass lead to compression of vascular supply, atrophy of hepatocyte parenchyma, and collapse of the portal tracts and septal fibrosis of the diseased liver to form a pseudocapsule. The histologic hallmark of these are the easy identification of the portal tract structures still remaining in the layers of the pseudocapsule (**Figs. 8** and **9**).

Mosaic Architecture and Nodule-In-Nodule Appearance

Radiology view

Mosaic architecture refers to randomly distributed internal nodules or compartments in a larger mass. This finding is usually associated with large HCCs, often larger than 3 cm.[40] Internally, each compartment's various imaging characteristics reflect foci of hemorrhage, necrosis, fat, and tumor heterogeneity.[41] Internal septations or capsules often exhibit delayed enhancement, suggesting their

fibrous nature[42] (**Fig. 10**). Nodular enhancing foci are suspicious for tumor tissue and possibly reflect clonal expansions of different cell lines at different stages of hepatocarcinogenesis.[42] Mosaic architecture is associated with high specificity of 99.0% and positive predictive value of 61.6% to 91.7% for HCC, especially among experienced radiologists.[43–45]

The nodule-in-nodule appearance is a subset of mosaic architecture in which a single smaller nodule is located within a larger nodule. The larger nodule is usually larger than 1 cm. The internal subnodule adopts different imaging characteristics from the parent nodule, suggesting dedifferentiation.[46] The internal subnodule imaging characteristics include arterial hyperenhancement, hyperintensity on T2W images, decreased fat or iron content, or hypointensity on the hepatobiliary phase.[47,48] As with mosaic architecture, nodule-in-nodule is uncommonly seen in non-HCC primary liver tumors, potentially helping to differentiate HCC from other hepatic neoplasms.

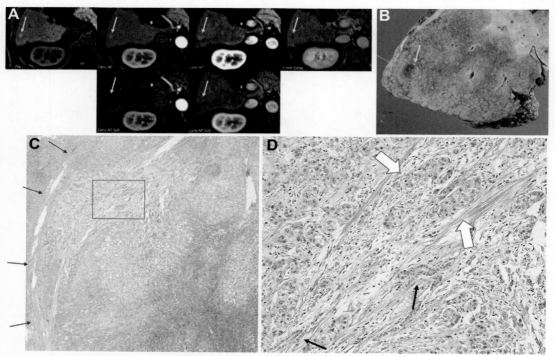

Fig. 11. Nodule-in-nodule/mosaic architecture of HCC. (*A*) T1-weighted fat-saturated images before and after contrast administration exhibits a segment 6 observation with arterial phase hyperenhancement. Washout appearance is only seen within a small portion of the nodule (*arrows*). (*B*) Gross pathology specimen shows a nodule-in-nodule appearance correlating to the imaging appearance. (*C*) Histology shows a round hepatocellular lesion (*arrows* define its round edge) (original magnification ×2). Pale areas within the nodules correspond to HCC defined by stromal invasion. (*D*) High magnification of the inset (original magnification ×10) shows well-differentiated hepatocytes within the stroma of a portal tract (*black arrows* highlight residual bile ducts). These represent HCC.

Pathology view

The diversity of subnodules is as seen radiographically. They may be one or few subnodules in a background lesion, such as emerging high-grade dysplasia or HCC in a background DN, or may be diversity of growth patterns, differentiate states, steatosis, focal necrosis, or relative congestion. When the lesion is small and likely to be a DN, the presence of a nodule-in-nodule pattern by imaging can be expected to represent the same in the DN and therefore confident diagnosis of an HGDN. If the entire lesion has LI-RADS 5 presentation, a nodule-in-nodule appearance suggests successive emergence of a more poorly differentiated/ higher grade HCC arising from the more well-differentiated earlier lesion (**Fig. 11**). When the lesion is larger and has a mosaic appearance, more than likely it has also already been diagnosed as an HCC by LI-RADS criteria.

However, one particular caution is important: combined hepatocellular-cholangiocarcinoma (cHCC-CCA) can also show a mosaic pattern. These tumors appear to be increasingly common, for various possible reasons; their treatment and prognosis differs significantly enough from HCC and from pure cholangiocarcinoma, such that it behooves radiologists to be aware of them in their imaging differential diagnosis and to target,[49] if possible, the different areas of the mosaic to better the chance of confirming cHCC-CCA by pathology.[50]

Key point

cHCC-CCAs share imaging characteristics with pure HCC and pure cholangiocarcinoma, including mosaic architecture, but have different treatment and prognosis from either of these types of malignancies. Radiologists should be aware and target different areas of the mosaic to increase the chance of confirming cHCC-CCA by pathology.

Intralesional Fat

Radiology view

Intralesional fat is defined as a nodule having increased lipid content when compared with the background liver. This feature is very rarely seen in non-HCC hepatic malignancies and is, thus, considered to be a feature that can help exclude intrahepatic cholangiocarcinoma.[47] The loss of signal on the out-of-phase images of the chemical shift gradient echo sequence is comparable to fine

needle aspiration for the detection of fatty change in hepatocellular nodules.[51] CT is less reliable in detecting intralesional fat, especially in small HCCs, due to partial volume effect.[52] Typically, intralesional fat content is homogeneous throughout the nodule and peaks in early HCC when the nodule is approximately 1.5 cm.[52,53]

As HCCs enlarge beyond 3.5 cm and the lesion continues to dedifferentiate, intratumoral fat, again, accumulates within the lesion. Although intralesional fat in early hepatocarcinogenesis exhibits a more homogeneous appearance throughout the nodule, intratumoral fat accumulation in this later stage is more heterogeneous throughout the lesion.[52] This second accumulation of fat is suspected to be related to a hypoxic environment as intratumoral arterial blood flow decreases, and the tumor converts from aerobic metabolism to glycolytic metabolism.[54]

Pathology view

As noted previously, intralesional fat peaks in HCC at approximately 1.5 cm,[53] but this is also seen in DNs that are diffusely steatotic or have a steatotic nodule-in-nodule not only in HCCs.[55] Kutami and colleagues[53] speculated that fat accumulation is hypoxia-induced given the relative decrease in vascular flow. As the hepatocellular nodule grows from 1.5 cm to 2.0 cm, the number of intranodular arteries increases and fatty change regresses until it becomes uncommon in HCCs larger than 3 cm. They point to small HCCs having relatively little angiogenesis compared with larger HCCs, whereas portal tracts have largely disappeared; the diminished portal blood flow with only moderately elevated arterial flow then may spur lipogenesis in the HCC.[53] In DNs, a similar process is suspected, although with greater variability. The persistence of portal tracts in dysplastic nodules with early stages of angiogenesis, similarly may reach this "sweet spot" of blood flow that spurs lipogenesis. The resulting HCC that might arise from the lesion may not necessarily be steatotic itself.[55]

SUMMARY

Hepatocarcinogenesis is a complex process resulting in predictable changes of the liver that can lead to HCC. Many of these pathologic changes result in characteristic imaging appearances. Thus, an understanding of hepatocarcinogenesis helps the radiologist to accurately characterize hepatic lesions in patients at increased risk for HCC and possibly identify those precursor lesions that are at a higher risk for malignancy.

CLINICS CARE POINTS

- LI-RADS categories do not correspond to histologic grade, but rather to the radiologist's degree of diagnostic suspicion for HCC.

- As progressed HCC becomes more advanced and infiltrative, these lesions may no longer exhibit APHE, possibly due to tumor cells converting to anaerobic metabolism.

- Hepatic observations with mosaic architecture may represent combined hepatocellular-cholangiocarcinoma and may warrant sampling of various areas within the mosaic for accurate diagnosis.

DISCLOSURE

A.F.: No disclosures. K.S.: No disclosures. M.T.: No disclosures. B.B.: No disclosure. N.T.: No disclosures.

REFERENCES

1. Marrero JA, Kulik LM, Sirlin CB, et al. Diagnosis, staging, and management of hepatocellular carcinoma: 2018 practice guidance by the American Association for the Study of Liver Diseases. Hepatology 2018;68(2):723–50.

2. Ding J, Wang H. Multiple interactive factors in hepatocarcinogenesis. Cancer Lett 2014;346(1):17–23.

3. Farazi PA, DePinho RA. Hepatocellular carcinoma pathogenesis: from genes to environment. Nat Rev Cancer 2006;6(9):674–87.

4. Chalasani N, Younossi Z, Lavine JE, et al. The diagnosis and management of nonalcoholic fatty liver disease: Practice guidance from the American Association for the Study of Liver Diseases. Hepatology 2018;67(1):328–57.

5. Marengo A, Rosso C, Bugianesi E. Liver cancer: connections with obesity, fatty liver, and cirrhosis. Annu Rev Med 2016;67:103–17.

6. Choi JY, Lee JM, Sirlin CB. CT and MR imaging diagnosis and staging of hepatocellular carcinoma: part I. development, growth, and spread: key pathologic and imaging aspects. Radiology 2014;272(3):635–54.

7. Narsinh KH, Cui J, Papadatos D, et al. Hepatocarcinogenesis and LI-RADS. Abdom Radiol (NY) 2018; 43(1):158–68.

8. Tsai WL, Chung RT. Viral hepatocarcinogenesis. Oncogene 2010;29(16):2309–24.

9. Galli A, Svegliati-Baroni G, Ceni E, et al. Oxidative stress stimulates proliferation and invasiveness of hepatic stellate cells via a MMP2-mediated mechanism. Hepatology 2005;41(5):1074–84.

10. Herath NI, Leggett BA, MacDonald GA. Review of genetic and epigenetic alterations in hepatocarcinogenesis. J Gastroenterol Hepatol 2006;21(1 Pt 1): 15–21.

11. Kim H, Oh BK, Roncalli M, et al. Large liver cell change in hepatitis B virus-related liver cirrhosis. Hepatology 2009;50(3):752–62.

12. Marchio A, Terris B, Meddeb M, et al. Chromosomal abnormalities in liver cell dysplasia detected by comparative genomic hybridisation. Mol Pathol 2001;54(4):270–4.

13. Plentz RR, Park YN, Lechel A, et al. Telomere shortening and inactivation of cell cycle checkpoints characterize human hepatocarcinogenesis. Hepatology 2007;45(4):968–76.

14. Watanabe S, Okita K, Harada T, et al. Morphologic studies of the liver cell dysplasia. Cancer 1983; 51(12):2197–205.

15. Gong L, Li YH, Su Q, et al. Clonality of nodular lesions in liver cirrhosis and chromosomal abnormalities in monoclonal nodules of altered hepatocytes. Histopathology 2010;56(5):589–99.

16. Arakawa M, Kage M, Sugihara S, et al. Emergence of malignant lesions within an adenomatous hyperplastic nodule in a cirrhotic liver. Observations in five cases. Gastroenterology 1986;91(1):198–208.

17. International Working P. Terminology of nodular hepatocellular lesions. Hepatology 1995;22(3):983–93.

18. Park YN, Yang CP, Fernandez GJ, et al. Neoangiogenesis and sinusoidal "capillarization" in dysplastic nodules of the liver. Am J Surg Pathol 1998;22(6): 656–62.

19. Park YN, Kojiro M, Di Tommaso L, et al. Ductular reaction is helpful in defining early stromal invasion, small hepatocellular carcinomas, and dysplastic nodules. Cancer 2007;109(5):915–23.

20. International Consensus Group for Hepatocellular Neoplasia; The International Consensus Group for Hepatocellular N. Pathologic diagnosis of early hepatocellular carcinoma: a report of the international consensus group for hepatocellular neoplasia. Hepatology 2009;49(2):658–64.

21. Hytiroglou P, Park YN, Krinsky G, et al. Hepatic precancerous lesions and small hepatocellular carcinoma. Gastroenterol Clin North Am 2007;36(4): 867–87, vii.

22. Kim TH, Kim SY, Tang A, et al. Comparison of international guidelines for noninvasive diagnosis of hepatocellular carcinoma: 2018 update. Clin Mol Hepatol 2019;25(3):245–63.

23. Hanna RF, Aguirre DA, Kased N, et al. Cirrhosis-associated hepatocellular nodules: correlation of histopathologic and MR imaging features. Radiographics 2008;28(3):747–69.

24. Hayashi M, Matsui O, Ueda K, et al. Correlation between the blood supply and grade of malignancy of hepatocellular nodules associated with liver cirrhosis: evaluation by CT during intraarterial injection of contrast medium. AJR Am J Roentgenol 1999;172(4):969–76.

25. Matsui O, Kadoya M, Kameyama T, et al. Benign and malignant nodules in cirrhotic livers: distinction based on blood supply. Radiology 1991;178(2):493–7.

26. Matsui O, Kobayashi S, Sanada J, et al. Hepatocelluar nodules in liver cirrhosis: hemodynamic evaluation (angiography-assisted CT) with special reference to multi-step hepatocarcinogenesis. Abdom Imaging 2011;36(3):264–72.

27. Asayama Y, Yoshimitsu K, Nishihara Y, et al. Arterial blood supply of hepatocellular carcinoma and histologic grading: radiologic-pathologic correlation. AJR Am J Roentgenol 2008;190(1):W28–34.

28. Tang A, Bashir MR, Corwin MT, et al. Evidence supporting LI-RADS major features for CT- and MR imaging-based diagnosis of hepatocellular carcinoma: a systematic review. Radiology 2018;286(1):29–48.

29. Tang Q, Ma C. Performance of Gd-EOB-DTPA-enhanced MRI for the diagnosis of LI-RADS 4 category hepatocellular carcinoma nodules with different diameters. Oncol Lett 2018;16(2):2725–31.

30. Abd Alkhalik Basha M, Abd El Aziz El Sammak D, El Sammak AA. Diagnostic efficacy of the liver imaging-reporting and data system (LI-RADS) with CT imaging in categorising small nodules (10-20 mm) detected in the cirrhotic liver at screening ultrasound. Clin Radiol 2017;72(10):901 e901–e911.

31. Hytiroglou P, Theise ND, Schwartz M, et al. Macroregenerative nodules in a series of adult cirrhotic liver explants: issues of classification and nomenclature. Hepatology 1995;21(3):703–8.

32. Theise ND, Jia J, Sun Y, et al. Progression and regression of fibrosis in viral hepatitis in the treatment era: the Beijing classification. Mod Pathol 2018;31(8):1191–200.

33. Chernyak V, Kobi M, Flusberg M, et al. Effect of threshold growth as a major feature on LI-RADS categorization. Abdom Radiol (NY) 2017;42(8):2089–100.

34. Wu H, Han X, Wang Z, et al. Prediction of the Ki-67 marker index in hepatocellular carcinoma based on CT radiomics features. Phys Med Biol 2020;65(23):235048.

35. Ishigami K, Yoshimitsu K, Nishihara Y, et al. Hepatocellular carcinoma with a pseudocapsule on gadolinium-enhanced MR images: correlation with histopathologic findings. Radiology 2009;250(2):435–43.

36. Santillan C, Fowler K, Kono Y, et al. LI-RADS major features: CT, MRI with extracellular agents, and MRI with hepatobiliary agents. Abdom Radiol (NY) 2018;43(1):75–81.

37. Kim B, Lee JH, Kim JK, et al. The capsule appearance of hepatocellular carcinoma in gadoxetic acid-enhanced MR imaging: correlation with pathology and dynamic CT. Medicine (Baltimore) 2018;97(25):e11142.

38. Cerny M, Chernyak V, Olivie D, et al. LI-RADS version 2018 ancillary features at MRI. Radiographics 2018;38(7):1973–2001.

39. Wald C, Russo MW, Heimbach JK, et al. New OPTN/UNOS policy for liver transplant allocation: standardization of liver imaging, diagnosis, classification, and reporting of hepatocellular carcinoma. Radiology 2013;266(2):376–82.

40. Huh J, Kim KW, Kim J, et al. Pathology-MRI correlation of hepatocarcinogenesis: recent update. J Pathol Transl Med 2015;49(3):218–29.

41. Li M, Xin Y, Fu S, et al. Corona enhancement and mosaic architecture for prognosis and selection between of liver resection versus transcatheter arterial chemoembolization in single hepatocellular carcinomas >5 cm without extrahepatic metastases: an imaging-based retrospective study. Medicine (Baltimore) 2016;95(2):e2458.

42. Stevens WR, Gulino SP, Batts KP, et al. Mosaic pattern of hepatocellular carcinoma: histologic basis for a characteristic CT appearance. J Comput Assist Tomogr 1996;20(3):337–42.

43. Cerny M, Bergeron C, Billiard JS, et al. LI-RADS for MR imaging diagnosis of hepatocellular carcinoma: performance of major and ancillary features. Radiology 2018;288(1):118–28.

44. Fraum TJ, Tsai R, Rohe E, et al. Differentiation of hepatocellular carcinoma from other hepatic malignancies in patients at risk: diagnostic performance of the liver imaging reporting and data system version 2014. Radiology 2018;286(1):158–72.

45. Horvat N, Nikolovski I, Long N, et al. Imaging features of hepatocellular carcinoma compared to intrahepatic cholangiocarcinoma and combined tumor on MRI using liver imaging and data system (LI-RADS) version 2014. Abdom Radiol (NY) 2018;43(1):169–78.

46. Efremidis SC, Hytiroglou P, Matsui O. Enhancement patterns and signal-intensity characteristics of small hepatocellular carcinoma in cirrhosis: pathologic basis and diagnostic challenges. Eur Radiol 2007;17(11):2969–82.

47. Choi JY, Lee JM, Sirlin CB. CT and MR imaging diagnosis and staging of hepatocellular carcinoma: part II. Extracellular agents, hepatobiliary agents, and

ancillary imaging features. Radiology 2014;273(1): 30–50.

48. Yu JS, Chung JJ, Kim JH, et al. Hypervascular focus in the nonhypervascular nodule ("nodule-in-nodule") on dynamic computed tomography: imaging evidence of aggressive progression in hepatocellular carcinoma. J Comput Assist Tomogr 2009;33(1): 131–5.

49. Brunt E, Aishima S, Clavien PA, et al. cHCC-CCA: consensus terminology for primary liver carcinomas with both hepatocytic and cholangiocytic differentation. Hepatology 2018;68(1):113–26.

50. Gigante E, Ronot M, Bertin C, et al. Combining imaging and tumour biopsy improves the diagnosis of combined hepatocellular-cholangiocarcinoma. Liver Int 2019;39(12):2386–96.

51. Martin J, Sentis M, Zidan A, et al. Fatty metamorphosis of hepatocellular carcinoma: detection with chemical shift gradient-echo MR imaging. Radiology 1995;195(1):125–30.

52. Balci NC, Befeler AS, Bieneman BK, et al. Fat containing HCC: findings on CT and MRI including serial contrast-enhanced imaging. Acad Radiol 2009; 16(8):963–8.

53. Kutami R, Nakashima Y, Nakashima O, et al. Pathomorphologic study on the mechanism of fatty change in small hepatocellular carcinoma of humans. J Hepatol 2000;33(2):282–9.

54. Asayama Y, Nishie A, Ishigami K, et al. Fatty change in moderately and poorly differentiated hepatocellular carcinoma on MRI: a possible mechanism related to decreased arterial flow. Clin Radiol 2016;71(12): 1277–83.

55. Nakanuma Y, Hirata K, Terasaki S, et al. Analytical histopathological diagnosis of small hepatocellular nodules in chronic liver disease. Histol Histopathol 1998;13(4):1077–87.

56. Kitao A, Zen Y, Matsui O, et al. Hepatocarcinogenesis: multistep changes of drainage vessels at CT during arterial portography and hepatic arteriography–radiologic-pathologic correlation. Radiology 2009;252(2):605–14.

57. Koh DM, Collins DJ. Diffusion-weighted MRI in the body: applications and challenges in oncology. AJR Am J Roentgenol 2007;188(6): 1622–35.

58. Terada T, Nakanuma Y. Iron-negative foci in siderotic macroregenerative nodules in human cirrhotic liver. A marker of incipient neoplastic lesions. Arch Pathol Lab Med 1989;113(8):916–20.

Liver Imaging Reporting and Data System Comprehensive Guide
MR Imaging Edition

Mohab M. Elmohr, MD[a],*, Victoria Chernyak, MD, MS[b],
Claude B. Sirlin, MD[c], Khaled M. Elsayes, MD, PhD[d]

KEYWORDS

- LI-RADS • Hepatocellular carcinoma • Magnetic resonance imaging • Major features
- Ancillary features

KEY POINTS

- The Liver Imaging Reporting and Data System (LI-RADS) is applicable to adult patients with cirrhosis, chronic hepatitis B infection, current or prior hepatocellular carcinoma (HCC), and none of the exclusion criteria.
- Late arterial-phase imaging is strongly preferred for HCC evaluation.
- Size greater than or equal to 10 mm and the presence of nonrim arterial-phase hyperenhancement are required for LR-5 (definite HCC) categorization.
- Ancillary features of malignancy cannot be used to upgrade LR-4 to LR-5.
- Targetoid morphology is 1 of the criteria for LR-M (probably malignant or definitely malignant, not HCC-specific) categorization.

INTRODUCTION

Hepatocellular carcinoma (HCC) is the most prevalent primary liver malignancy and the sixth most commonly diagnosed cancer.[1] With its progressively increasing mortality, liver cancer currently is the fourth-leading cause of cancer-related deaths worldwide.[2] For the most part, HCC tends to develop in a background of cirrhosis due to chronic hepatitis B or hepatitis C virus infection or alcoholic liver disease.[3] Imaging plays a pivotal role in the evaluation of HCC. By using a combination of imaging features, HCC can be diagnosed confidently on the basis of imaging alone with a specificity of more than 90%, often without a need for tissue sampling.[4] Given the particular importance of imaging in HCC, the need for consistency and clarity in radiological interpretation and reporting has become more evident.

LIVER IMAGING REPORTING AND DATA SYSTEM

The Liver Imaging Reporting and Data System (LI-RADS) was developed in 2011 by a multidisciplinary team of diagnostic and interventional radiologists, hepatologists, hepatobiliary surgeons, and hepatopathologists—with the support of the American College of Radiology—to standardize the terminology, technique, interpretation, reporting, and data collection of liver imaging.[5] LI-RADS underwent a series of significant updates before reaching the current algorithms: computed tomography (CT)/MR imaging for HCC diagnosis

a Department of Radiology, Baylor College of Medicine, One Baylor Plaza, BCM360, Houston, TX 77030, USA;
b Department of Radiology, Beth Israel Deaconess Medical Center, 330 Brookline Avenue, Boston, MA 02215, USA; c Liver Imaging Group, Department of Radiology, University of California, San Diego, 9500 Gilman Drive, La Jolla, CA 92093, USA; d Department of Abdominal Imaging, Division of Diagnostic Imaging, The University of Texas MD Anderson Cancer Center, 1515 Holcombe Boulevard, Houston, TX 77030, USA
* Corresponding author.
E-mail address: mohab.elmohr@bcm.edu

Magn Reson Imaging Clin N Am 29 (2021) 375–387
https://doi.org/10.1016/j.mric.2021.05.012
1064-9689/21/© 2021 Elsevier Inc. All rights reserved.

(version 2018), ultrasound (US) for HCC screening (version 2017), contrast-enhanced US (CEUS) for HCC diagnosis (version 2017), and CT/MR imaging for treatment response assessment (version 2018).[6] These algorithms are to be used only in adult patients at high risk for developing HCC, namely those with cirrhosis, chronic hepatitis B or hepatitis C viral infection, or current or prior HCC, including adult liver transplant candidates and recipients post-transplant, as per LI-RADS inclusion criteria.[6,7]

In LI-RADS, each liver observation is categorized according to its relative probability of benignity, general malignancy, and HCC. LR-1 is definitely benign, LR-2 is probably benign, LR-3 is intermediate probability for HCC, LR-4 is probably HCC, and LR-5 is definitely HCC. LR-M is probably malignant or definitely malignant, but not HCC-specific, and LR-TIV is definitely tumor in vein. LR-NC is assigned to observations that cannot be categorized owing to image degradation or omission. The categories LR-3, LR-4, and LR-5 are assigned on the basis of a combination of major imaging features (MFs). The MFs are used to assign the initial category, which can be adjusted up or down by a single category using the ancillary imaging features (AFs). A crucial exception is that AFs of malignancy cannot be used to upgrade from LR-4 to LR-5. Instead, the criteria for LR-5 must be met on the basis of MFs. In addition to adjusting categories, AFs can increase confidence in diagnosis.[8]

This article discusses the LI-RADS CT/MR imaging diagnostic algorithm, with particular emphasis on MR imaging, and highlights the recommended MR imaging technical requirements, explains the diagnosis algorithm, and defines the MFs and AFs pertaining to liver MR imaging.

MR IMAGING TECHNIQUE

Since the debut of LI-RADS, version 2013, technical recommendations regarding modalities and contrast media have been revised continuously to define the minimum technical requirements.[9] These technical parameters are meant to guide radiologists and technologists in avoiding suboptimal studies. For example, image degradation or omission may result in a study that is inadequate for accurate diagnosis and lead to subsequent repeat imaging and delayed management.[10]

LI-RADS was developed to be applied to multiphase CT or MR imaging studies performed with either an extracellular or a hepatobiliary contrast agent. Gadoxetate disodium and gadobenate dimeglumine are the 2 hepatobiliary MR imaging agents used routinely in clinical practice.[11]

LI-RADS recommends that all MR imaging examinations be done using a 1.5T or 3T MR imaging scanner with a torso phased-array coil for improved liver-to-lesion contrast-to-noise ratios.[12] Required MR imaging sequences include unenhanced T1-weighted in-phase and out-of-phase imaging, enhanced multiphase T1-weighted imaging, and T2-weighted imaging with or without fat saturation (**Table 1**). Multiphase T1-weighted imaging is performed initially in the precontrast phase, followed by the arterial, portal venous, and delayed (2–5 minutes postinjection) contrast-enhanced phases. It is strongly recommended that arterial-phase imaging be done in the late arterial phase when the portal veins but not the hepatic veins are enhanced, that is, 35 seconds to 40 seconds postinjection versus 15 seconds to 20 seconds postinjection for the early arterial phase when the portal vein is not yet enhanced.[13] Transitional-phase imaging (2–5 minutes postinjection) replaces delayed-phase imaging for gadoxetate disodium, a hepatobiliary agent, owing to its relatively early hepatocellular uptake.[11] Hepatobiliary-phase imaging during the excretion of hepatobiliary contrast agents into the biliary system is required when using gadoxetate disodium (approximately 20 minutes postinjection) and optional with gadobenate dimeglumine (1–3 hours postinjection). Diffusion-weighted imaging, subtraction imaging, and multiplanar reformatted images are optional in LI-RADS but are considered routine images in many academic institutions and community centers.[14]

APPROACH TO LIVER IMAGING REPORTING AND DATA SYSTEM, VERSION 2018, DIAGNOSTIC ALGORITHM

Upon encountering an untreated liver observation on a liver MR imaging study in a patient at high risk for HCC, the CT/MR imaging LI-RADS, version 2018, diagnostic algorithm should be applied.[7] This algorithm uses a stepwise approach in assigning categories, where each of the preceding categories must be excluded before proceeding down the decision tree. In the initial step, quality assurance is performed to ensure the technical adequacy of the acquired images. If technical limitations are such that an observation cannot be assessed as likely benign (LR-1/2) versus likely malignant (LR-4/5/M), the LR-NC category is assigned. In the next 2 steps, the imaging features are assessed to determine whether the observation is interpreted as definitely benign (LR-1) or probably benign (LR-2), respectively, and 1 of these categories is assigned, if appropriate. If the observation is not definitely benign or probably

Table 1
Technical recommendations for MR imaging phases

Contrast Agent	Precontrast	Arterial Phase	Portal Venous Phase	Delayed Phase or Transitional Phase	Hepatobiliary Phase
ECA	Required	Required	Required	Required; delayed	—
Gadobenate dimeglumine (HBA)	Required	Required	Required	Required; transitional	Optional
Gadoxetate disodium (HBA)	Required	Required	Required	Required; transitional	Required

Abbreviations: ECA, extracellular agent; HBA, hepatobiliary agent.

benign, the next step is to assess the observation for the presence of targetoid imaging features, in which case the LR-M category is assigned (**Fig. 1**). Note that the presence of at least 1 targetoid feature is sufficient for LR-M category assignment, an approach that helps to achieve high specificity of the LR-5 category for the diagnosis of HCC.[15] Targetoid features include rim arterial-phase hyperenhancement (APHE), peripheral washout, delayed central enhancement, targetoid diffusion restriction, and targetoid morphology visible in the transitional/hepatobiliary phase.[15] The latter 2 features can be assessed only on MR imaging.

Once the LR-NC, LR-TIV, LR-1, LR-2, and LR-M categories have been excluded, the CT/MR imaging diagnostic table is applied to categorize the observation as LR-3, LR-4, or LR-5 (**Fig. 2**).

The final category then can be adjusted, at the radiologist's discretion, on the basis of the presence of AFs. The category can be upgraded or downgraded by 1 in the presence of greater than or equal to 1 AF, indicating malignancy, or greater than or equal to 1 AF, indicating benignity, respectively. In cases of greater than or equal to 1 AF, indicating malignancy, and greater than or equal to 1 AF, indicating benignity, the initially assigned category is not changed. In order to maintain the required high specificity of LR-5 for the diagnosis of HCC, AFs cannot be used to upgrade from the LR-4 to LR-5 category.

MAJOR IMAGING FEATURES

Classically, HCC is a hypervascular tumor that typically sources almost 100% of its blood supply from the hepatic arteries instead of the portal vein, which supplies normal hepatic parenchyma. This vascular shift leads to the characteristic appearance of HCC: early enhancement and washout on enhanced cross-sectional imaging. In LI-

RADS, HCC is diagnosed on the basis of a combination of 5 MFs with a specificity of 94% in cases of LR-5 observations.[16] MFs are required for LR-3, LR-4, and LR-5 category assignments and comprise the following: nonrim APHE, nonperipheral washout, enhancing capsule, size greater than 10 mm, and threshold growth (**Fig. 3**).

Nonrim Arterial-phase Hyperenhancement

APHE is defined as enhancement in arterial phase greater than liver, resulting in brightness greater than liver. Nonrim APHE is a subtype of APHE in which APHE is not most pronounced in the periphery of observation.[17] The reported sensitivity of non-rim APHE is as high as 96% for progressed HCC, surpassing the rest of the MFs, although it lacks the specificity to be used alone.[18] Nonrim APHE is required for LR-5 category assignment.

Nonperipheral Washout

Washout is defined as reduction in enhancement from earlier to later phase resulting in hypoenhancement relative to liver. This can have 1 of the following patterns on MR imaging: hyperenhancing to hypoenhancing or isoenhancing to hypoenhancing. Nonperipheral washout is the subtype of washout in which the appearance of washout is not most pronounced in the observation periphery.[17] The washout must be assessed in the extracellular phase, which includes the portal venous phase and delayed phase when extracellular agents and gadobenate dimeglumine are used and the portal venous phase only when gadoxetate disodium is used. Transitional-phase hypointensity and hepatobiliary-phase hypointensity do not qualify as washout but count as AFs favoring malignancy in general.[19] APHE does not have to be present to characterize washout. The hypoenhancement of either a portion of observation or its entirety qualifies for washout.

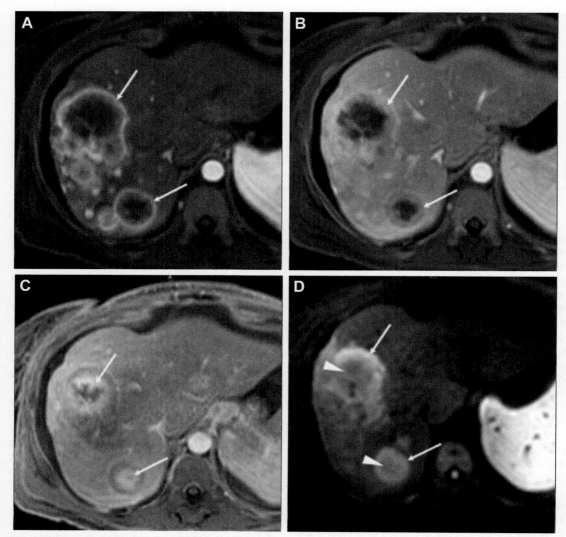

Fig. 1. Illustration of LR-M targetoid features in a 66-year-old woman with cryptogenic cirrhosis. Arterial phase (*A*) demonstrates rim APHE, seen as hyperenhancement in the periphery of observations (*arrows*). On the portal venous–phase (*B*) and delayed-phase (*C*) images, there is peripheral washout (*arrows* [*B*]) and delayed central enhancement (*arrows* [*C*]). The observations demonstrate targetoid restricted diffusion, where the periphery of the observations (*arrows* [*D*]) is more hyperintense than the center (*arrowheads* [*D*]). The presence of targetoid morphology results in LR-M categorization. Pathology confirmed multifocal intrahepatic cholangiocarcinoma.

Washout has a specificity of 62% to 100% and a positive predictive value (PPV) of 55% to 100% for HCC. When combined with nonrim APHE, the specificity increases to 75% to 100% and PPV to 87% to 100% for HCC in at-risk patients.[20]

Enhancing Capsule

Capsule is defined as smooth, uniform, sharp border around most or all of an observation. If the liver parenchyma visually consists of both nodules and fibrosis, then the capsule must be thicker or more conspicuous than the fibrotic tissue around background nodules. An enhancing capsule is the subtype of capsule visible as an enhancing rim in the portal venous phase, delayed phase, or transitional phase.[17] In addition to a true fibrous tumor capsule, which is a characteristic histopathologic feature of HCC, a pseudocapsule due to compressed surrounding hepatic parenchyma also can have the appearance of a capsule on imaging.[21]

Enhancing capsule can be confused with corona enhancement, an AF favoring malignancy. These 2 features can be differentiated from each other based on their temporal pattern after

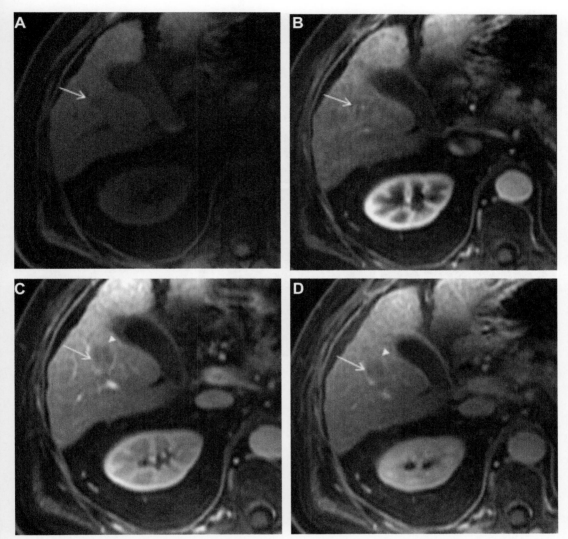

Fig. 2. Example of LR-5 observation in a 65-year-old man with pathology-proved HCC. Axial MR images of the abdomen in the precontrast (*A*), late arterial phase (*B*), portal venous phase (*C*), and delayed phase (*D*) demonstrate a 2.1-cm T1-hypointense (*arrow* [*A*]) observation in hepatic segment V. This observation is categorized as LR-5 based on size (≥20 mm), nonrim APHE (*arrow* [*B*]), non-peripheral washout (*arrow* [*C, D*]), and enhancing capsule (*arrowhead* [*C, D*]).

contrast injection. Capsule appearance is appreciated best in the portal venous phase, delayed phase, or transitional phase. In contrast, corona enhancement, due to perilesional venous drainage from the tumor, is seen in the late arterial phase or early portal venous phase.[22] Capsule has a specificity of 86% to 96% for HCC in at-risk patients.[18]

Size

Size is an independent predictor of malignancy.[18] In LI-RADS, size is defined as the largest outer-to-outer-edge dimension of an observation and should

be measured on the phase or image in which the margins are demarcated most sharply without anatomic distortion or surrounding perfusion alteration. Arterial-phase images and diffusion-weighted images should not be used if the observation is seen clearly in other phases.[7] Anatomic distortion on diffusion-weighted imaging hinders the accurate measurement of an observation, whereas size overestimation due to perilesional enhancement reduces the reliability of measurement in the arterial phase. Any perfusion alteration contiguous with the observation should be excluded from measurement. If the observation

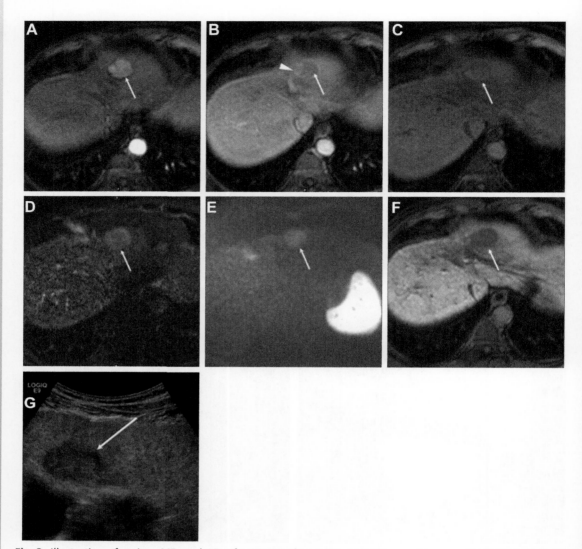

Fig. 3. Illustration of various MFs and AFs of a 27-mm observation in a 67-year-old man with cirrhosis. Arterial-phase image (*A*) demonstrates nonrim APHE (*arrow*). Portal venous–phase image (*B*) demonstrates nonperipheral washout (*arrow*) and enhancing capsule (*arrowhead*). Note that the capsule also is seen as a hypointense rim on precontrast T1-weighted image (*arrow* [*C*]). When a rim is seen on both non-contrast and postcontrast images, it should be characterized as an enhancing capsule. This combination of MFs allows LR-5 (definite HCC) categorization. The observation also demonstrates multiple AFs of malignancy (*arrows*): mild T2 hyperintensity (*D*), mildly restricted diffusion (*E*), hepatobiliary-phase hypointensity (*F*), and US visibility as a solid nodule (*G*).

has a capsule or nodule-in-nodule appearance, the entirety of the observation, including the capsule, should be included in the measurement.[23]

In LI-RADS, size is divided into 3 strata: less than 10 mm, 10 mm to 20 mm, and greater than 20 mm. Size greater than or equal to 10 mm is required for LR-5 category assignment.

Threshold Growth

Threshold growth is defined as size increase of a mass by greater than or equal to 50% in less than or equal to 6 months. When evaluating for threshold growth on prior CT or MR imaging studies, it is essential to use the same sequence, phase, and plane. Threshold growth cannot be assessed by comparing MR imaging with a prior US or CEUS. Growth not meeting the threshold growth criteria is considered subthreshold growth, an AF favoring malignancy. Examples include a size increase of less than 50%, greater than or equal to 100% size increase in greater than 6 months, and a new greater than or equal to 10-mm observation.

ANCILLARY IMAGING FEATURES

AFs are optional imaging features used in LI-RADS for increased confidence and improved detection and characterization. In contrast to MFs, AFs alone cannot be used to diagnose HCC because of their imperfect specificity. Still, they can be applied alongside a combination of MFs to enhance the overall diagnostic sensitivity for HCC. LI-RADS classifies AFs into 3 categories: AFs that favor HCC in particular, AFs that favor malignancy in general, and AFs that favor benignity (**Table 2**) (see **Fig. 3**). AFs are used at the radiologist's discretion to adjust the initially assigned category; AFs that favor malignancy and those that favor HCC can be used to upgrade by a single category (up to LR-4), and AFs that favor benignity can be used to downgrade by a single category.

Ancillary Features Favoring Hepatocellular Carcinoma in Particular

Five AFs indicate HCC in particular but lack the specificity required to be considered an MF. Among these 5 features, all can be detected on MR imaging and include the following: nonenhancing capsule, nodule-in-nodule appearance, mosaic appearance, fat in mass, and blood products in mass (**Fig. 4**).

Nonenhancing capsule

A nonenhancing capsule is a subtype of capsule that does not show enhancement on any image.[17] A fibrous capsule is a histopathologic feature of HCC that can be detected on MR imaging as a rim of hypointensity on both T1-weighted and T2-weighted images.[21] Although capsule appearance also can result from tumor growth compressing the surrounding parenchyma (pseudocapsule), both etiologies share the same MR imaging appearance.

Nodule-in-nodule appearance

Nodule-in-nodule appearance is defined as the presence of a smaller inner nodule within a larger outer nodule or mass.[17] This appearance can be explained by a growing focus of HCC, the inner nodule, within an outer dysplastic nodule during the process of hepatocarcinogenesis.[24] The inner nodule usually exhibits imaging features of HCC, such as APHE, whereas the outer nodule is hypovascular and, therefore, does not enhance in the arterial phase.[25]

Mosaic appearance

The presence of any combination of internal nodules, compartments, or septations within a mass is referred to as a mosaic appearance.[17] This

---

Table 2
Ancillary features in the Liver Imaging Reporting and Data System, version 2018

Ancillary Features Favoring Hepatocellular Carcinoma in Particular	Ancillary Features Favoring Malignancy in General	Ancillary Features Favoring Benignity
Nonenhancing capsule	US visibility as discrete nodule	Size stability ≥ 2 y
Nodule-in-nodule architecture	Subthreshold growth	Size reduction
Mosaic architecture	Corona enhancement	Parallels blood pool enhancement
Fat in mass, more than adjacent liver	Fat sparing in solid mass	Undistorted vessels
Blood products in mass	Restricted diffusion	Iron in mass, more than liver
	Mild–moderate T2 hyperintensity	Marked T2 hyperintensity
	Iron sparing in solid mass	Hepatobiliary-phase isointensity; *MR imaging HBA*[a]
	Transitional-phase hypointensity; *MR imaging HBA*[a]	
	Hepatobiliary-phase hypointensity; *MR imaging HBA*[a]	

[a] Transitionalphase hypointensity, hepatobiliary-phase hypointensity, and hepatobiliary-phase isointensity are seen only on MR imaging with hepatobiliary contrast agent.

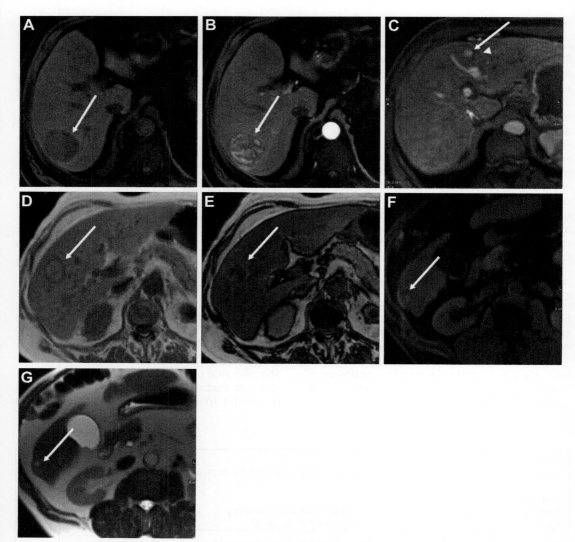

Fig. 4. Illustration of AFs favoring HCC in particular. Unenhanced T1-weighted image (*A*) in a patient with HCC demonstrates an observation with a non-enhancing capsule (*arrow*). Arterial-phase T1WI contrast-enhanced C+ (*B*) in the same patient shows mosaic architecture (*arrow*) of the observation. Arterial-phase T1-weighted image C+ (*C*) in another patient with HCC demonstrates nodule-in-nodule appearance, seen as an enhancing nodule (*arrow*) within an outer nonenhancing nodule (*arrowhead*). In-phase and out-of-phase gradient-echo images (*D, E*) in a patient with HCC demonstrate fat in mass more than adjacent liver (*arrows*), seen as loss of signal intensity on out-of-phase compared with in-phase images. Unenhanced T1-weighted image (*F*) and T2-weighted image (*G*) in a patient with HCC demonstrate blood products in mass, seen as high signal intensity in an observation on both T1-weighted and T2-weighted sequences.

mosaic appearance occurs when there are multiple histologic components (fat, necrosis, or hemorrhage) and usually is seen in large progressed HCCs. On MR imaging, a large mass with multiple internal components of different signal intensities and enhancement patterns is appreciated.[26] Nodule-in-nodule appearance is a subtype of mosaic appearance.

Fat in mass

Fat in mass refers to a greater amount of fat within a mass relative to the adjacent liver.[17] The presence of intracellular fat in HCC has been speculated to occur in high-grade dysplastic nodules and early HCC in response to tumor hypoxia.[27] MR imaging is more specific than CT for the detection of intravoxel fat.[28] Intravoxel fat generally is characterized on MR imaging as a loss in signal intensity on out-of-phase imaging compared with in-phase imaging or signal loss on fat-suppressed imaging compared with non–fat-suppressed imaging.

Blood products in mass

Hemorrhage inside a lesion in the absence of biopsy, trauma, or intervention is another AF indicative of HCC.[17] Spontaneous hemorrhage is an uncommon but characteristic imaging finding in HCC and is thought to occur when high-flow fragile arteries in the tumor rupture.[29] Varying degrees of signal intensities are seen on MR imaging, depending on the age of the blood products: hyperintense in the acute stage and hypointense in the chronic stage on both T1-weighted and T2-weighted sequences. Hemorrhage rarely is seen with non-HCC malignancies.[8]

Ancillary Features Favoring Malignancy in General

The second group of AFs are imaging features on CT and MR imaging that are suggestive of malignancy but not specific to HCC. Many of these

AFs can be seen only on MR imaging (eg, mild T2 hyperintensity and restricted diffusion). Transitional-phase hypointensity and hepatobiliary-phase hypointensity require MR imaging with a hepatobiliary contrast agent.

Ultrasound visibility as nodule

The unenhanced US visibility as discrete nodule or mass corresponding to CT-detected or MR imaging–detected observation is considered an AF for general malignancy.[17]

Subthreshold growth

Size increase of a mass less than threshold growth is referred to as subthreshold growth.[17]

Corona enhancement

Venous drainage from a tumor can result in corona enhancement, which is periobservational enhancement in the late arterial phase or early portal venous phase[17] (**Fig. 5**). The temporal pattern of enhancement helps to differentiate corona enhancement from an enhancing capsule.

Fat sparing in solid mass

Paucity of fat in solid mass relative to steatotic liver.[17] Fat sparing can be seen in an inner nodule

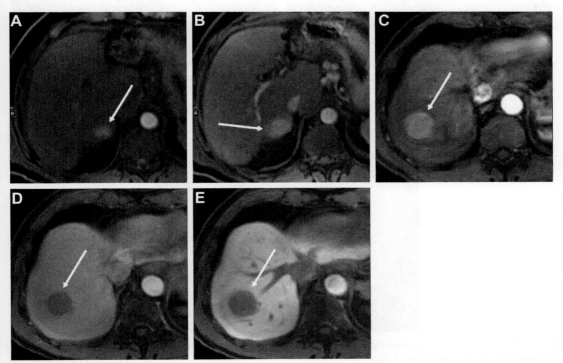

Fig. 5. Illustration of AFs favoring malignancy in general. T1-weighted images C+ (*A, B*) in a patient with HCC demonstrate corona enhancement (*arrows*), seen as a rim of periobservation enhancement in the late arterial phase (*A*) or portal venous phase (*B*) surrounding an APHE mass. T1-weighted images C+ (*C–E*) in a different patient with confirmed HCC demonstrate an APHE observation (*arrow* [*C*]) exhibiting transitional-phase hypointensity (*arrow* [*E*]) and hepatobiliary-phase hypointensity (*arrow* [*E*]).

relative to the outer nodule. Focal fat sparing usu-ally occurs in areas of regionally decreased portal blood flow, for example, during hepatocarcino-genesis.[30] When compared with the steatotic background liver, the mass shows less signal loss on out-of-phase gradient-echo imaging compared with in-phase gradient-echo imaging or on fat-suppressed imaging compared with non–fat-suppressed imaging.[31]

Restricted diffusion

Restricted diffusion refers to intensity higher than liver on moderately or highly diffusion-weighted images not attributed to T2 shine-through.[17] T2 shine-through can be excluded if the apparent diffusion coefficient is similar to or lower than liver. Restricted diffusion is characteristic of malignant neoplasms and is thought to be due to increased tumor cellularity.[32]

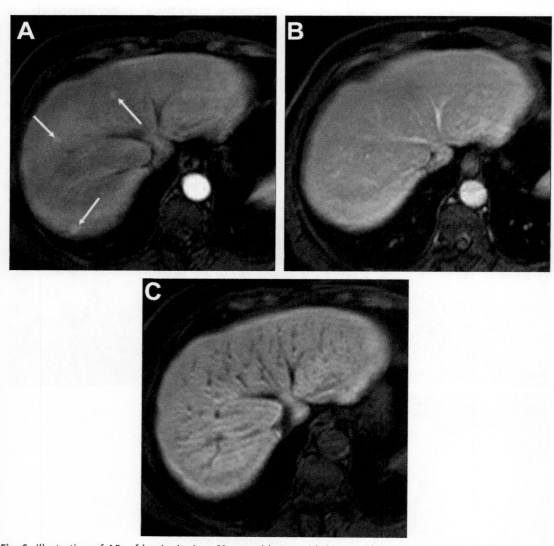

Fig. 6. Illustration of AFs of benignity in a 69-year-old man with history of HCC. Arterial-phase (A) image demonstrates several rounded observations (arrows), all less than 10 mm, with nonrim APHE and no washout or capsule on the portal venous phase (B). Based on the MFs, the observations are categorized as LR-3 (intermediate probability of malignancy). The observations are uniformly isointense to the parenchyma in the hepatobiliary phase (C) and demonstrate no AFs of malignancy on any other sequences (not shown). Application of AF favoring benignity allows the category to be downgraded to LR-2 (probably benign). The observations represent probable vascular shunts.

Mild to moderate T2 hyperintensity

Intensity on T2-weighted imaging that is higher than liver and similar to or less than non–iron-overloaded spleen is considered mild to moderate T2 hyperintensity.[17] This feature is common in most hepatic malignancies, including metastases.[33]

Iron sparing in solid mass

Paucity of iron in solid mass relative to iron-overloaded liver.[17] MR imaging is more sensitive and specific for the detection of iron sparing compared with CT.[34] On most commercial 1.5T scanners, the mass shows less signal loss on the in-phase compared with the out-of-phase gradient-echo imaging, and the mass is less hypointense on T2-weighted spin-echo/fast spin-echo and T2*-weighted gradient-echo imaging. In such cases, signal loss on in-phase gradient-echo imaging is nonspecific, because it could be confounded largely by the presence of steatosis.[35]

Transitional-phase hypointensity

Intensity in the transitional phase less than liver[17] (see **Fig. 5**). Transitional-phase hypointensity is evaluated on MR imaging with a hepatobiliary contrast agent only.

Hepatobiliary-phase hypointensity

Intensity in the hepatobiliary phase less than liver (see **Fig. 5**)[17] also is evaluated on MR imaging with a hepatobiliary contrast agent only.

Ancillary Features Favoring Benignity

Several imaging features seen in benign liver masses favor benignity in an observation (**Fig. 6**).

Size stability greater than or equal to 2 years

No significant change in observation size measured on examinations greater than or equal to 2 years apart in absence of treatment.[17]

Size reduction

Spontaneous decrease in size over time that cannot be attributed only to artifact, technique differences, measurement error, or resorption of blood products.[17]

Parallels blood pool enhancement

Temporal pattern in which enhancement eventually reaches and then matches that of blood pool.[17] This enhancement pattern typically is seen with hemangioma and, therefore, is suggestive of benignity.[36]

Undistorted vessels

Vessels traversing an observation without displacement, deformation, or other alteration.[17] Because distortion of vessels usually is seen in space-occupying tumors, the absence of distorted vessels is highly suggestive of benignity.

Iron in mass, more than liver

Excess iron in a mass relative to background liver[17] Intralesional iron content can be evaluated through chemical shift MR imaging showing loss of signal on the in-phase imaging compared with the out-of-phase imaging. Siderotic nodules, which are iron-rich regenerative or dysplastic nodules, are common in cirrhotic patients and usually have a benign course.[37] Therefore, excess iron in an observation is indicative of siderotic nodules and indirectly indicative of benignity.

Marked T2 hyperintensity

Intensity on T2-weighted images greater than non–iron-overloaded spleen is considered marked T2 hyperintensity.[17] T2 hyperintensity commonly is seen in benign hepatic lesions, including biliary hamartomas, cysts, and abscesses.[38]

Hepatobiliary phase isointensity

Uniform intensity in hepatobiliary phase identical or nearly identical to liver is another indication of benignity.[17] Hepatic malignancies, including HCC, typically are hypointense in the hepatobiliary phase because of their altered perfusion. HCC, however, can be isointense or even hyperintense the hepatobiliary phase in less than 8% of cases.[8] Generally, hepatobiliary-phase isointensity is considered suggestive of benignity.

SUMMARY

LI-RADS is a comprehensive system for HCC diagnosis providing a standardized lexicon, technical recommendations, and diagnostic algorithms for CT, MR imaging, and CEUS in high-risk patients. By using a combination of imaging MFs and AFs, liver observations can be categorized on the basis of the probability of their being HCC, from LR-1 to LR-5, with high specificity of LR-5 category assignment for a diagnosis of HCC.

CLINICS CARE POINTS

- Washout must be assessed in the extracellular phase. Transitional phase hypointensity and hepatobiliary phase hypointensity do not qualify as washout but count as ancillary features (AFs) favoring malignancy in general.

- Size should not be measured on the arterial phase and diffusion-weighted images if the observation is clearly seen in other phases.

- In contrast with corona enhancement, capsule appearance is best appreciated in the portal venous, delayed, or transitional phase.
- The presence of at least one targetoid feature is sufficient for LR-M category assignment.

DISCLOSURE

The authors have no relevant disclosures.

REFERENCES

1. Jemal A, Ward EM, Johnson CJ, et al. Annual report to the nation on the status of cancer, 1975–2014, featuring survival. J Natl Cancer Inst 2017;109(9):djx030.
2. Bray F, Ferlay J, Soerjomataram I, et al. Global cancer statistics 2018: GLOBOCAN estimates of incidence and mortality worldwide for 36 cancers in 185 countries. CA Cancer J Clin 2018;68(6):394–424.
3. Villanueva A. Hepatocellular Carcinoma. N Engl J Med 2019;380(15):1450–62.
4. Roberts LR, Sirlin CB, Zaiem F, et al. Imaging for the diagnosis of hepatocellular carcinoma: a systematic review and meta-analysis. Hepatology 2018;67(1):401–21.
5. Elsayes KM, Kielar AZ, Chernyak V, et al. LI-RADS: a conceptual and historical review from its beginning to its recent integration into AASLD clinical practice guidance. J Hepatocell Carcinoma 2019;6:49.
6. Elsayes KM, Kielar AZ, Elmohr MM, et al. White paper of the Society of Abdominal Radiology hepatocellular carcinoma diagnosis disease-focused panel on LI-RADS v2018 for CT and MRI. Abdom Radiol 2018;43(10):2625–42.
7. (ACR) ACoR. Liver Imaging Reporting and Data System (LI-RADS) v2018. ACR; 2018. Available at: https://www.acr.org/-/media/ACR/Files/RADS/LI-RADS/LI-RADS-2018-Core.pdf?la=en. Accessed 12/01, 2019.
8. Chernyak V, Tang A, Flusberg M, et al. LI-RADS® ancillary features on CT and MRI. Abdom Radiol 2018;43(1):82–100.
9. Santillan CS, Tang A, Cruite I, et al. Understanding LI-RADS: a primer for practical use. Magn Reson Imaging Clin N Am 2014;22(3):337–52.
10. Tang A, Cruite I, Sirlin CB, et al. Toward a standardized system for hepatocellular carcinoma diagnosis using computed tomography and MRI. Expert Rev Gastroenterol Hepatol 2013;7(3):269–79.
11. Hope TA, Fowler KJ, Sirlin CB, et al. Hepatobiliary agents and their role in LI-RADS. Abdom Imaging 2015;40(3):613–25.
12. Schwartz LH, Panicek DM, Thomson E, et al. Comparison of phased-array and body coils for MR imaging of liver. Clin Radiol 1997;52(10):745–9.
13. Murakami T, Kim T, Takamura M, et al. Hypervascular hepatocellular carcinoma: detection with double arterial phase multi-detector row helical CT. Radiology 2001;218(3):763–7.
14. Shankar S, Kalra N, Bhatia A, et al. Role of Diffusion Weighted Imaging (DWI) for Hepatocellular Carcinoma (HCC) detection and its grading on 3t mri: a prospective study. J Clin Exp Hepatol 2016;6(4):303–10.
15. Chernyak V, Fowler KJ, Kamaya A, et al. Liver Imaging Reporting and Data System (LI-RADS) version 2018: imaging of hepatocellular carcinoma in at-risk patients. Radiology 2018;289(3):816–30.
16. Van der Pol CB, Lim CS, Sirlin CB, et al. Accuracy of the liver imaging reporting and data system in computed tomography and magnetic resonance image analysis of hepatocellular carcinoma or overall malignancy—a systematic review. Gastroenterology 2019;156(4):976–86.
17. American College of Radiology website. The LI-RADS lexicon. 2018. Available at: www.acr.org/-/media/ACR/Files/RADS/LI-RADS/Lexicon-Table-2020.pdf. Accessed September 2020.
18. Tang A, Bashir MR, Corwin MT, et al. Evidence supporting LI-RADS major features for CT- and MR imaging–based diagnosis of hepatocellular carcinoma: a systematic review. Radiology 2018;286(1):29–48.
19. Santillan C, Fowler K, Kono Y, et al. LI-RADS major features: CT, MRI with extracellular agents, and MRI with hepatobiliary agents. Abdom Radiol 2018;43(1):75–81.
20. Sangiovanni A, Manini MA, Iavarone M, et al. The diagnostic and economic impact of contrast imaging techniques in the diagnosis of small hepatocellular carcinoma in cirrhosis. Gut 2010;59(5):638–44.
21. Ishigami K, Yoshimitsu K, Nishihara Y, et al. Hepatocellular carcinoma with a pseudocapsule on gadolinium-enhanced MR images: correlation with histopathologic findings. Radiology 2009;250(2):435–43.
22. Ito K. Hepatocellular carcinoma: conventional MRI findings including gadolinium-enhanced dynamic imaging. Eur J Radiol 2006;58(2):186–99.
23. Kojiro M. 'Nodule-in-nodule' appearance in hepatocellular carcinoma: its significance as a morphologic marker of dedifferentiation. Intervirology 2004;47(3–5):179–83.
24. Giambelluca D, Cannella R, Caruana G, et al. "Nodule-in-nodule" architecture of hepatocellular carcinoma. Abdom Radiol 2019;44(7):2671–3.
25. Cerny M, Chernyak V, Olivié D, et al. LI-RADS version 2018 ancillary features at MRI. Radiographics 2018;38(7):1973–2001.

26. Cannella R, Furlan A. Mosaic architecture of hepatocellular carcinoma. Abdom Radiol 2018;43(7):1847–8.

27. Kojiro M, Roskams T. Early hepatocellular carcinoma and dysplastic nodules. In: Paper presented at: seminars in liver disease. 2005.

28. Venkataraman S, Braga L, Semelka RC. Imaging the fatty liver. Magn Reson Imaging Clin 2002;10(1):93–103.

29. Kim PT, Su JC, Buczkowski AK, et al. Computed tomography and angiographic interventional features of ruptured hepatocellular carcinoma: pictorial essay. Can Assoc Radiol J 2006;57(3):159.

30. Grossholz M, Terrier F, Rubbia L, et al. Focal sparing in the fatty liver as a sign of an adjacent space-occupying lesion. AJR Am J Roentgenol 1998;171(5):1391–5.

31. Hamer OW, Aguirre DA, Casola G, et al. Fatty liver: imaging patterns and pitfalls. Radiographics 2006;26(6):1637–53.

32. White NS, McDonald C, Farid N, et al. Diffusion-weighted imaging in cancer: physical foundations and applications of restriction spectrum imaging. Cancer Res 2014;74(17):4638–52.

33. Albiin N. MRI of focal liver lesions. Curr Med Imaging Rev 2012;8(2):107–16.

34. İdilman İS, Akata D, Özmen MN, et al. Different forms of iron accumulation in the liver on MRI. Diagn Interv Radiol 2016;22(1):22.

35. Sirlin CB, Reeder SB. Magnetic resonance imaging quantification of liver iron. Magn Reson Imaging Clin N Am 2010;18(3):359–ix.

36. Semelka RC, Brown ED, Ascher SM, et al. Hepatic hemangiomas: a multi-institutional study of appearance on T2-weighted and serial gadolinium-enhanced gradient-echo MR images. Radiology 1994;192(2):401–6.

37. Krinsky GA, Lee VS, Nguyen MT, et al. Siderotic nodules at MR imaging: regenerative or dysplastic? J Comput Assist Tomogr 2000;24(5):773–6.

38. Mortelé KJ, Ros PR. Cystic focal liver lesions in the adult: differential CT and MR imaging features. Radiographics 2001;21(4):895–910.

Evaluation of Hepatocellular Carcinoma Treatment Response After Locoregional Therapy

Rony Kampalath, MD[a], Karen Tran-Harding, MD[a],
Richard K.G. Do, MD, PhD[b,c],*, Mishal Mendiratta-Lala, MD[d],
Vahid Yaghmai, MD, MS[e]

KEYWORDS

- LI-RADS • HCC • Locoregional therapy • Response assessment • mRECIST

KEY POINTS

- The purpose of imaging after locoregional therapy is primarily to assess treatment response of targeted lesions but also to assess untreated liver tumors, identify complications of therapy, detect extrahepatic progression, and to direct patient prognosis and management.
- Liver Imaging Reporting and Data System (LI-RADS) treatment response algorithm is distinct from modified response evaluation criteria in solid tumors by providing response assessment at the individual treated lesion and by including washout appearance as an imaging finding consistent with viable tumor.
- After locoregional therapy, if a lesion is evaluable on imaging, the radiologist can choose from 1 of the 3 LI-RADS response categories: LR-TR Viable, LR-TR Equivocal, and LR-TR Nonviable.

INTRODUCTION

Hepatocellular carcinoma (HCC) is the fifth most common cancer in the world and the third highest cause of cancer-related mortality. More than 80% of patients diagnosed with HCC have preexisting cirrhosis. Although most of the cases are diagnosed in developing countries, the incidence of HCC has been rapidly increasing in the United States over the last few decades.[1]

Historically, surgical resection or liver transplantation offered the only chance for cure in patients with HCC. Over the last 30 years, therapies such as percutaneous ablation, transarterial chemoembolization, and intraarterial and external beam radiotherapy have evolved rapidly. These locoregional therapies now offer selected patients a nonsurgical treatment option for downstaging, bridging to transplant, or even cure.[2,3]

Increased adoption of locoregional therapy for HCC has prompted the need for better ways to assess treatment response. Well-established response evaluation criteria, such as the World Health Organization (WHO) and Response Evaluation Criteria in Solid tumors (RECIST), were designed primarily for the evaluation of patients in clinical trials on cytotoxic chemotherapy.[4,5] These criteria, which quantify tumor response by a change in lesion size, are less well suited to assess response in patients who have undergone locoregional therapy, especially for HCC, which can remain unchanged in size despite loss of

[a] Department of Radiological Sciences, University of California Irvine, 101 The City Drive South, Orange, CA 92868, USA; [b] Radiology, Memorial Sloan Kettering Cancer Center, New York, NY, USA; [c] Radiology, Weill Medical College of Cornell University, New York, NY, USA; [d] Radiology, University of Michigan School of Medicine, 1500 East Medical Center Drive, UH B2A209R, Ann Arbor, MI 48109-5030, USA; [e] University of California, Irvine, 101 The City Drive South, Orange, CA 92868, USA
* Corresponding author. Memorial Sloan Kettering Cancer Center, 1275 York Avenue, H-710, New York, NY 10065.
E-mail address: dok@mskcc.org

Magn Reson Imaging Clin N Am 29 (2021) 389–402
https://doi.org/10.1016/j.mric.2021.05.013
1064-9689/21/© 2021 Elsevier Inc. All rights reserved.

enhancement, and this has led to the development of new response criteria, including modified Response Evaluation Criteria in Solid tumors (mRECIST), European Association for the Study of the liver (EASL), and the Liver Imaging Reporting and Data System (LI-RADS) treatment response algorithm (TRA).

This chapter reviews different locoregional treatment strategies for HCC and discuss the treatment response criteria that have evolved to address the unique appearance of locally treated disease.

THERAPY FOR HEPATOCELLULAR CARCINOMA
Classification of Therapy Based on Intent

The choice of treatment of HCC depends on a complex interplay of factors including transplant candidacy, tumor size and location, multiplicity, liver function, performance status, and stage of disease.[6,7] Therefore, determining the most effective treatment plan can be challenging and requires expertise from several different specialties in a multidisciplinary tumor board setting, which includes hepatologists, hepatobiliary surgeons, transplant surgeons, radiation oncologists, medical oncologists, and diagnostic and interventional radiologists.[8]

Curative

Curative treatment options for hepatocellular carcinoma include liver transplantation, surgical resection, and thermal ablation.[9]

The Milan criteria determines the eligibility criteria for transplantation as a single lesion smaller than 5 cm or 2 to 3 lesions, none larger than 3 cm, without macrovascular invasion.[10] Liver transplantation removes hepatic tumor burden and gives the most reasonable expectation for curative treatment.[11] Deceased donor liver transplant is used for those with disease within Milan criteria or are downstaged to meet Milan criteria. Living donor liver transplantation (LDLT) is offered to patients beyond Milan criteria so that they may undergo transplantation or to patients within Milan criteria to shorten their wait time on the transplant list. Although LDLT does enable a potentially lifesaving procedure, there is a higher rate of recurrence with LDLT than after deceased donation, after adjusting for HCC characteristics.[12]

Long-term survival rates after a liver resection (LR) are only slightly inferior to the survival rates after liver transplantation.[13] Intrahepatic tumor recurrence occurs in half of the cases at 3 years after LR or ablation.[13] Anatomic LR involves en-bloc removal of a liver segment fed by a branch of the hepatic artery and portal vein. Nonanatomic or wedge resections spare a larger margin of liver parenchyma, preserving a larger liver remnant, optimal for patients with impaired liver function, but may leave behind potential intrahepatic satellite micrometastases.[14]

Laparoscopic resection of tumor has demonstrated similar recurrence rates and overall survival (OS) as conventional HCC resection, with quicker postoperative recovery, reduced blood loss, and fewer postoperative complications.[15]

Downstaging/Debulking

Tumor downstaging uses systemic or locoregional therapies to meet selection criteria for liver transplantation by decreasing the size/burden of HCC lesions. Studies have shown that tumor size reduction and downstaging to Milan criteria before transplantation results in improved outcomes.[16] Downstaging is considered successful if a tumor remains stable after a follow-up period of at least 3 months.[17] It has been hypothesized that tumors with a favorable biology will have a superior recurrence-free survival after transplantation due to superior response to locoregional therapies.[18]

Bridging

Locoregional therapies may also be used to achieve local tumor control and reduce wait-list drop out and recurrence after liver transplantation.[18] According to the Scientific Registry of Transplant Recipients from the United States, patients who received pretransplant treatments (mostly transcatheter arterial chemoembolization [TACE] and radiofrequency ablation [RFA]) had greater adjusted 3-year posttransplant survival than those who did not receive pretransplant treatment.[19] In the current literature, the study populations received differing treatment modalities before transplantation, depending on institutional preference,[19] and superiority of a single technique as a bridge to transplantation has not yet been shown.

Palliative

Approximately 70% of patients are not surgical candidates.[20] For these patients, locoregional therapy may reduce the rate of tumor progression or prolong survival.[21] They may be applied more than once for patients with untreated tumor.

Locoregional Therapies for Hepatocellular Carcinoma

Locoregional therapy (LRT) can be used alone or in combination with other therapies to improve overall and disease-free survival in patients who are unable to undergo resection.[22]

Ablative Therapy

The first ablative therapy used for HCC was percutaneous ethanol injection (PEI), where under image guidance, ethanol is injected directly into the tumor to achieve tumor death by ischemia and coagulative necrosis.[23] PEI has been shown to have good efficacy and low complication rates, but limitations include prolonged treatment times and the need for repeat treatment.[24] In 1999, the first thermal ablation was performed, demonstrating a 5-year survival rate similar to surgical resection for tumors less than 3 cm in size with good efficacy and a high safety profile.[25]

Thermal ablation modalities include both radiofrequency and microwave ablation. Thermal ablation can be performed under image guidance or laproscopically and involves percutaneous or direct insertion of an electrode into the tumor, which then creates high temperatures by using different frequencies of energy with rapidly oscillating field strength, resulting in coagulation necrosis of tumor.[26] In contrast, cryoablation, although also performed via percutaneous placement of probes, uses a cold energy source to cause ischemic cell death.

Multiple randomized controlled trials have demonstrated that RFA is superior to PEI in terms of OS, complete response, and local recurrence.[27] The outcomes of RFA seem to be similar to those of microwave ablation and cryoablation, particularly in small tumors. In larger tumors, microwave ablation and cryoablation may have higher rates of complete tumor ablation and lower rates of local tumor recurrence,[28] but more studies are needed to confirm these findings.

Percutaneous ablation can be curative in patients with very early stage HCC (BCLC stage 0). In these patients, ablation seems to be as effective as surgical resection and is more cost-effective.[29] As discussed earlier, ablation may also be used to prevent progression in patients with more advanced disease awaiting transplant (bridging therapy).

Transarterial-Based Therapy

Arterial-based therapy provides intraarterial delivery of either bland (transarterial embolization or TAE) or chemotherapy coated (transarterial chemoembolization or TACE/drug-eluting bead transarterial chemoembolization or DEB-TACE) embolic material into the HCC arterial blood supply, eliminating arterial inflow to the tumor and causing cell death.[30] Bland TAE uses gelatin sponge and microparticles to occlude the arterial supply.[31] Conventional TACE uses embolic particles (iodized oil) coated with chemotherapeutic agent, whereas DEB-TACE uses hydrogel beads coated with chemotherapeutic agent to increase the efficacy of treatment with more prolonged delivery.[32,33]

During a TACE procedure, tumor cell death occurs with a dual effect of chemotoxic injury and ischemic injury.[34] Although the decision for TACE is often made in a multidisciplinary setting, TACE is typically offered to patients with intermediate stage HCC without metastatic disease or vascular invasion (BCLC stage B). TACE may also be used as bridging therapy or to downstage patients to meet transplant criteria.[29,32]

The presence of portal vein thrombus is a relative contraindication to arterial-based therapy as both the arterial and portal venous flow to the liver would be compromised.[35]

Radiation-Based Therapy

Transarterial radioembolization (TARE) and stereotactic body radiotherapy (SBRT) are the most common radiation-based treatment modalities used today.[36] Patient assessment, including disease burden, biochemical parameters including bilirubin and albumin levels, and performance status determine which form of therapy is preferred. TARE is ideal if the disease is limited to less than half of the liver.[37] TARE consists of injection of yttrium-90 (Y-90) microspheres with a small diameter (20–60 microns) into the hepatic arteries to deliver targeted radiation and a small microembolic effect.[38]

Unlike TAE/TACE, portal vein thrombus is not a contraindication for TARE, because this form of intraarterial therapy does not result in complete arterial embolization.[37,38]

SBRT involves the use of multiple tightly focused high-energy beams of radiation to deliver higher doses of radiation to the tumor, with relative sparing of adjacent parenchyma, thus significantly reducing the risk for radiation-induced liver injury when compared with older methods of external beam radiation therapy.

Systemic Therapy

Underlying liver disease has traditionally severely limited the applicability of most chemotherapy regimens.[18] Because HCC is a very chemotherapy-resistant tumor, standard systemic care was not a treatment choice for patients with advanced HCC over an extended period of time.[39] However, in 2006, the first multikinase inhibitor sorafenib (Nexavar) demonstrated survival benefit in those with advanced HCC.[40] In the last few years, multiple new systemic agents have been shown to improve outcomes.[41] For example, Lenvatinib is a new first-line agent for HCC; second-line agents include regorafenib, cabozantinib, ramucirumab, and nivolumab.

Multimodal Approaches

After LRT or hepatic resection, salvage orthotopic liver transplant has been offered for patients with recurrent hepatocellular carcinoma or compromised liver function. Most of the patients with recurrent disease present within criteria for transplantation, so that salvage orthotopic liver transplantation may lower the risk of wait-list drop out and improve management of liver allografts.[42,43]

LRT can also aid surgical resection in patients with deteriorating liver function. Not only does therapy involving Y-90 reduce tumor size, it also has the advantage of leading to a compensatory hypertrophy of the contralateral liver lobe.[44]

This 2-stage approach of Y-90–induced local control and hepatic volume changes in patients with functionally irresectable HCC may result in the patient reaching secondary resectability criteria, facilitating surgical resection of previously unresectable tumors.[45]

A combination of RFA and TACE has been proposed for tumors with a maximum diameter of 3 to 5 cm. This treatment results in extension of area of ablation and reducing local tumor progression by limiting arterial hepatic blood flow and perfusion-mediated tissue cooling, reducing the number of required future interventions.[46]

Assessment of Hepatocellular Carcinoma After Treatment

After local therapy for HCC, follow-up imaging should be performed with multiphase computed tomography (CT) or MR imaging, including precontrast, arterial phase, portal venous phase, and delayed phase images. The choice of modality depends on institutional preference and other patient- and treatment-related factors. The purpose of follow-up imaging is to identify complications of therapy, assess treatment response (including whether viable tumor is present), identify and stage other untreated liver tumors, detect extrahepatic progression, and to direct patient prognosis and management.

The follow-up schedule may vary depending on institutional protocol and depends on what treatment was used, what future treatments are planned, and the results of multidisciplinary discussion. A typical schedule may call for imaging at 1 month, followed by repeat imaging at 3-month intervals.[47,48]

Expected Posttreatment Appearance

As discussed earlier, LRT for HCC can be broadly categorized into ablative therapies, transarterial-based nonradiation therapies, or radiation-based therapy. Radiation-based therapies can be subdivided into TARE and SBRT. The imaging appearance of HCC after LRT varies with the general treatment category, with treated tumor appearing similar for ablative therapies and catheter-based therapies without radiation (TACE). Radiation-based therapies create more complex posttreatment appearances for HCC that vary over time.[48–53]

Ablative Therapy

After ablation therapy, foci of gas may be seen in the treated area and may persist for days or weeks. These are thought to represent nitrogen gas from contracting tumor and do not necessarily imply infection.[47,54,55] Segmental or lobar bile duct dilatation often develops after cryoablation.[47]

A nonenhancing ablation zone should be seen at the site of treatment. Because adequate ablation requires a treatment margin of 5 to 10 mm around the tumor, the ablation zone should be larger than the original lesion (**Fig. 1**). The ablation zone typically begins to shrink at about 6 months after therapy, then stabilizes. A small ablation zone may persist indefinitely.[47]

Tumor ablation results in coagulation necrosis in the treated area, which may seem hyperintense on T1-weighted MR images and hyperdense on precontrast CT.[47,49,55,56] This hyperintensity or high density should not be confused for residual viable tumor, and comparison with precontrast images and MR imaging subtraction images is critical to prevent misinterpretation. In contrast, tumors treated with cryoablation often demonstrate decreased T1 signal in the ablation zone after therapy.[47]

A thin, uniform rim of enhancement along the periphery of the ablation zone is expected, and geographic arterial phase hyperenhancement (APHE) may also be seen in the adjacent liver parenchyma. These transient hepatic intensity/attenuation differences (THIDS/THADS) are thought to be related to arterioportal shunts created during the procedure and usually resolve over time. The lack of mass effect, washout, or capsule can help distinguish between THIDS/THADS and residual viable tumor.[48,49,57]

On diffusion-weighted images (DWI), the ablation zone is centrally hypointense, with hyperintensity around the periphery of the lesion. This hyperintense rim may be due to hyperemia and edema and may be difficult to distinguish from viable tumor using DWI alone.[58]

Transarterial-Based Therapies

After catheter-based therapies (without radiation), imaging findings are similar to those following ablation therapy. When successful, a nonenhancing treatment zone is seen, with a thin peripheral rim of enhancement that may persist for months

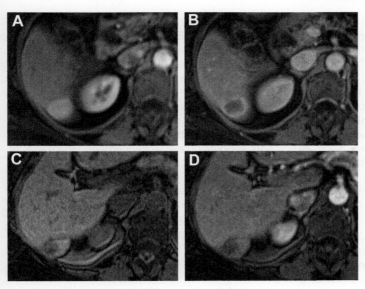

Fig. 1. An 85-year-old woman with biopsy-proven HCC. Pretreatment MR imaging shows a 2.7 cm segment 6 lesion with APHE (*A*), venous phase washout and an enhancing capsule (*B*), LI-RADS 5. MR imaging 1 month post-RFA. T1 precontrast shows central high signal, secondary to coagulation necrosis (*C*). Arterial phase shows no evidence of enhancement (confirmed by subtraction imaging) (*D*). The ablation zone is larger than the original HCC, as expected. This is consistent with successfully treated disease, LR-TR Nonviable.

or years (**Fig. 2**).[48,51,54] Because of postprocedural edema and blood products, the treatment zone may be slightly larger than the original tumor but should shrink over time. Because of the presence of necrosis and blood products, signal is variable on unenhanced T1-weighted (T1W) and T2W images.[51,58] Geographic enhancement may be seen in the surrounding liver parenchyma, likely related to perfusional changes from inflammation and arterial embolization.

A special consideration after catheter-based therapies is the use of iodinated oil that is hyperdense on precontrast CT. On short-term follow-up, increased uptake of iodinated oil is associated with higher rates of technical success.[47,49,51] However, hyperdense oil may obscure arterial phase enhancement on CT, thereby limiting the evaluation for residual viable tumor. In these situations, MR imaging is an attractive alternative for follow-up, as iodinated oil is not visible on MR images, and thus would not obscure evaluation for subtle areas of APHE within and along the treatment margin.[47,51]

Suspicious imaging findings suggesting viable tumor are similar after ablation or catheter-based therapies without radiation. Thick peripheral

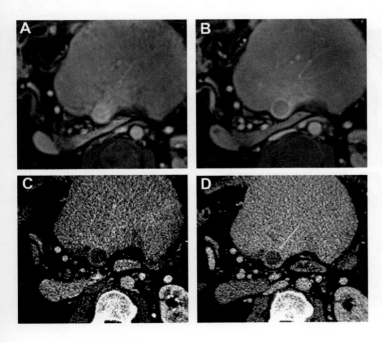

Fig. 2. A 53-year-old woman with alcoholic cirrhosis. Dynamic contrast-enhanced MR imaging shows a 2.3 cm lesion in segment 2 of the liver with arterial enhancement (*A, B*), washout and capsule (*red arrows*) (*C, D*), LI-RADS 5. After embolization, only a thin rim of enhancement (*yellow arrow*) is present, an expected posttreatment finding, which is consistent with LR-TR Nonviable.

irregular or nodular areas of arterial phase enhancement, with or without washout appearance, implies residual tumor (**Fig. 3**).[48] Other suspicious findings include washout alone or enhancement characteristics similar to those of the pretreatment tumor. Discontinuity in the smooth peripheral rim of enhancement after ablation also suggests recurrent disease.[47,48,54] Although the use of ancillary features, such as T2W hyperintense signal, restricted diffusion, or hepatobiliary phase hypointensity, is not part of the TRA, they may help in posttreatment assessment for equivocal cases of viability or nonviability.

Radiation-Based Therapies

The expected imaging findings after radiation-based therapies differ from those seen after other LRT.[48,51] The tumor responds to radiation in a slow and prolonged manner, as radiation causes DNA and stromal damage and activates proinflammatory pathways. The therapeutic effects of TARE depend more on the effects of radiation, with the embolic effect playing a lesser role.[47,51,54] Therapeutic effect may thus be delayed with a slow evolution of changes both at a cellular and radiographic level. For this reason, interpretation of follow-up scans within 6 months of treatment is challenging and should be performed with caution (**Fig. 4**).[47,51]

Persistent tumoral APHE may be seen for 3 to 6 months after TARE (and even longer in some cases) and may not represent residual viable tumor, but rather senescent cancer cells undergoing radiation-related changes. Ill-defined regions of geographic peritumoral arterial phase enhancement may be seen and may be difficult to distinguish from infiltrative tumor. Benign peritumoral enhancement usually resolves within 5 months.[47,48]

Effects on tumor size after TARE may also be relatively slow. In fact, the treated zone may increase in size immediately after treatment. Shrinkage is often delayed, with decreases in size expected over the course of several months.[47,48] Posttreatment fibrosis may develop, with venous phase enhancement, shrinkage of the treated lobe, capsular retraction, and hypertrophy of the contralateral lobe.[47,48]

Successfully treated tumors will eventually lose their arterial phase enhancement. Rim enhancement may be present for several months and most likely represent inflammatory changes related to treatment (**Fig. 5**).[47,50,55] New or increasing nodular or masslike arterial enhancement in or around the treated tumor should raise suspicion for residual or recurrent tumor. Hyperintensity on DWIs may be helpful to detect recurrence in cases where the enhancement pattern is equivocal.[49–51,55]

As with TARE, posttreatment changes after SBRT evolve over a prolonged period. Arterial phase tumoral enhancement with or without washout may persist or even increase, particularly in the first few months.[47,48,52,53] Enhancement should gradually decrease over time but may not completely disappear.[43,48,49] Size can be stable or decrease over time; however, increase in size suggests tumor progression.[53]

The response of the surrounding liver to radiation also evolves over months. Shortly after treatment, peritumoral edema is often seen. Microvascular changes may result in altered liver enhancement and foci of hemorrhage.[47] In the early

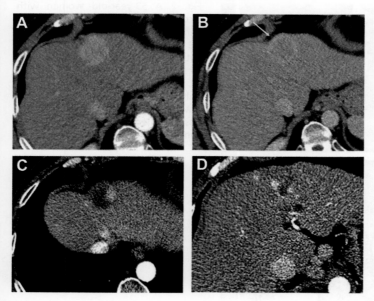

Fig. 3. A 69-year-old patient with cirrhosis. CT shows a 4.0 cm segment 2 mass with APHE (*A*), washout and capsule (*yellow arrow*) (*B*), LIRADS 5. (*C, D*) CT 1 month post-TACE demonstrates areas of peripheral nodular APHE (*red arrows*), consistent with residual disease, LR-TR Viable.

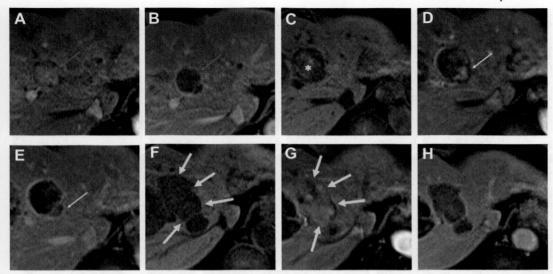

Fig. 4. A 77-year-old man with hepatitis B cirrhosis, status post-TACE and MWA for multiple prior HCCs, presenting for follow-up imaging. There is a new lesion within segment 8 with APHE (*red arrow, A*), washout and capsule (*red arrow, B*), LIRADS 5. MR imaging 1 month post-TARE. T1 precontrast imaging demonstrates central hyperintense signal (*asterisk*) (*C*). Arterial phase imaging shows persistent areas of nodular APHE along the medial aspect of the treated lesion (*yellow arrow*) (*D*), which demonstrates washout on the PV phase (*E*). These can be expected post-TARE imaging findings that can last for up to 6 months or longer, LR-TR Equivocal. MR imaging 6 months after TARE. T1 precontrast images show an increasing hypointense lesion with no central hyperintensity as was seen on the 1-month post-TARE MR imaging (*yellow arrow, F*). Arterial phase MR imaging shows persistent and increasing size of APHE (*yellow arrow, G*), with washout appearance (*H*). Overall, the lesion has significantly increased in size with new and increasing enhancement, LR-TR Viable.

posttreatment period, these changes manifest as geographic areas of arterial phase enhancement around the tumor that evolve to areas of progressive delayed enhancement as fibrosis develops **(Fig. 6)**.[47,48] Other fibrosis-related findings may include liver capsular retraction and peripheral intrahepatic biliary ductal dilatation.[44]

Of note, treatment-related hepatocyte damage may impair the uptake of hepatobiliary agents, causing decreased signal intensity on hepatobiliary phase images; this may be erroneously interpreted as viable tumor.[47]

Findings suspicious for recurrent disease includes increased intensity of arterial phase enhancement within the tumor, especially if this occurs after a period of favorable response. Increased size of a treated tumor also suggests recurrent disease.[52,53] Because of the confounding treatment-related changes, the interpreting radiologist should assess treatment response by accounting for the evolution of imaging findings over time rather than interpret findings in isolation at any one particular time point.

Complications of Therapy

Each category of LRT is associated with specific complications that should be recognized by the radiologist. Ablation procedures can cause damage to adjacent structures, including the pleura, bile ducts, vessels, or bowel. Hematomas or bilomas can develop within or around the treatment zone. Abscesses can form in the ablation zone, although gas in the treated region may be an expected finding for weeks after ablation.[47,48,59] Vascular complications include arterial or venous thrombosis or arteriovenous shunts along the probe tract.[47,48] Fracture of the hepatic capsule is one of the most serious complications of cryoablation and can cause severe hemorrhage.[47,60]

Catheter-based therapies are typically well tolerated, and the most common complication is postembolization syndrome, characterized by nausea, fatigue, fever, and abdominal pain in the days after the procedure.[48,61] Nontarget embolization may occur and may result in pancreatitis, pulmonary emboli, or ischemic cholecystitis.[47,61] Patients with arteriovenous shunts are at increased risk for nontarget embolization, and these vascular abnormalities may need embolization before treatment; this is particularly a concern with TARE, where the consequences of nontarget embolization to the lungs or gastrointestinal tract are especially serious.[47] Hepatic angiography and intraarterial Tc99m-MAA scintigraphy are routinely performed before therapy in order to identify shunts.

Other unusual complications of catheter-based therapies include hepatic abscess or infarction.[61] Radiation-induced biliary complications such as cholecystitis, bilomas, biliary strictures, or

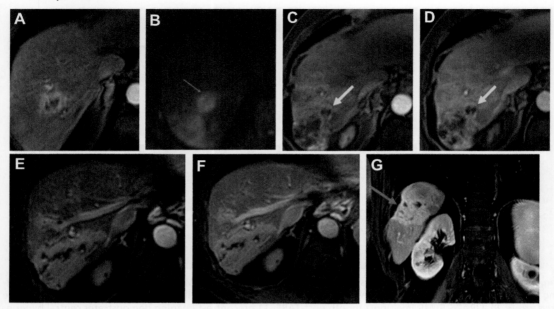

Fig. 5. A 77-year-old man with biopsy-proved HCC, 1 year post-TACE. Follow-up MR imaging demonstrates a treated lesion in the right hepatic lobe with thick, irregular, and nodular peripheral enhancement (*A*) demonstrating restricted diffusion on DWI (*red arrow*) (*B*). Findings are compatible with disease recurrence, LR-TR viable. MR imaging 4 months post-TARE. There is faint peripheral rim APHE around the treated lesion (*yellow arrows*) seen on arterial phase (*C*) and persisting on delayed phase (*D*), with a thin linear area of central enhancement. These findings are compatible with expected post-TARE imaging findings and can persist for up to 1 year. Thus, these findings are classified as LR-TR Equivocal. Note, there is geographic and heterogeneous APHE surrounding the treated lesion, upstream from the tumor, with areas of parenchymal hypoenhancement, expected postradiation changes within the parenchyma. Follow-up MR imaging 8 months after TARE. The treated lesion is no longer visible. Persistent geographic parenchymal enhancement seen on arterial (*E*) and PV (*F*) phase imaging with liver capsular retraction (*red arrow*) (*G*) and intrahepatic biliary ductal dilatation in the treatment zone suggest segmental fibrosis, which are expected postradiation findings. LR-TR Nonviable.

abscesses may occur rarely after TARE. These complications often respond to conservative therapy, although percutaneous drainage or cholecystectomy may be required in more severe cases.[50]

Most complications of external beam radiation are related to radiation-related injury to the surrounding liver. Radiation-induced liver disease (RILD) can be severe and is an important limitation to the total therapeutic dose that can be delivered. Hepatic dysfunction related to RILD usually responds to supportive therapy, but some patients may develop progressive liver failure.[50,62] These risks have been significantly mitigated by the advent of SBRT, in which the radiation dose is focused to the target with minimal dose to the adjacent parenchyma with careful patient selection, procedural planning, and intratreatment monitoring.[63,64] After treatment, with SBRT, normal liver parenchyma around the tumor may undergo scarring, with capsular retraction and biliary dilatation apparent on follow-up imaging.[47]

Treatment Response Evaluation

Standardizing the assessment and reporting of response to cancer therapy is critical for appropriate patient management and for the conduct of well-designed clinical trials. In 1979, the WHO took important steps toward this goal, publishing the WHO criteria for the evaluation of cancer treatment response.[5] The RECIST, first introduced in 2000, represented an evolution of the WHO criteria and has since been extensively validated and adopted worldwide.[4]

The WHO and RECIST guidelines rely on changes in tumor size to assess treatment response. Unfortunately, they are poorly suited to assess HCC locoregional response because, as discussed earlier, successfully treated lesions may be unchanged in size or even become larger after therapy. Subsequently, EASL and mRECIST proposed measuring only the enhancing portion of the residual liver lesion, a better indicator of the degree of remaining viable tumor after LRT.[65–67]

The LI-RADS TRA was introduced in 2017 by the American College of Radiology, as part of the LI-RADS. LI-RADS TRA was developed to guide the interpretation and reporting of imaging findings of HCC after locoregional therapy. Earlier versions of LI-RADS before 2017 included an "LI-RADS Treated"

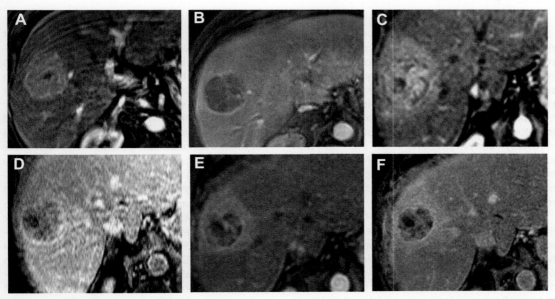

Fig. 6. A 62-year-old man with cirrhosis, presenting with a 4.7 cm right lobe lesion demonstrating APHE (*A*), washout and capsule (*B*), LIRADS 5 HCC. Three months post-SBRT, the lesion demonstrates persistent APHE similar to pretreatment imaging (*C*), washout and capsule (*D*), and no change in size. There is surrounding geographic parenchymal enhancement in the radiation treatment zone, which becomes isoenhancing on the delayed phase of imaging. These findings are "expected" post-SBRT findings early posttreatment. The importance is to evaluate the evolution of changes over time. LR-TR Equivocal. MR imaging 6 months post-SBRT shows significantly decreasing central APHE (*E*), with no change on the delayed phase (*F*). The lesion has also decreased in size, now measuring 3.9 cm. Surrounding geographic parenchymal APHE now persists on the delayed phase, compatible with radiation fibrosis, expected. Although the imaging findings are expected post-SBRT, given that it is still less than 1 year, this would be considered LR-TR Equivocal.

category that indicated that treatment had been performed but did not provide guidance to assess response.[68,69]

LI-RADS TRA differs from other criteria in a few important ways. The RECIST and mRECIST systems were designed to evaluate total tumor burden in patients on clinical trials. Although the LI-RADS TR algorithm integrates concepts from mRECIST, it was specifically designed to evaluate individual treated lesions, to provide guidance for routine clinical management.[68,69] The LI-RADS TRA also expanded on mRECIST by providing categories for nonevaluable, equivocal, or nonviable disease. The LI-RADS TR algorithm further adds imaging features of washout and enhancement similar to pretreatment appearance as findings that support the presence of residual viable disease.[47] All of these features are designed to help clinical management on a lesion-by-lesion basis, because HCC treatment is so heterogeneous even within the same patient.

The LI-RADS TRA can be applied to pathologically proved or presumed liver malignancy treated by local ablation, transcatheter ablation, or external radiation therapy. It does not apply to patients undergoing systemic therapy, and the American College of Radiology (ACR) urges caution when using the algorithm in patients treated with a combination of systemic and locoregional therapy.[47]

The LI-RADS TR algorithm, as the mRECIST system, uses APHE as the main indicator of viable tumor. LI-RADS TR also includes additional imaging criteria to identify viable tumor.[22] For example, washout appearance alone can be seen in viable disease, particularly in tumors that do not have APHE before treatment. Also, some untreated tumors show atypical enhancement patterns, such as peripheral or targetoid enhancement. Similar enhancement to pretreatment imaging after treatment should be interpreted as viable disease.[47]

When applying the algorithm, the radiologist must decide whether treatment response is evaluable. If the treated observation cannot be evaluated because of image artifacts, poor timing of contrast injection, or lack of multiphase imaging, it is assigned the LR-TR Nonevaluable category.[22,47,69]

For each treated observation that can be assessed, the LI-RADS TR algorithm classifies treatment response into 1 of 3 categories. LR-TR viable treated observations have tissue in or around the treatment cavity that is nodular, mass-like, or thick and irregular. This tissue may have APHE, washout appearance, or enhancement similar to the pretreatment appearance. The size of the viable tumor should be measured in the longest dimension of the enhancing area, without including the nonenhancing area.[69]

LR-TR nonviable observations have no enhancement or an enhancement pattern expected for the treatment in question; this is important in HCC treated with radiation-based therapy, because the tumors can demonstrate persistent APHE for months or longer after treatment, not necessarily indicating viable tumor. In these cases, misinterpretation of APHE as viable tumor could lead to unnecessary early retreatment in patients with underlying chronic liver disease. Note that the lack of enhancement does not imply pathologic necrosis, and the use of the term "nonviable" is preferred over "necrotic."[47]

LR-TR equivocal observations have imaging characteristics that may represent treatment response or viable tumor. This category is used if there is lesional enhancement, which is atypical for the treatment used, but does not meet the criteria for viable disease,[47,69] and this can often be seen after nonradiation-based intraarterial therapy, when the embolic effects may result in perfusional aberrations in the parenchyma adjacent to the tumor, thus confounding viable tumor from treatment related changes. In addition, as discussed earlier, the distinction between treatment-related enhancement and viable disease can be especially difficult soon after radiation-based therapy. In the first few months after radiation, the most commonly assigned LR-TR category is LR-TR equivocal.[69] If the radiologist is unsure of what category to assign, the ACR recommends assignment of the category reflecting less certainty, specifically LR-TR equivocal.[47]

Validation

When compared with histopathological findings, early studies have shown that the LI-RADS TR algorithm has good predictive value in determining the presence of incomplete or complete necrosis in lesions treated with bland embolization or ablation.[70,71] The ability to detect residual tumor varies significantly with tumor size, with improved sensitivity for larger lesions.[72] After RFA, Zhang and colleagues showed that patients with LR-TR viable lesions had lower OS than those with LR-TR nonviable or LR-TR equivocal lesions.[73] After RFA, Zhang and colleagues showed no significant difference in OS between patients with LR-TR equivocal or nonviable disease.[74]

Most lesions rated LR-TR equivocal after ablation are incompletely necrotic on histopathological examination.[70,71] Cools and colleagues found that including lesions rated LR-TR equivocal into the LR-TR viable category improved the sensitivity for the presence of residual tumor on pathologic examination.[72] These findings are not surprising, considering older studies that show that

microscopic foci of viable tumor may be present in treated lesions that do not have enhancement.[57,74,75] It is possible that ablation disrupts blood flow to the treatment cavity, resulting in decreased enhancement and a decreased ability to detect small volume residual viable disease.[72]

Different studies have shown moderate or good interreader reliability when assigning LIRADS treatment response categories.[70,72,73] Interreader reliability is better for LR-TR viable and nonviable categories than it is for the LR-TR equivocal category.[76] Although radiologists may have a good grasp of the imaging findings of frankly viable disease, it is possible that the expected findings after treatment are less familiar, leading to misapplication of the LR-TR algorithm.[73] As treatment models for HCC evolve, with increased adoption of newer modalities, it is important that radiologists remain abreast of the different posttreatment appearances of HCC.

Future Directions

The LI-RADS TRA is acknowledged to be a dynamic document, expected to be revised and expanded as knowledge accrues. Further research is needed to determine whether certain treatments need their own specific TRAs.[22] As discussed, HCC has a unique appearance after radiation-based locoregional treatment, and a new algorithm may be better suited to evaluate response after these therapies. Posttreatment management implications must also be taken into account in this cohort of radiation-treated patients.

Also, further study is required concerning the assessment of HCC treatment response in patients undergoing systemic therapy with or without concurrent LRT. The use of systemic therapy in patients with advanced HCC is rapidly evolving, as new treatments have been approved in recent years. The addition of systemic therapy to LRT, expected to become more common with time, complicates the assessment of treatment response. The ACR currently urges caution in the application of the LR-TRA in patients treated with both systemic and locoregional therapy.

The optimal follow-up schedule to address treatment response is another area of uncertainty. Cools and colleagues noted in their study that having more surveillance MR imagings was significantly associated with higher odds of correct classification by LR-TR.[72] The ACR suggests a follow-up CT or MR imaging at 3-month intervals. The actual follow-up schedule is often determined by institutional preference, the type of treatment used, and future treatment plans. Follow-up is often limited by imaging reimbursement guidelines by health insurance providers.[22]

All the major systems for the assessment of HCC locoregional treatment response rely on the presence of contrast enhancement and washout. However, there is growing evidence that ancillary features on MR imaging improve the sensitivity for the detection of viable tumor on imaging after treatment response. Specifically hepatobiliary phase hypointensity, diffusion restriction, and intermediate hyperintensity on T2W images seem to be particularly useful in the assessment of treatment response.[77–79] As MR imaging becomes more widespread, more study is needed to determine whether these ancillary features should be incorporated into future response assessment algorithms.

Although recently introduced in 2017, LI-RADS TRA is increasingly adopted in routine clinical practice, and the early validation results are promising. Just as the LI-RADS CT/MR imaging diagnostic algorithm has improved over time with a growing body of research in this field, the TRA will probably evolve for the better in the near future. Finally, the impact of LI-RADS TRA should be addressed beyond the prediction of residual viable tumor, to the more challenging aspect of patient benefit in the form of OS in the clinical trial setting.

CLINICS CARE POINTS

- A thin and uniform peripheral rim of enhancement is often seen along the ablation zone after locoablative therapy, a finding that will resolve over time. Equivocal findings after ablative therapy often indicate incomplete necrosis when compared with histopathologic examination.

- Thick peripheral irregular or nodular areas of arterial phase hyperenhancement, with or without washout appearance, indicates viable tumor after transarterial-based locoregional therapy.

- Persistent arterial phase hyperenhancement of targeted tumors may be seen for several months after transarterial radioembolization or external beam radiation therapy due to the prolonged response to radiation. In the early posttreatment period, LR-TR Equivocal is often used, as response to radiation treatment continues to evolve.

- Complications to locoregional therapy seen on posttreatment imaging include hepatic abscesses, bile duct injury, and infarcts.

ACKNOWLEDGMENTS

Dr R.K.G. Do: NIH/NCI Cancer Center Support Grant P30 CA008748.

DISCLOSURE

The authors have nothing to disclose.

REFERENCES

1. Marrero JA, Kulik LM, Sirlin CB, et al. Diagnosis, staging, and management of hepatocellular carcinoma: 2018 practice guidance by the American Association for the Study of Liver Diseases. Hepatology 2018;68(2):723–50. https://doi.org/10.1002/hep.29913.

2. Lope CR, Tremosini S, Forner A, et al. Management of HCC. J Hepatol 2012;56. https://doi.org/10.1016/s0168-8278(12)60009-9.

3. Nishikawa H, Kimura T, Kita R, et al. Radiofrequency ablation for hepatocellular carcinoma. Int J Hyperthermia 2013;29(6):558–68. https://doi.org/10.3109/02656736.2013.821528.

4. Therasse P, Arbuck SG, Eisenhauer EA, et al. New guidelines to evaluate the response to treatment in solid tumors. J Natl Cancer Inst 2000;92(3):205–16.

5. Miller A, Hoogstraten B, Staquet M, et al. Reporting results of cancer treatment. Cancer 1981;47(1):207–14.

6. Mora RA, Ali R, Gabr A, et al. Pictorial essay: imaging findings following Y90 radiation segmentectomy for hepatocellular carcinoma. Abdom Radiol (NY) 2018;43(7):1723–38. https://doi.org/10.1007/s00261-017-1391-1. PMID: 29147766.

7. Galun D, Basaric D, Zuvela M, et al. Hepatocellular carcinoma: from clinical practice to evidence-based treatment protocols. World J Hepatol 2015;7(20):2274–91. https://doi.org/10.4254/wjh.v7.i20.2274. PMID: 26380652; PMCID: PMC4568488.

8. Gadsden MM, Kaplan DE. Multidisciplinary approach to HCC management: how can this be done? Dig Dis Sci 2019;64(4):968–75. https://doi.org/10.1007/s10620-019-05593-8.

9. Cho YK, Rhim H, Noh S. Radiofrequency ablation versus surgical resection as primary treatment of hepatocellular carcinoma meeting the Milan criteria: a systematic review. J Gastroenterol Hepatol 2011;26(9):1354–60.

10. Mazzaferro V, Regalia E, Doci R, et al. Liver transplantation for the treatment of small hepatocellular carcinomas in patients with cirrhosis. N Engl J Med 1996;334(11):693–9. https://doi.org/10.1056/NEJM199603143341104. PMID: 8594428.

11. Byam J, Renz J, Millis JM. Liver transplantation for hepatocellular carcinoma. Hepatobiliary Surg Nutr 2013;2(1):22–30.

12. Kulik LM, Fisher RA, Rodrigo DR, et al. Outcomes of living and deceased donor liver transplant recipients with hepatocellular carcinoma: results of the A2ALL cohort. Am J Transplant 2012;12(11): 2997–3007. https://doi.org/10.1111/j.1600-6143. 2012.04272.x. PMID: 22994906; PMCID: PMC3523685.

13. Llovet JM, Schwartz M, Mazzaferro V. Resection and liver transplantation for hepatocellular carcinoma. Semin Liver Dis 2005;25(2):181–200.

14. Chen J, Huang K, Wu J, et al. Survival after anatomic resection versus nonanatomic resection for hepatocellular carcinoma: a meta-analysis. Dig Dis Sci 2011;56(6):1626–33. https://doi.org/10.1007/ s10620-010-1482-0. PMID: 21082347.

15. Mirnezami R, Mirnezami AH, Chandrakumaran K, et al. Short- and long-term outcomes after laparoscopic and open hepatic resection: systematic review and meta-analysis. HPB (Oxford) 2011;13(5): 295–308. https://doi.org/10.1111/j.1477-2574.2011. 00295.x.

16. Yao FY, Kerlan RK Jr, Hirose R, et al. Excellent outcome following down-staging of hepatocellular carcinoma prior to liver transplantation: an intention-to-treat analysis. Hepatology 2008;48(3): 819–27. https://doi.org/10.1002/hep.22412. PMID: 18688876; PMCID: PMC4142499.

17. Pomfret EA, Washburn K, Wald C, et al. Report of a national conference on liver allocation in patients with hepatocellular carcinoma in the United States. Liver Transpl 2010;16(3):262–78. https://doi.org/10. 1002/lt.21999. PMID: 20209641.

18. Lurje I, Czigany Z, Bednarsch J, et al. Treatment strategies for hepatocellular carcinoma - a multidisciplinary approach. Int J Mol Sci 2019;20(6):1465. https://doi.org/10.3390/ijms20061465. PMID: 30909504; PMCID: PMC6470895.

19. Freeman RB Jr, Steffick DE, Guidinger MK, et al. Liver and intestine transplantation in the United States, 1997-2006. Am J Transplant 2008;8(4 Pt 2): 958–76. https://doi.org/10.1111/j.1600-6143.2008. 02174.x. PMID: 18336699.

20. Belghiti J, Kianmanesh R. Surgical treatment of hepatocellular carcinoma. HPB (Oxford) 2005;7(1): 42–9. https://doi.org/10.1080/13651820410024067.

21. Llovet JM, Burroughs A, Bruix J. Hepatocellular carcinoma. Lancet 2003;362(9399):1907–17. https:// doi.org/10.1016/s0140-6736(03)14964-1.

22. Kielar A, Fowler KJ, Lewis S, et al. Locoregional therapies for hepatocellular carcinoma and the new LI-RADS treatment response algorithm. Abdom Radiol (NY) 2018;43(1):218–30. https://doi.org/10.1007/ s00261-017-1281-6. PMID: 28780679; PMCID: PMC5771991.

23. Guan YS, Sun L, Zhou XP, et al. Hepatocellular carcinoma treated with interventional procedures: CT and MRI follow-up. World J Gastroenterol 2004; 10(24):3543–8. https://doi.org/10.3748/wjg.v10.i24. 3543.

24. Shiina S, Tagawa K, Niwa Y, et al. Percutaneous ethanol injection therapy for hepatocellular carcinoma: results in 146 patients. AJR Am J Roentgenol 1993;160(5):1023–8. https://doi.org/10.2214/ajr.160. 5.7682378. PMID: 7682378.

25. Ishikawa T. Strategy for improving survival and reducing recurrence of HCV-related hepatocellular carcinoma. World J Gastroenterol 2013;19(37): 6127–30.

26. Ahmed M, Solbiati L, Brace CL, et al, International Working Group on Image-guided Tumor Ablation, Interventional Oncology Sans Frontières Expert Panel, Technology Assessment Committee of the Society of Interventional Radiology, Standard of Practice Committee of the Cardiovascular and Interventional Radiological Society of Europe. Image-guided tumor ablation: standardization of terminology and reporting criteria–a 10-year update. Radiology 2014; 273(1):241–60. https://doi.org/10.1148/radiol. 14132958. PMID: 24927329; PMCID: PMC4263618.

27. Shiina S, Teratani T, Obi S, et al. A randomized controlled trial of radiofrequency ablation with ethanol injection for small hepatocellular carcinoma. Gastroenterology 2005;129(1):122–30. https://doi. org/10.1053/j.gastro.2005.04.009. PMID: 16012942.

28. Luo W, Zhang Y, He G, et al. Effects of radiofrequency ablation versus other ablating techniques on hepatocellular carcinomas: a systematic review and meta-analysis. World J Surg Oncol 2017;15(1). https://doi.org/10.1186/s12957-017-1196-2.

29. Bruix J, Reig M, Sherman M. Evidence-based diagnosis, staging, and treatment of patients with hepatocellular carcinoma. Gastroenterology 2016;150(4): 835–53. https://doi.org/10.1053/j.gastro.2015.12. 041.

30. Gaba RC, Lewandowski RJ, Hickey R, et al, Society of Interventional Radiology Technology Assessment Committee. Transcatheter therapy for hepatic malignancy: standardization of terminology and reporting criteria. J Vasc Interv Radiol 2016;27(4):457–73. https://doi.org/10.1016/j.jvir.2015.12.752. PMID: 26851158.

31. Tsochatzis EA, Fatourou E, O'Beirne J, et al. Transarterial chemoembolization and bland embolization for hepatocellular carcinoma. World J Gastroenterol 2014;20(12):3069–77. https://doi.org/10.3748/wjg. v20.i12.3069.

32. Lammer J, Malagari K, Vogl T, et al, PRECISION V Investigators. Prospective randomized study of doxorubicin-eluting-bead embolization in the treatment of hepatocellular carcinoma: results of the PRECISION V study. Cardiovasc Intervent Radiol 2010;33(1):41–52. https://doi.org/10.1007/s00270- 009-9711-7. PMID: 19908093; PMCID: PMC2816794.

33. Meza-Junco J, Montano-Loza AJ, Liu DM, et al. Locoregional radiological treatment for hepatocellular carcinoma; Which, when and how? Cancer Treat Rev 2012;38(1):54–62. https://doi.org/10.1016/j.ctrv.2011.05.002. PMID: 21726960.

34. Huppert P. Current concepts in transarterial chemoembolization of hepatocellular carcinoma. Abdom Imaging 2011;36(6):677–83.

35. Piscaglia F, Ogasawara S. Patient selection for transarterial chemoembolization in hepatocellular carcinoma: importance of benefit/risk assessment. Liver Cancer 2018;7(1):104–19.

36. Hickey RM, Lewandowski RJ, Salem R. Yttrium-90 radioembolization for hepatocellular carcinoma. Semin Nucl Med 2016;46(2):105–8.

37. Lau WY, Sangro B, Chen PJ, et al. Treatment for hepatocellular carcinoma with portal vein tumor thrombosis: the emerging role for radioembolization using yttrium-90. Oncology 2013;84(5):311–8. https://doi.org/10.1159/000348325. PMID: 23615394.

38. Iñarrairaegui M, Thurston KG, Bilbao JI, et al. Radioembolization with use of yttrium-90 resin microspheres in patients with hepatocellular carcinoma and portal vein thrombosis. J Vasc Interv Radiol 2010;21(8):1205–12. https://doi.org/10.1016/j.jvir.2010.04.012. PMID: 20598574.

39. Jiang W, Lu Z, He Y, et al. Dihydropyrimidine dehydrogenase activity in hepatocellular carcinoma: implication in 5-fluorouracil-based chemotherapy. Clin Cancer Res 1997;3(3):395–9. PMID: 9815697.

40. Abou-Alfa GK, Schwartz L, Ricci S, et al. Phase II study of sorafenib in patients with advanced hepatocellular carcinoma. J Clin Oncol 2006;24(26):4293–300. https://doi.org/10.1200/JCO.2005.01.3441. PMID: 16908937.

41. Llovet JM, Montal R, Sia D, et al. Molecular therapies and precision medicine for hepatocellular carcinoma. Nat Rev Clin Oncol 2018;15(10):599–616. https://doi.org/10.1038/s41571-018-0073-4.

42. Orcutt ST, Anaya DA. Liver resection and surgical strategies for management of primary liver cancer. Cancer Control 2018;25(1). 1073274817744621.

43. Cherqui D, Laurent A, Mocellin N, et al. Liver resection for transplantable hepatocellular carcinoma: long-term survival and role of secondary liver transplantation. Ann Surg 2009;250(5):738–46. https://doi.org/10.1097/SLA.0b013e3181bd582b. PMID: 19801927.

44. Theysohn JM, Ertle J, Müller S, et al. Hepatic volume changes after lobar selective internal radiation therapy (SIRT) of hepatocellular carcinoma. Clin Radiol 2014;69(2):172–8. https://doi.org/10.1016/j.crad.2013.09.009. PMID: 24209871.

45. Garlipp B, de Baere T, Damm R, et al. Left-liver hypertrophy after therapeutic right-liver radioembolization is substantial but less than after portal vein embolization. Hepatology 2014;59(5):1864–73.

https://doi.org/10.1002/hep.26947.   PMID: 24259442.

46. Morimoto M, Numata K, Kondou M, et al. Midterm outcomes in patients with intermediate-sized hepatocellular carcinoma: a randomized controlled trial for determining the efficacy of radiofrequency ablation combined with transcatheter arterial chemoembolization. Cancer 2010;116(23):5452–60. https://doi.org/10.1002/cncr.25314. PMID: 20672352.

47. American College of Radiology. Liver Imaging Reporting and Data System version 2018 Manual. 2018. Available at: https://www.acr.org/-/media/ACR/Files/Clinical-Resources/LIRADS/LI-RADS-2018-Manual-5Dec18.pdf?la=en. Accessed June 25, 2020.

48. Voizard N, Cerny M, Assad A, et al. Assessment of hepatocellular carcinoma treatment response with LI-RADS: A pictorial review. Insights Imaging 2019;10(1). https://doi.org/10.1186/s13244-019-0801-z.

49. Crocetti L, Della Pina C, Cioni D, et al. Peri-intraprocedural imaging: US, CT, and MRI. Abdom Radiol (NY) 2011;36(6):648–60. https://doi.org/10.1007/s00261-011-9750-9.

50. Ibrahim SM, Nikolaidis P, Miller FH, et al. Radiologic findings following Y90 radioembolization for primary liver malignancies. Abdom Imaging 2009;34(5):566–81. https://doi.org/10.1007/s00261-008-9454-y. PMID: 18777189.

51. Kallini JR, Miller FH, Gabr A, et al. Hepatic imaging following intra-arterial embolotherapy. Abdom Radiol (NY) 2016;41(4):600–16. https://doi.org/10.1007/s00261-016-0639-5.

52. Mendiratta-Lala M, Gu E, Owen D, et al. Imaging findings within the first 12 months of hepatocellular carcinoma treated with stereotactic body radiation therapy. Int J Radiat Oncol Biol Phys 2018;102(4):1063–9. https://doi.org/10.1016/j.ijrobp.2017.08.022. PMID: 29029891; PMCID: PMC5826807.

53. Mendiratta-Lala M, Masch W, Owen D, Aslam A, et al. Natural history of hepatocellular carcinoma after stereotactic body radiation therapy. Abdom Radiol (NY) 2020. https://doi.org/10.1007/s00261-020-02532-4.

54. Adam SZ, Miller FH. Imaging of the liver following interventional therapy for hepatic neoplasms. Radiol Clin North Am 2015;53(5):1061–76. https://doi.org/10.1016/j.rcl.2015.05.009.

55. Kim KW, Lee JM, Choi BI. Assessment of the treatment response of HCC. Abdom Imaging 2011;36(3):300–14.

56. Minami Y. Therapeutic response assessment of RFA for HCC: Contrast-enhanced US, CT and MRI. World J Gastroenterol 2014;20(15):4160. https://doi.org/10.3748/wjg.v20.i15.4160.

57. Ehman EC, Umetsu SE, Ohliger MA, et al. Imaging prediction of residual hepatocellular carcinoma after locoregional therapy in patients undergoing liver

transplantation or partial hepatectomy. Abdom Radiol (NY) 2016;41(11):2161–8. https://doi.org/10.1007/s00261-016-0837-1.

58. Hussein RS, Tantawy W, Abbas YA. MRI assessment of hepatocellular carcinoma after locoregional therapy. Insights Imaging 2019;10(1). https://doi.org/10.1186/s13244-019-0690-1.

59. Mendiratta-Lala M, Brook OR, Midkiff BD, et al. Quality initiatives: strategies for anticipating and reducing complications and treatment failures in hepatic radiofrequency ablation. RadioGraphics 2010; 30(4):1107–22. https://doi.org/10.1148/rg.304095202.

60. Xu K. Percutaneous cryoablation in combination with ethanol injection for unresectable hepatocellular carcinoma. World J Gastroenterol 2003;9(12):2686. https://doi.org/10.3748/wjg.v9.i12.2686.

61. Tsurusaki M, Murakami T. Surgical and locoregional therapy of HCC: TACE. Liver Cancer 2015;4(3): 165–75. https://doi.org/10.1159/000367739.

62. Gerum S, Heinz C, Belka C, et al. Stereotactic body radiation therapy (SBRT) in patients with hepatocellular carcinoma and oligometastatic liver disease. Radiation Oncol 2018;13(1). https://doi.org/10.1186/s13014-018-1048-4.

63. Rim CH, Seong J. Application of radiotherapy for hepatocellular carcinoma in current clinical practice guidelines. Radiat Oncol J 2016;34(3):160–7. https://doi.org/10.3857/roj.2016.01970.

64. Lee S, Kim H, Ji Y, et al. Evaluation of hepatic toxicity after repeated stereotactic body radiation therapy for recurrent hepatocellular carcinoma using deformable image registration. Sci Rep 2018;8(1). https://doi.org/10.1038/s41598-018-34676-1.

65. Gordic S, Corcuera-Solano I, Stueck A, et al. Evaluation of HCC response to locoregional therapy: validation of MRI-based response criteria versus explant pathology. J Hepatol 2017;67(6):1213–21. https://doi.org/10.1016/j.jhep.2017.07.030.

66. Bruix J, Sherman M, Llovet JM, et al. Clinical management of hepatocellular carcinoma. Conclusions of the Barcelona-2000 EASL Conference. J Hepatol 2001;35(3):421–30. https://doi.org/10.1016/s0168-8278(01)00130-1.

67. Lencioni R, Llovet J. Modified RECIST (mRECIST) assessment for hepatocellular carcinoma. Semin Liver Dis 2010;30(01):052–60. https://doi.org/10.1055/s-0030-1247132.

68. Elsayes KM, Kielar AZ, Chernyak V, et al. LI-RADS: a conceptual and historical review from its beginning to its recent integration into AASLD clinical practice guidance. J Hepatocell Carcinoma 2019;6:49–69. https://doi.org/10.2147/JHC.S186239. PMID: 30788336; PMCID: PMC6368120.

69. Tang A, Singal AG, Mitchell DG, et al. Introduction to the liver imaging reporting and data system for hepatocellular carcinoma. Clin Gastroenterol Hepatol 2019;17(7):1228–38. https://doi.org/10.1016/j.cgh.2018.10.014. PMID: 30326302.

70. Shropshire EL, Chaudhry M, Miller CM, et al. LI-RADS treatment response algorithm: performance and diagnostic accuracy. Radiology 2019;292(1): 226–34. https://doi.org/10.1148/radiol.2019182135.

71. Chaudhry M, Mcginty KA, Mervak B, et al. The LI-RADS Version 2018 MRI treatment response algorithm: evaluation of ablated hepatocellular carcinoma. Radiology 2020;294(2):320–6. https://doi.org/10.1148/radiol.2019191581.

72. Cools KS, Moon AM, Burke LM, et al. Validation of the liver imaging reporting and data system treatment response criteria after thermal ablation for hepatocellular carcinoma. Liver Transpl 2019;26(2): 203–14. https://doi.org/10.1002/lt.25673.

73. Zhang Y, Wang J, Li H, et al. Performance of LI-RADS version 2018 CT treatment response algorithm in tumor response evaluation and survival prediction of patients with single hepatocellular carcinoma after radiofrequency ablation. Ann Transl Med 2020;8(6): 388. https://doi.org/10.21037/atm.2020.03.120.

74. Chung W, Lee K, Park M, et al. Enhancement patterns of hepatocellular carcinoma after transarterial chemoembolization using drug-eluting beads on arterial phase CT images: a pilot retrospective study. Am J Roentgenol 2012;199(2):349–59. https://doi.org/10.2214/ajr.11.7563.

75. Hunt SJ, Yu W, Weintraub J, et al. Radiologic monitoring of hepatocellular carcinoma tumor viability after transhepatic arterial chemoembolization: estimating the accuracy of contrast-enhanced cross-sectional imaging with histopathologic correlation. J Vasc Interv Radiol 2009;20(1):30–8. https://doi.org/10.1016/j.jvir.2008.09.034.

76. Abdel Razek A, El-Serougy L, Saleh G, et al. Reproducibility of LI-RADS treatment response algorithm for hepatocellular carcinoma after locoregional therapy. Diagn Interv Imaging 2020. https://doi.org/10.1016/j.diii.2020.03.008.

77. Kim SW, Joo I, Kim H, et al. LI-RADS treatment response categorization on gadoxetic acid-enhanced MRI: diagnostic performance compared to mRECIST and added value of ancillary features. Eur Radiol 2020;30(5):2861–70. https://doi.org/10.1007/s00330-019-06623-9.

78. Park S, Joo I, Lee DH, et al. Diagnostic performance of LI-RADS treatment response algorithm for hepatocellular carcinoma: adding ancillary features to MRI compared with enhancement patterns at CT and MRI. Radiology 2020;192797. https://doi.org/10.1148/radiol.2020192797.

79. Do RK, Mendiratta-Lala M. Moving away from uncertainty: a potential role for ancillary features in LI-RADS treatment response. Radiology 2020; 202637. https://doi.org/10.1148/radiol.2020202637.

Magnetic Resonance Imaging of Nonhepatocellular Malignancies in Chronic Liver Disease

Roberto Cannella, MD[a,b], Guilherme Moura Cunha, MD[c],
Roberta Catania, MD[d], Kalina Chupetlovska, MD[e], Amir A. Borhani, MD[d],
Kathryn J. Fowler, MD[f], Alessandro Furlan, MD[g],*

KEYWORDS

- Magnetic resonance imaging • Cirrhosis • Hepatocellular carcinoma
- Intrahepatic cholangiocarcinoma • Combined hepatocellular-cholangiocarcinoma • Metastasis
- Liver imaging reporting and data system

KEY POINTS

- Intrahepatic cholangiocarcinoma (iCCA) is the most common non-hepatocellular carcinoma (non-HCC) primary hepatic malignancy. On MR imaging, iCCA typically demonstrates targetoid appearance with rim arterial phase hyperenhancement, peripheral washout, and/or central delayed enhancement.
- Combined hepatocellular-cholangiocarcinoma most commonly presents with similar imaging features to iCCA (targetoid appearance), although tumors with predominant HCC components may be misdiagnosed as HCC.
- Hepatic metastases and lymphoma are rare in cirrhosis, but they should be considered in the differential diagnosis in patients with extrahepatic primary cancers or systemic lymphomas.
- The LR-M category applies to observations that are probably or definitively malignant, but not specific for HCC, in patients at high risk for HCC.
- Management of patients with LR-M lesions should be discussed in multidisciplinary meetings. Lesion biopsy may be considered as an option to establish the diagnosis.

INTRODUCTION

Liver cancer is the third most common cancer and the second most frequent cause of cancer-related mortality worldwide.[1] Hepatocellular carcinoma (HCC) accounts for 90% of all primary liver cancers and is the fifth most common cancer worldwide.[1,2]

[a] Section of Radiology - Department of Biomedicine, Neuroscience and Advanced Diagnostics (BiND), University Hospital "Paolo Giaccone", Via del Vespro 129, Palermo 90127, Italy; [b] Department of Health Promotion, Mother and Child Care, Internal Medicine and Medical Specialties (PROMISE), University of Palermo, Via del Vespro, 129, Palermo 90127, Italy; [c] Department of Radiology, University of Washington, 1959 NE Pacific Street, NW011, Seattle, WA 98195-7115, USA; [d] Department of Radiology, Division of Abdominal Imaging, Northwestern University Feinberg School of Medicine, 676 North St.Clair Street, Chicago, IL 60611, USA; [e] Department of Radiology, University Hospital Saint Ivan Rilski, Ivan Geshov Blvd 15, Sofia 1431, Bulgaria; [f] Liver Imaging Group, Department of Radiology – University of California San Diego, 6206 Lakewood Street, San Diego, CA 92122, USA; [g] Department of Radiology, Abdominal Imaging Division, University of Pittsburgh, 200 Lothrop Street, UPMC Presbyterian Suite 200, Pittsburgh, PA 15213, USA
* Corresponding author.
E-mail address: furlana@upmc.edu

Magn Reson Imaging Clin N Am 29 (2021) 403–417
https://doi.org/10.1016/j.mric.2021.05.009

HCC and other primary liver carcinomas arise most commonly in the setting of chronic liver disease. Cirrhosis caused by viral hepatitis, alcohol abuse, nonalcoholic fatty liver disease, and chronic hepatitis B virus (HBV) infection is considered a higher risk for the development of primary liver cancers. The estimated risk for HCC development in patients with these conditions is greater than 1.5% per year.[2]

Although HCC is the most common, almost 10% of hepatic malignancies in patients with chronic liver disease are non-HCC primary liver carcinomas, or, rarely, metastases from extrahepatic malignancies.[1] The treatment options for HCC and for non-HCC malignancies significantly differ. Locoregional therapies (eg, radiofrequency ablation, transarterial chemoembolization), and/or liver transplantation are often performed with curative intent for HCC, while surgical resection is the only curative option for patients with non-HCC primary liver carcinomas. Moreover, non-HCC malignancies are currently considered a contraindication for liver transplantation because of the high rate of recurrence and worse prognosis.[3] Imaging plays a crucial role in differentiating HCCs from non-HCC malignancies and is a primary driver of management decisions in patients with focal liver lesions arising in the context of chronic liver disease. Observations presenting with imaging features of definitive HCC (ie, size ≥10 mm, arterial phase hyperenhancement, and portal venous washout in combination) may undergo tumor staging and treatment planning without histopathological confirmation.[1,2] Conversely, observations with imaging features of non-HCC malignancies may still require additional workup (eg, tissue biopsy) for definite diagnosis and management determination.

This article discusses the role of imaging in the diagnosis of non-HCC malignancies, with emphasis on the MR imaging features useful to differentiate of these lesions from HCC in patients with chronic liver disease.

PATHOLOGY AND CLASSIFICATION OF NON-HEPATOCELLULAR CARCINOMA MALIGNANCIES

Non-HCC primary liver malignancies most commonly encountered in patients with chronic liver disease include intrahepatic cholangiocarcinoma (iCCA) and combined hepatocellular-cholangiocarcinomas (cHCC-CCAs). Lymphoma and metastases account for less than 1% of liver malignancies in cirrhosis.[4]

Intrahepatic Cholangiocarcinoma

Intrahepatic cholangiocarcinoma is the most common primary non-HCC malignancy, accounting for up to 10% to 15% of all primary liver carcinomas in patients with chronic liver disease.[4–6] iCCA originates from the intrahepatic bile ducts (ie, bile ducts distal to second-order branches).[7] About 90% of iCCAs are adenocarcinomas made of tubular glandular structures surrounded by abundant desmoplastic stroma.[8] According to the most recent World Health Organization (WHO) classification published in 2019, iCCAs are divided into 2 subtypes[6,9]: large-duct iCCA located distal to the secondary-order branches of bile ducts, presenting with a periductal-infiltrating pattern[10,11]; and small-duct iCCA, the most common type accounting for 80% of cases, presenting as a discrete mass (previously described as mass-forming iCCA).[8] On gross pathologic examination, mass-forming iCCA presents as a homogeneous white sclerotic mass with irregular lobulated margins and components of dense fibrosis (**Fig. 1**). At diagnosis, iCCA may be large because of the lack of symptoms at early stages, especially in patients with unrecognized or mild chronic liver disease who are not undergoing routine ultrasound surveillance for HCC.[10,11] On histopathological examination, the viable tumor cells are usually located at the periphery of the tumor, forming invasive glandular structures surrounded by abundant fibrotic stroma (see **Fig. 1**). The central core of the mass is mainly composed of dense desmoplastic stroma and coagulative necrosis.[11] On immunohistochemistry, iCCAs are typically positive for cytokeratin (CK) 7 and CK 19.[6]

Combined Hepatocellular-Cholangiocarcinoma

Combined hepatocellular-cholangiocarcinoma is a rare primary liver carcinoma, accounting for less than 5% of all primary hepatic malignancies.[12] cHCC-CCA shows pathologic features of both HCC and iCCA.[13,14] These tumors are thought to originate from hepatic progenitor cells, which are liver stem cells capable of differentiating into hepatocytes or cholangiocytes. In prior WHO classifications, cHCC-CCAs were divided into classical subtype and the subtype with a predominance of stem cell features.[15] This classification has been abandoned, as other primary liver tumors may also exhibit features of progenitor/stem cells.[12] Yet, to be considered a true combined tumor and not a collision tumor, transitional zones with cells exhibiting intermediate morphology need to be observed between the 2 tumor lineages.[13] Distinctive degrees of tumor differentiation can be seen within the same lesion and in both the HCC and iCCA components. The immunohistochemistry profile shows the presence of both

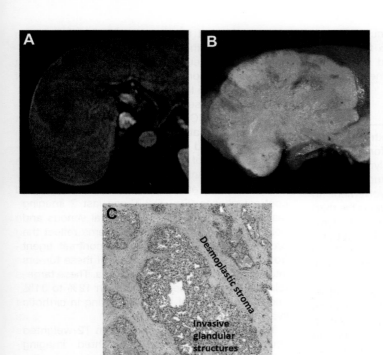

Fig. 1. 63-year-old man with intrahepatic mass-forming cholangiocarcinoma. (*A*) Gadoxetate disodium-enhanced MR imaging during portal venous phase shows a 12.7 cm liver mass with peripheral washout. (*B*) Macroscopic specimens after left liver resection demonstrates a white-tan solid mass with lobulated margins and dense central fibrotic stroma. (*C*) Example of histopathological specimen shows tubular glandular structures of adenocarcinoma in a background of abundant desmoplastic stroma. (*Image courtesy* (1*C*): Dr. M.I. Minervini, University of Pittsburgh.)

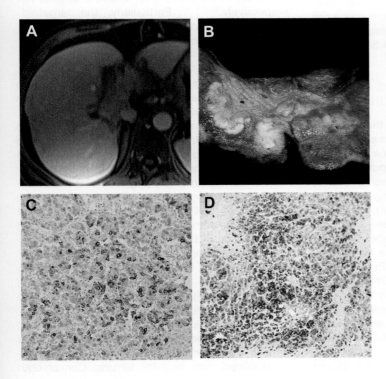

Fig. 2. 61-year-old woman with combined hepatocellular-cholangiocarcinoma. (*A*) Gadoxetate disodium-enhanced MR imaging during portal venous phase shows a 9.0 cm liver mass with peripheral washout and retraction of the liver capsule. (*B*) Macroscopic specimen after central hepatectomy shows a large heterogeneous mass with irregular margins and early cirrhotic changes in the background liver parenchyma. The immunohistochemically stains were positive for α-fetoprotein (*C*), a hepatocytes marker, and for CK7 (*D*), a marker of biliary cells. (*Image courtesy* (2*C-D*): Dr. M.I. Minervini, University of Pittsburgh.)

phenotypes (**Fig. 2**), with markers including, but not limited to, hepatocyte paraffin 1, α-fetoprotein, CD-10, glypican-3, CK7, CK19, and markers of stem/progenitor cells (neural cell adhesion molecule, CD-133, and c-Kit).[12,15]

Other Non-HCC Malignancies

Primary hepatic lymphoma is an extremely rare non-HCC malignancy, accounting for less than 1% of all extranodal non-Hodgkin lymphomas.[4] Hence, most cases of hepatic lymphoma are caused by secondary hepatic involvement in setting of systemic lymphoma. The liver is the third most common abdominal organ involved by lymphoma, preceded by the spleen and the gastrointestinal tract. Non-Hodgkin diffuse large B-cell lymphoma is the most common histopathological pattern.[4]

The liver is a common site of metastatic involvement of extrahepatic malignancies. Most common tumors metastasizing to the liver are primary from the colon, lung, breast, pancreas, stomach, and melanoma. Yet, the prevalence of hepatic metastases in patients with chronic liver disease appears to be significantly lower than that in patients with normal liver.[16,17] Although the underlying reason is not yet clear, the unfavorable liver microenvironment (unfavorable soil) and altered hemodynamics associated with chronic liver disease have been suggested as hypotheses.[18] Metastases would occur less frequently in cirrhosis because of background hepatic fibrosis/regeneration, immune cell activation in inflammation, and increased portal venous pressure or reversed portal flow caused by portosystemic shunts.

MAGNETIC RESONANCE IMAGING OF INTRAHEPATIC CHOLANGIOCARCINOMA

Intrahepatic cholangiocarcinoma is the main differential diagnosis for HCC in patients with chronic liver disease. The imaging appearance of iCCA on multiphasic contrast-enhanced computed tomography (CT) and MR imaging can overlap that of HCC and make the diagnosis challenging.

On contrast-enhanced MR imaging, iCCA typically demonstrates a targetoid appearance with peripheral enhancement on the images acquired during the late hepatic arterial phase (rim arterial phase hyperenhancement – rim APHE). This imaging feature has been described in 80% to 93% of iCCA larger than 3 cm,[19–22] and likely reflects the histopathological distribution of tumor components; viable tumoral cells and invasive glands mainly located at the periphery of the tumor and the desmoplastic stroma are more prominent in the center of the lesion (**Fig. 3**). Rim APHE should

be differentiated from other types of peripheral APHE, such as the peripheral nodular discontinuous enhancement typical of hepatic hemangiomas and the corona enhancement (perilesional enhancement on late arterial phase fading on the subsequent phases) that may be encountered in progressed HCCs.[23] The targetoid dynamic enhancement pattern also includes peripheral washout, defined as more pronounced washout at the periphery of the lesion (**Fig. 4**), and targetoid delayed central enhancement, defined as progressive centripetal enhancement on delayed postcontrast phases (**Fig. 5**).[5] These last 2 imaging features can be observed on portal venous and delayed phase images. Both patterns reflect the progressive shift of extracellular contrast agent from the highly cellular periphery of these tumors into the central desmoplastic stroma. These targetoid features have been reported in 12% to 31% and 45% to 60% of iCCAs occurring in cirrhotic livers, respectively.[19,22,24]

The appearance of the lesion on T2-weighted sequences and diffusion weighted imaging (DWI) may provide additional information for the characterization of non-HCC malignancies. iCCA usually demonstrates heterogeneous mild-to-moderate T2 hyperintensity and true diffusion restriction, with low values on apparent diffusion coefficient (ADC) maps. A targetoid appearance is reported in 18% to 43% and 25% to 68% of cases on T2-weighted (**Fig. 6**) and DWI (**Fig. 7**), respectively.[22,24–26] Particularly, the targetoid restricted diffusion is thought to represent the increased cellularity at the periphery of the tumor, as opposed to the central hypocellularity and necrotic areas. When using the hepatobiliary contrast agent (eg, gadoxetate disodium), there may be additional features observed during the transitional phase (TP) and hepatobiliary phase (HBP). iCCA may demonstrate hypointensity compared with the background hepatic parenchyma or targetoid appearance with moderate-to-marked peripheral hypointensity and possible central iso-hypointensity (**Fig. 8**) on TP and HBP images. This targetoid appearance on HBP is seen in 47% to 90% of iCCAs when using gadoxetate disodium and reflects the lack of hepatocellular function in the tumor periphery associated with accumulation of contrast in the loose extracellular space in the central desmoplastic stroma.[24,27–30]

Additional imaging features that may favor the diagnosis of iCCA over HCC are hepatic capsular retraction (**Fig. 9**), presence of satellite nodules because of intrahepatic tumoral spread, and intrahepatic bile duct dilatation, the latter mostly encountered with perihilar tumors. Conversely,

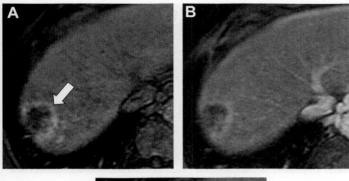

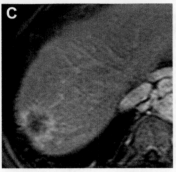

Fig. 3. 80-year-old man with HCV-related cirrhosis and biopsy-proven intrahepatic cholangiocarcinoma. Gadobenate dimeglumine-enhanced MR imaging shows a 5.0 cm liver mass with rim arterial phase hyperenhancement (*A, arrow*) and persistent peripheral enhancement on portal venous (*B*) and delayed (*C*) phases.

presence of an enhancing capsule and nonperipheral washout on portal venous or delayed phases, as well as intralesional fat, are helpful features favoring the diagnosis of progressed HCC.[31] The

authors believe that another key feature for the differential diagnosis of primary liver carcinomas is the relationship with the intrahepatic vessels. In the authors' experience, iCCA demonstrates

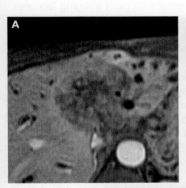

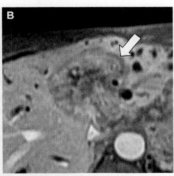

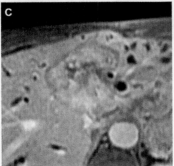

Fig. 4. 73-year-old woman with biopsy-proven intrahepatic cholangiocarcinoma. Gadobenate dimeglumine-enhanced MR imaging shows a 6.0 cm liver mass with heterogeneous enhancement on arterial phase (*A*) and peripheral washout on portal venous (*B, arrow*) and delayed (*C*) phases. Note the marked dilatation of the intrahepatic bile ducts.

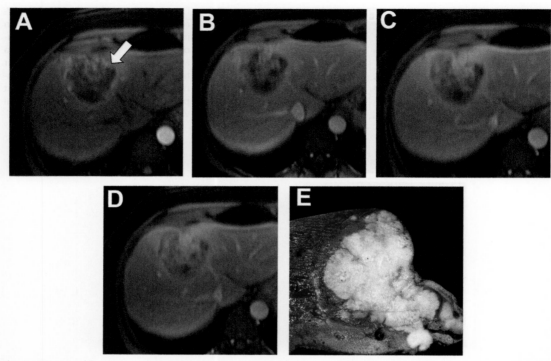

Fig. 5. 55-year-old woman with intrahepatic cholangiocarcinoma. Gadobenate dimeglumine-enhanced MR imaging demonstrates a 6.8 cm liver mass (*arrow*) with rim arterial phase hyperenhancement (*A*) and progressive centripetal enhancement on portal venous (*B*), 3 minutes (*C*), and 5 minutes (*D*) delayed phases. Specimen after hepatic resection (*E*) confirms the diagnosis of intrahepatic cholangiocarcinoma with mild fibrosis in the background liver parenchyma.

higher frequency of intrahepatic vascular involvement compared to HCC, with encasement of portal vein or hepatic veins without definitive evidence of tumor in vein (**Fig. 10**).[20,32] In iCCA, macrovascular invasion with tumor-in-vein is less commonly encountered than in HCC, with reported frequency ranging from 17% to 22%.[24,33] These different vascular involvements may reflect the origin of iCCA from perivascular cholangiocytes and the infiltrative tumor growth as opposed to the nodular growth and origin from parenchymal hepatocytes of HCC.

In patients with advanced fibrosis and cirrhosis, iCCA may demonstrate atypical imaging features. Recent studies have demonstrated that the presence of cirrhosis, which leads to alteration of the hepatic flow, tends to alter the imaging appearance of iCCA.[34,35] iCCA arising in this population may lack the typical features of iCCA, challenging the differential diagnosis from HCC on imaging. On postcontrast dynamic imaging, small iCCAs (<3 cm) detected in patients with cirrhosis more frequently exhibit imaging features of HCC, such as nonrim APHE (**Fig. 11**) and nonperipheral

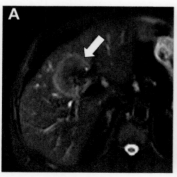
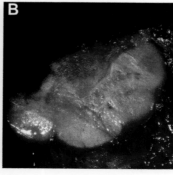

Fig. 6. 60-year-old man with history of nonalcoholic fatty liver disease and intrahepatic cholangiocarcinoma. T2-weighted MR imaging (*A*) shows a 5.0 cm liver mass with targetoid appearance characterized by peripheral hyperintensity and central iso-hypointensity (*arrow*). Specimen after hepatic resection (*B*) confirms the diagnosis of intrahepatic cholangiocarcinoma.

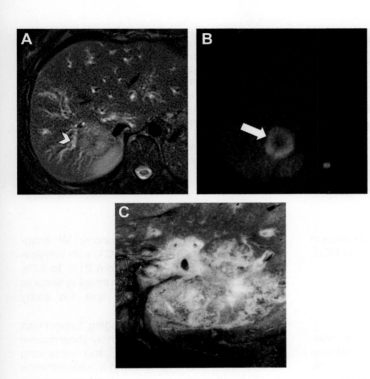

Fig. 7. 33-year-old woman with primary sclerosing cholangitis and intrahepatic cholangiocarcinoma. T2-weighted MR imaging (*A*) shows a 5.0 cm liver mass with mild-to-moderate T2 hyperintensity and dilatation of the adjacent intrahepatic bile duct (*arrowhead*). Diffusion weighted imaging (*B*) demonstrates targetoid restricted diffusion (*arrow*). Specimen after hepatic resection (*C*) confirms the diagnosis of intrahepatic cholangiocarcinoma with encasement of the intrahepatic biliary duct.

washout on portal venous or delayed phase.[34–36] This appearance has been related to the smaller amount of fibrotic stroma and central necrosis and a relatively larger amount of viable neoplastic tissue in these small tumors that are fortuitously diagnosed early in cirrhotic patients undergoing surveillance for HCC.[22,34] Lesion features on other sequences (ie, DWI and HBP), as described

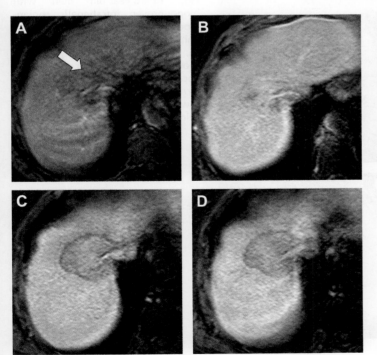

Fig. 8. 84-year-old woman with HCV-related cirrhosis and biopsy-proven intrahepatic cholangiocarcinoma. Gadoxetate disodium-enhanced MR imaging shows a 5.5 cm liver mass with mild heterogeneous enhancement during hepatic arterial phase (*A*, *arrow*), and progressive targetoid appearance on 5 minutes (*B*), 10 minutes (*C*) transitional phases and 20 minutes hepatobiliary phase (*D*). Note the suboptimal hepatobiliary phase caused by the impaired liver function.

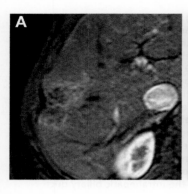
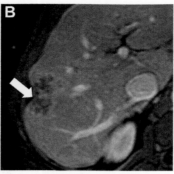

Fig. 9. 56-year-old man with HBV-related cirrhosis and biopsy-proven intrahepatic cholangiocarcinoma. Gadobenate dimeglumine-enhanced MR imaging demonstrates a 4.2 cm liver mass (*arrow*) with rim arterial phase hyperenhancement (*A*) and heterogeneous enhancement on portal venous phase (*B*). Note the associated retraction of the adjacent liver capsule (*arrow*).

previously, may help increasing the confidence in the differential diagnosis between iCCA and HCC.

MAGNETIC RESONANCE IMAGING OF COMBINED HEPATOCELLULAR-CHOLANGIOCARCINOMA

The imaging diagnosis of cHCC-CCA is challenging because of its heterogeneous constitution and appearance. Serum tumor markers can be helpful for the diagnosis, particularly when the imaging presentation and tumor markers are discordant (eg, imaging features of cholangiocarcinoma associated with elevated AFP would suggest cHCC-CCA).[37] Limited data are available regarding the diagnostic performance of MR imaging for the diagnosis of cHCC-CCA, with sensitivities and specificities varying from 21% to 57% and 79% to 100%, depending on imaging features considered for the diagnosis and the study population.[37,38]

On contrast-enhanced MR imaging, tumors with a predominant HCC component may show nonrim APHE, nonperipheral washout, and enhancing capsule. Conversely, tumors with a predominance of iCCA often have a targetoid appearance (**Fig. 12**) and may show capsular retraction and biliary dilatation. When targetoid features are present, rim APHE is the most commonly observed feature.[37] A third presentation is also described,

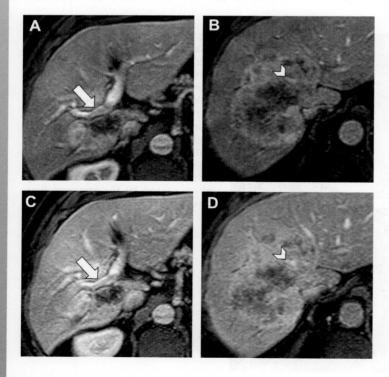

Fig. 10. 78-year-old man with biopsy-proven intrahepatic cholangiocarcinoma. Gadoxetate disodium-enhanced MR imaging on arterial (*A*, *B*) and portal venous (*C*, *D*) phase shows a 10.0 cm liver mass with encasement of both right portal vein (*arrows*) and right hepatic vein (*arrowheads*) and absence of tumor in vein.

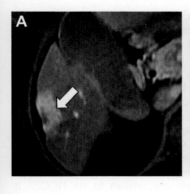 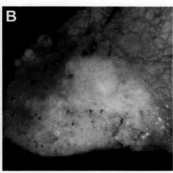

Fig. 11. 61-year-old woman with cirrhosis secondary to nonalcoholic steatohepatitis and intrahepatic cholangiocarcinoma. Gadobutrol-enhanced MR imaging (*A*) shows a 4.0 cm liver mass with nonrim arterial phase hyperenhancement (*arrow*). Specimen after hepatic resection (*B*) was consistent with the diagnosis of intrahepatic cholangiocarcinoma in a background cirrhotic liver parenchyma.

when 2 distinct tumor components can be clearly identified, one resembling the classical appearance of HCC and the other following an iCCA pattern. Although this latter presentation is the most suggestive of cHCC-CCA, studies examining the imaging features of cHCC-CCA have found that iCCA features (ie, targetoid appearance) tend to predominate.[37–40] However, the frequency of tumors with imaging features of HCC (nonrim APHE, washout, and capsule) is not negligible. Hence, it is important to assess for the presence of concomitant ancillary features that suggest non-HCC malignancies, as these may provide important clues to the diagnosis.[41,42]

MR imaging has the advantage of superior contrast resolution and tissue differentiation compared with CT and may better support the diagnosis. On T1-weighted images cHCC-CCAs are mildly heterogeneous and are predominantly hypointense. On T2-weighted sequences, these tumors demonstrate predominantly intermediate to high signal intensity, although hypointense foci can be seen within the tumor due to the presence of fibrotic components. Most cHCC-CCAs show restricted diffusion, which, when more pronounced in the periphery, results in a targetoid appearance, similar to an iCCA.[38,41] On gadoxetate-disodium-enhanced MR imaging, cHCC-CCAs are virtually always hypointense on HPB, as the reduced expression of membrane organic-anion-transporting polypeptides (OATP1B3) results in lack of uptake of

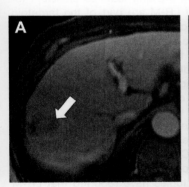 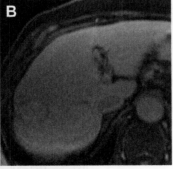

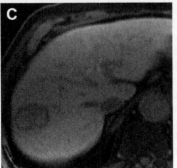

Fig. 12. 77-year-old man with cirrhosis and combined hepatocellular-cholangiocarcinoma. Gadoxetate disodium-enhanced MR imaging shows a 4.5 cm mass (*arrow*) with rim arterial phase hyperenhancement (*A*), peripheral washout on portal venous phase (*B*), and targetoid appearance on hepatobiliary phase (*C*).

hepatobiliary contrast agent. Similar to iCCA, cHCC-CCAs may show a targetoid appearance on HBP images, more pronounced hypointensity in the periphery than in the center of the lesion.[38]

MAGNETIC RESONANCE IMAGING OF OTHER NONHEPATOCELLULAR CARCINOMA MALIGNANCIES

Hepatic lymphomas have heterogeneous imaging appearances, although there are no reported differences in the imaging presentation compared to patients without chronic liver disease. These tumors may present as solitary or multiple focal masses or have an infiltrative pattern. On MR imaging, hepatic lymphoma usually demonstrates hypointensity on T1-weighted images, hyperintensity on T2-weighted sequences, restricted diffusion, and low values on ADC maps. On postcontrast images, lymphomas are typically hypovascular in all phases, and demonstrate hypointensity on HBP images acquired after the injection of gadoxetate disodium.[43–45] In secondary hepatic lymphomas, extrahepatic findings such as splenomegaly, multiple hypovascular splenic lesions and enlarged lymph nodes support the diagnosis (**Fig. 13**). Other primary non-HCC malignant tumors are extremely rare in the setting of chronic liver disease and include epithelioid hemangioendothelioma and angiosarcoma, with few described in cirrhotic patients.[46,47]

The imaging appearance of metastases in cirrhotic livers is not different from that of metastases in noncirrhotic livers. The targetoid appearance with rim APHE is the most frequently observed pattern of liver metastasis in patients with chronic liver disease.[48] Tumor multiplicity, presence of enlarged lymph nodes, and history of extrahepatic primary cancers are additional findings to suggest the diagnosis of hepatic metastases (**Fig. 14**), while some ancillary features such as nodule-in-nodule or mosaic architecture, blood byproducts in the mass, and intralesional fat should favor the diagnosis of HCC.[48]

LIVER IMAGING REPORTING AND DATA SYSTEM: THE LR-M CATEGORY

The Liver Imaging Reporting and Data System (LI-RADS) has designed a specific category for liver observations that are probably or definitely malignant, but not HCC specific (LR-M).[49,50] In the latest LI-RADS version, which has been integrated into the American Association for the Study of Liver Diseases (AASLD) practice guidance, an observation detected in patients at high risk for HCC (ie, with cirrhosis, chronic hepatitis B even

without cirrhosis, or current or prior history of HCC) may be categorized as LR-M if demonstrating targetoid appearance or other features of malignancy but not meeting criteria for LR-5 (definitively HCC).[2,49] However, the LR-M category does not exclude the diagnosis of HCC since atypical HCCs may lack the typical imaging features of LR-5 (ie, nonrim APHE, nonperipheral washout, and enhancing capsule) or have targetoid features similar to non-HCC malignancies.

A recent meta-analysis reported that 93% of the observations categorized as LR-M are malignant and 36% of them are proven to be HCC.[51] It should be noted that 7% of LR-M observations are benign lesions, such as atypical hemangiomas in cirrhosis, which may be miscategorized because of the presence of rim APHE and delayed progressive enhancement in lesions lacking marked T2 hyperintensity.[51] Other studies reported sensitivity of 65% to 89% and specificity of 48% to 89% for the LR-M category for the diagnosis of non-HCC malignancies.[52,53] The management of patients with LR-M observations should be discussed in multidisciplinary meetings, considering other clinical and laboratory parameters (ie, serum tumor markers). Histopathological confirmation is often recommended to reach the final diagnosis and provide the most appropriate treatment.[5]

LI-RADS lists several imaging features that are suggestive of the diagnosis of non-HCC malignancies (**Fig. 15**). Imaging features sufficient for categorization of LR-M are part of the targetoid appearance spectrum (ie, rim APHE, peripheral washout, delayed central enhancement, targetoid restriction, and targetoid TP or HPB appearance).[5,49] In addition, LI-RADS describes other nontargetoid imaging features that are suggestive of malignancies other than HCC. These include infiltrative mass without tumor in vein, marked diffusion restriction, necrosis or severe ischemia, and other features that in radiologist's judgment suggest non-HCC malignancies (ie, hepatic capsule retraction, biliary dilatation, multiplicity).[5,49] Recent studies have reported that LR-M imaging features have a good specificity (range, 83% to 97%) for the diagnosis of non-HCC malignancies, although the sensitivity of these imaging features widely ranges (35% to 71%).[52] Particularly, rim APHE has been reported as the most sensitive feature for the diagnosis of non-HCC malignancies (55%–78%).[52,53] The inter-reader agreement ranges from fair to moderate (k values 0.36–0.55) for LI-RADS categorization of non-HCC primary liver carcinomas, and only slight to moderate (k values 0.05–0.58) for individual LR-M imaging features.[54–56]

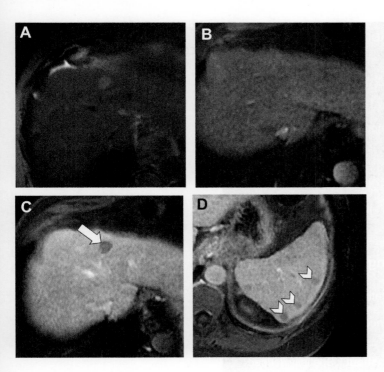

Fig. 13. 68-year-old woman with HCV-related cirrhosis and biopsy-proven hepatic non-Hodgkin B-cell lymphoma. Gadoxetate disodium-enhanced MR imaging shows a 2 cm liver lesions with moderate T2 hyper-intensity (*A*), isoenhancing in the hepatic arterial phase (*B*), and with washout on portal venous phase (*C, arrow*). Multiple other hypovascular lesions are noted in the spleen (*D, arrowheads*).

Similar to HCCs, patients with non-HCC primary liver carcinomas may also present with macrovascular invasion.[55] When tumor in vein (TIV) is detected on imaging (unequivocal enhancing soft tissue within the vein), radiologists should favor the LR-TIV category over LR-M, as the presence of vascular invasion may alter management determinations, independent of the tumor etiology. However, LI-RADS recognizes the possibility of LR-TIV occurring in conjunction with an LR-M

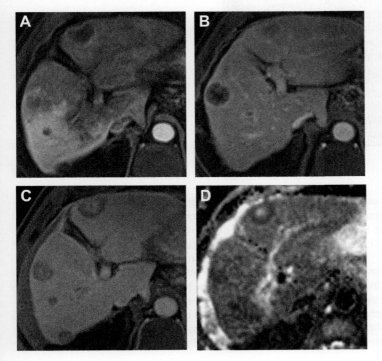

Fig. 14. 63-year-old man with hepatitis C virus (HCV)-related cirrhosis. Gadoxetate disodium-enhanced MR imaging shows multiple bilobar hepatic lesions with rim arterial phase hyperenhancement (*A*), peripheral washout on portal venous phase (*B*), targetoid appearance on hepatobiliary phase (*C*), and targetoid restricted diffusion on ADC map (*D*). Biopsy of liver lesion showed poorly differentiated large-cell type neuroendocrine tumor.

LR-M Criteria

Targetoid mass

OR

Nontargetoid mass with one or more of the following (not meeting LR-5 or LR-TIV criteria):

- Infiltrative appearance.
- Marked diffusion restriction.
- Necrosis or severe ischemia.
- Other feature that in radiologist's judgment suggests non non-HCC malignancy.

Targetoid imaging features

Rim APHE: Spatially defined subtype of APHE in which arterial phase enhancement is most pronounced in observation periphery.

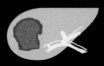
Peripheral "washout": Spatially defined subtype of "washout" in which apparent washout is most pronounced in observation periphery.

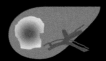
Delayed central enhancement: Central area of progressive postarterial phase enhancement.

Targetoid restriction: Concentric pattern on DWI characterized by restricted diffusion in observation periphery with less restricted diffusion in observation center.

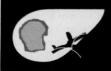
Targetoid TP or HBP appearance: Concentric pattern in TP or HBP characterized by moderate-to-marked hypointensity in observation periphery with milder hypointensity in center.

Fig. 15. LI-RADS criteria for probably or definitively malignant, but not HCC-specific (LR-M) observations.

mass, and suggests that when TIV is adjacent to a mass with a targetoid imaging appearance, the observation should be categorized as LR-TIV and the most likely etiology reported (ie, "may be due to non-HCC malignancy").[49]

The LR-M category intends to preserve the specificity for the diagnosis of HCC in patients at high risk, without compromising the sensitivity for the diagnosis of malignancy in general. Notably, cHCC-CCA represents most of the false-positive non-HCC malignancies miscategorized as LR-5, due to the overlap in imaging features with HCC.[40,55] Radiologists should be watchful for the presence of ancillary features or additional patterns such as tumor in vein, a feature most commonly seen in HCCs, and lymph node metastasis, more common to CCAs, herein increasing the suspicion for the diagnosis of a combined tumor. Indeed, when a c-HCC-CCA presents with major features of definite HCC (LR-5), about 90% will exhibit at least 1 ancillary feature suggestive of non-HCC malignancy.[41] In this case, or when any other imaging features raises suspicion for malignancies other than HCC, radiologists should favor the least specific LI-RADS category (LR-M) to correctly consider the possibility of cHCC-CCA.

Finally, emerging data suggest that LI-RADS categorization may also provide prognostic information in patients with chronic liver disease and primary liver malignancies. A few studies have reported that HCCs categorized as LR-M because of the presence of atypical imaging features are associated with more aggressive histopathological subtypes and worse outcomes than HCCs categorized as LR-5.[57] Similarly, non-HCC malignancies categorized as LR-M have significantly worse recurrence-free survival and overall survival after surgical resection when compared with observations showing imaging features of LR-5 or LR-4.[40,58,59] Further research is needed to validate these findings and to further investigate the role of LR-M imaging features in patient prognostication.

SUMMARY

Non-HCC malignancies should be always considered in the differential diagnosis of focal liver lesions encountered in patients with chronic liver disease. Although non-HCC malignancies typically present with targetoid imaging features, there remains considerable overlap in imaging findings of HCC and non-HCC malignancies. Attention to ancillary imaging features and tumor markers may aid with better differentiation of these 2 entities. When using the LI-RADS system, observations with imaging features suggesting non-HCC malignancies are categorized as LR-M and are discussed in multidisciplinary meetings to guide the most appropriate management.

CLINICS CARE POINTS

- 10% of hepatic malignancies in patients with chronic liver disease are non-HCC primary liver carcinomas.
- Rim arterial phase hyperenhancement has been described in 80% to 93% of intrahepatic cholangiocarcinomas larger than 3 cm. Peripheral washout and targetoid delayed central enhancement have been reported in 12% to 31% and 45% to 60% of intrahepatic cholangiocarcinomas occurring in cirrhotic livers, respectively.
- Small intrahepatic cholangiocarcinoma arising in patients with cirrhosis may demonstrate atypical enhancement pattern, with nonrim arterial phase hyperenhancement and nonperipheral washout on portal venous or delayed phase.

- Sensitivities and specificities of MRI diagnosis of combined hepatocellular-cholangiocarcinoma varying from 21% to 57% and 79% to 100%, respectively.
- When using the LI-RADS, the LR-M category has a sensitivity of 65% to 89% and specificity of 48% to 89% for the diagnosis of non-HCC malignancies.

REFERENCES

1. European Association for the Study of the Liver. EASL clinical practice guidelines: management of hepatocellular carcinoma. J Hepatol 2018;69: 182–236.
2. Marrero JA, Kulik LM, Sirlin CB, et al. Diagnosis, staging, and management of hepatocellular carcinoma: 2018 practice guidance by the American Association for the Study of Liver Diseases. Hepatology 2018;68:723–50.
3. Wald C, Russo MW, Heimbach JK, et al. New OPTN/ UNOS policy for liver transplant allocation: standardization of liver imaging, diagnosis, classification, and reporting of hepatocellular carcinoma. Radiology 2013;266:376–82.
4. Ronot M, Dioguardi Burgio M, Purcell Y, et al. Focal lesions in cirrhosis: not always HCC. Eur J Radiol 2017;93:157–68.
5. Fowler KJ, Potretzke TA, Hope TA, et al. Definite or probable malignancy, not specific for hepatocellular carcinoma. Abdom Radiol (NY) 2018;43:149–57.
6. Kim JH, Yoon JH, Joo I, et al. Evaluation of primary liver cancers using hepatocyte-specific contrast-enhanced MRI: pitfalls and potential tips. J Magn Reson Imaging 2020. https://doi.org/10.1002/jmri.27213.
7. Lee WJ, Lim HK, Jang KM, et al. Radiologic spectrum of cholangiocarcinoma: emphasis on unusual manifestations and differential diagnoses. Radiographics 2001;21(Spec No):S97–116.
8. Lim JH. Cholangiocarcinoma: morphologic classification according to growth pattern and imaging findings. AJR Am J Roentgenol 2003;181: 819–27.
9. Nagtegaal ID, Odze RD, Klimstra D, et al. The 2019 WHO classification of tumours of the digestive system. Histopathology 2020;76:182–8.
10. Han JK, Choi BI, Kim AY, et al. Cholangiocarcinoma: pictorial essay of CT and cholangiographic findings. Radiographics 2002;22:173–87.
11. Chung YE, Kim MJ, Park YN, et al. Varying appearances of cholangiocarcinoma: radiologic-pathologic correlation. Radiographics 2009;29: 683–700.
12. Brunt E, Aishima S, Clavien PA, et al. cHCC-CCA: consensus terminology for primary liver carcinomas

with both hepatocytic and cholangiocytic differentiation. Hepatology 2018;68:113–26.

13. Stavraka C, Rush H, Ross P. Combined hepatocellular cholangiocarcinoma (cHCC-CC): an update of genetics, molecular biology, and therapeutic interventions. J Hepatocell Carcinoma 2019;6:11.

14. Ramai D, Ofosu A, Lai JK, et al. Combined hepatocellular cholangiocarcinoma: a population-based retrospective study. Am J Gastroenterol 2019;114:1496–501.

15. Sasaki M, Sato H, Kakuda Y, et al. Clinicopathological significance of "subtypes with stem-cell feature" in combined hepatocellular-cholangiocarcinoma. Liver Int 2015;35:1024–35.

16. Augustin G, Bruketa T, Korolija D, et al. Lower incidence of hepatic metastases of colorectal cancer in patients with chronic liver diseases: meta-analysis. Hepatogastroenterology 2013;60:1164–8.

17. Cai B, Liao K, Song XQ, et al. Patients with chronically diseased livers have lower incidence of colorectal liver metastases: a meta-analysis. PLoS One 2014;9:e108618.

18. Wang L, Sun Y, Yi M, et al. IEO model: a novel concept describing the complete metastatic process in the liver microenvironment. Oncol Lett 2020;19:3627–33.

19. Kim SJ, Lee JM, Han JK, et al. Peripheral mass-forming cholangiocarcinoma in cirrhotic liver. AJR Am J Roentgenol 2007;189:1428–34.

20. Mamone G, Marrone G, Caruso S, et al. Intrahepatic mass-forming cholangiocarcinoma: enhancement pattern on Gd-BOPTA-MRI with emphasis of hepatobiliary phase. Abdom Imaging 2015;40:2313–22.

21. Quaia E, Angileri R, Arban F, et al. Predictors of intrahepatic cholangiocarcinoma in cirrhotic patients scanned by gadobenate dimeglumine-enhanced magnetic resonance imaging: diagnostic accuracy and confidence. Clin Imaging 2015;39:1032–8.

22. Ni T, Shang XS, Wang WT, et al. Different MR features for differentiation of intrahepatic mass-forming cholangiocarcinoma from hepatocellular carcinoma according to tumor size. Br J Radiol 2018;91:20180017.

23. Cannella R, Fowler KJ, Borhani AA, et al. Common pitfalls when using the Liver Imaging Reporting and Data System (LI-RADS): lessons learned from a multi-year experience. Abdom Radiol (NY) 2019;44:43–53.

24. Joo I, Lee JM, Lee SM, et al. Diagnostic accuracy of Liver Imaging Reporting and Data System (LI-RADS) v2014 for intrahepatic mass-forming cholangiocarcinomas in patients with chronic liver disease on gadoxetic acid-enhanced MRI. J Magn Reson Imaging 2016;44:1330–8.

25. Sheng RF, Zeng MS, Rao SX, et al. MRI of small intrahepatic mass-forming cholangiocarcinoma and atypical small hepatocellular carcinoma (≤3 cm) with cirrhosis and chronic viral hepatitis: a comparative study. Clin Imaging 2014;38:265–72.

26. Fattach HE, Dohan A, Guerrache Y, et al. Intrahepatic and hilar mass-forming cholangiocarcinoma: qualitative and quantitative evaluation with diffusion-weighted MR imaging. Eur J Radiol 2015;84:1444–51.

27. Jeong HT, Kim MJ, Chung YE, et al. Gadoxetate disodium-enhanced MRI of mass-forming intrahepatic cholangiocarcinomas: imaging-histologic correlation. AJR Am J Roentgenol 2013;201:W603–11.

28. Kim R, Lee JM, Shin CI, et al. Differentiation of intrahepatic mass-forming cholangiocarcinoma from hepatocellular carcinoma on gadoxetic acid-enhanced liver MR imaging. Eur Radiol 2016;26:1808–17.

29. Choi SH, Lee SS, Kim SY, et al. Intrahepatic cholangiocarcinoma in patients with cirrhosis: differentiation from hepatocellular carcinoma by using gadoxetic acid-enhanced MR imaging and dynamic CT. Radiology 2017;282:771–81.

30. Min JH, Kim YK, Choi SY, et al. Differentiation between cholangiocarcinoma and hepatocellular carcinoma with target sign on diffusion-weighted imaging and hepatobiliary phase gadoxetic acid-enhanced MR imaging: Classification tree analysis applying capsule and septum. Eur J Radiol 2017;92:1–10.

31. Asayama Y, Nishie A, Ishigami K, et al. Distinguishing intrahepatic cholangiocarcinoma from poorly differentiated hepatocellular carcinoma using pre-contrast and gadoxetic acid-enhanced MRI. Diagn Interv Radiol 2015;21:96–104.

32. Tsunematsu S, Chuma M, Kamiyama T, et al. Intratumoral artery on contrast-enhanced computed tomography imaging: differentiating intrahepatic cholangiocarcinoma from poorly differentiated hepatocellular carcinoma. Abdom Imaging 2015;40:1492–9.

33. Zhao YJ, Chen WX, Wu DS, et al. Differentiation of mass-forming intrahepatic cholangiocarcinoma from poorly differentiated hepatocellular carcinoma: based on the multivariate analysis of contrast-enhanced computed tomography findings. Abdom Radiol (NY) 2016;41:978–89.

34. Kim SA, Lee JM, Lee KB, et al. Intrahepatic mass-forming cholangiocarcinomas: enhancement patterns at multiphasic CT, with special emphasis on arterial enhancement pattern–correlation with clinicopathologic findings. Radiology 2011;260:148–57.

35. Fraum TJ, Cannella R, Ludwig DR, et al. Assessment of primary liver carcinomas other than hepatocellular carcinoma (HCC) with LI-RADS v2018: comparison of the LI-RADS target population to patients without LI-RADS-defined HCC risk factors. Eur Radiol 2020;30:996–1007.

36. Huang B, Wu L, Lu XY, et al. Small intrahepatic cholangiocarcinoma and hepatocellular carcinoma in

cirrhotic livers may share similar enhancement patterns at multiphase dynamic MR imaging. Radiology 2016;281:150–7.

37. Fowler KJ, Sheybani A, Parker RA 3rd, et al. Combined hepatocellular and cholangiocarcinoma (biphenotypic) tumors: imaging features and diagnostic accuracy of contrast-enhanced CT and MRI. AJR Am J Roentgenol 2013;201:332–9.

38. Lee HS, Kim MJ, An C. How to utilize LR-M features of the LI-RADS to improve the diagnosis of combined hepatocellular-cholangiocarcinoma on gadoxetate-enhanced MRI? Eur Radiol 2019;29: 2408–16.

39. de Campos RO, Semelka RC, Azevedo RM, et al. Combined hepatocellular carcinoma-cholangiocarcinoma: report of MR appearance in eleven patients. J Magn Reson Imaging 2012;36:1139–47.

40. Jeon SK, Joo I, Lee DH, et al. Combined hepatocellular cholangiocarcinoma: LI-RADS v2017 categorisation for differential diagnosis and prognostication on gadoxetic acid-enhanced MR imaging. Eur Radiol 2019;29:373–82.

41. Potretzke TA, Tan BR, Doyle MB, et al. Imaging features of biphenotypic primary liver carcinoma (hepatocholangiocarcinoma) and the potential to mimic hepatocellular carcinoma: LI-RADS analysis of CT and MRI features in 61 cases. Am J Roentgenol 2016;207:25–31.

42. Park SH, Lee SS, Yu E, et al. Combined hepatocellular-cholangiocarcinoma: gadoxetic acid-enhanced MRI findings correlated with pathologic features and prognosis. J Magn Reson Imaging 2017;46:267–80.

43. Rajesh S, Bansal K, Sureka B, et al. The imaging conundrum of hepatic lymphoma revisited. Insights Imaging 2015;6:679–92.

44. Tomasian A, Sandrasegaran K, Elsayes KM, et al. Hematologic malignancies of the liver: spectrum of disease. Radiographics 2015;35:71–86.

45. Colagrande S, Calistri L, Grazzini G, et al. MRI features of primary hepatic lymphoma. Abdom Radiol (NY) 2018;43:2277–87.

46. Baron PW, Amankonah T, Cubas RF, et al. Diffuse hepatic epithelioid hemangioendothelioma developed in a patient with hepatitis C cirrhosis. Case Rep Transplant 2014;2014:694903.

47. Sánchez Rodríguez E, Pinilla Pagnon I, Ríos Leon R, et al. Hepatic angiosarcoma in a patient with liver cirrhosis. Gastroenterol Hepatol 2019;42:304–5.

48. Cho MJ, An C, Aljoqiman KS, et al. Diagnostic performance of Liver Imaging Reporting and Data System in patients at risk of both hepatocellular carcinoma and metastasis. Abdom Radiol (NY) 2020. https://doi.org/10.1007/s00261-020-02581-9.

49. American College of Radiology. CT/MRI Liver imaging reporting and data system v2018 Core.

Available at: https://www.acr.org/Clinical-Resources/Reporting-and-Data-Systems/LI-RADS/CT-MRI-LI-RADS-v2018. Accessed October 10, 2020.

50. Chernyak V, Fowler KJ, Kamaya A, et al. Liver Imaging Reporting and Data System (LI-RADS) version 2018: imaging of hepatocellular carcinoma in at-risk patients. Radiology 2018;289:816–30.

51. van der Pol CB, Lim CS, Sirlin CB, et al. Accuracy of the liver imaging reporting and data system in computed tomography and magnetic resonance image analysis of hepatocellular carcinoma or overall malignancy-a systematic review. Gastroenterology 2019;156:976–86.

52. Kim YY, Kim MJ, Kim EH, et al. Hepatocellular carcinoma versus other hepatic malignancy in cirrhosis: performance of LI-RADS version 2018. Radiology 2019;291:72–80.

53. Ludwig DR, Fraum TJ, Cannella R, et al. Hepatocellular carcinoma (HCC) versus non-HCC: accuracy and reliability of Liver Imaging Reporting and Data System v2018. Abdom Radiol (NY) 2019;44: 2116–32.

54. Horvat N, Nikolovski I, Long N, et al. Imaging features of hepatocellular carcinoma compared to intrahepatic cholangiocarcinoma and combined tumor on MRI using liver imaging and data system (LI-RADS) version 2014. Abdom Radiol (NY) 2018;43: 169–78.

55. Fraum TJ, Tsai R, Rohe E, et al. Differentiation of hepatocellular carcinoma from other hepatic malignancies in patients at risk: diagnostic performance of the Liver Imaging Reporting and Data System Version 2014. Radiology 2018;286:158–72.

56. Ludwig DR, Fraum TJ, Cannella R, et al. Expanding the Liver Imaging Reporting and Data System (LI-RADS) v2018 diagnostic population: performance and reliability of LI-RADS for distinguishing hepatocellular carcinoma (HCC) from non-HCC primary liver carcinoma in patients who do not meet strict LI-RADS high-risk criteria. HPB (Oxford) 2019;21: 1697–706.

57. Mulé S, Galletto Pregliasco A, Tenenhaus A, et al. Multiphase liver mri for identifying the macrotrabecular-massive subtype of hepatocellular carcinoma. Radiology 2020;295:562–71.

58. An C, Park S, Chung YE, et al. Curative resection of single primary hepatic malignancy: liver imaging reporting and data system category LR-M portends a worse prognosis. AJR Am J Roentgenol 2017;209: 576–83.

59. Choi SH, Lee SS, Park SH, et al. LI-RADS classification and prognosis of primary liver cancers at gadoxetic acid-enhanced MRI. Radiology 2019;290: 388–97.

Errors and Misinterpretations in Imaging of Chronic Liver Diseases

Ali Morshid, MD[a],*, Janio Szklaruk, MD, PhD[b], Joseph H. Yacoub, MD[c],
Khaled M. Elsayes, MD, PhD[b]

KEYWORDS

• Magnetic resonance imaging • Cirrhosis • Pitfalls • Misinterpretations

KEY POINTS

- Chronic liver disease complicates liver imaging, producing many imaging mimics and potential pitfalls.
- MR imaging of the liver is a powerful diagnostic tool impacted by multiple technical artifacts.
- Awareness of technical artifacts and imaging pitfalls and ways to mitigate them is essential for accurate and safe reporting.

INTRODUCTION

Magnetic resonance imaging (MRI) provides a sensitive and specific modality for liver imaging. Tailored imaging protocols and the advent of hepatobiliary contrast agents established MR imaging as an important problem-solving tool for accurate characterization of liver lesions. Despite the classic MR imaging characteristics of many benign and malignant liver lesions, imaging mimics and technical artifacts are commonly encountered and can lead to interpretation errors. These pitfalls are often accentuated in the setting of a chronically diseased liver and radiologist awareness is essential for accurate reporting and patient safety. Understanding liver-specific MR imaging acquisition techniques is important for recognizing and addressing these pitfalls. In this article, we discuss liver MR imaging techniques, technical artifacts, and the spectrum of misdiagnoses commonly encountered in chronic liver disease. We will also discuss pitfalls specific to the use of hepatobiliary contrast agents.

NORMAL ANATOMY AND ANATOMIC CONSIDERATIONS

Evaluation of biliary and vascular anatomy as well as the presence of anatomic variants is essential for surgical planning and radiologic intervention. Computed tomography angiogram (CTA) is a noninvasive modality for the evaluation of liver vascular anatomy and provides excellent three-dimensional (3D) reconstructions. MR angiography has an inferior resolution to both CTA and conventional angiography and is reverted to when there is a contraindication to iodinated contrast material. The liver has a unique dual blood supply through the hepatic artery (20%) and portal vein (80%). Arterial and venous blood then mix within the hepatic sinusoids and drains into the central veins then into the hepatic veins.[1] The common hepatic artery arises from the celiac

[a] Department of Diagnostic Radiology, The University of Texas Medical Branch, 301 University Boulevard, Galveston, TX 77555, USA; [b] Department of Diagnostic Radiology, The University of Texas MD Anderson Cancer Center, 1400 Pressler Street, Houston, TX 77030, USA; [c] Department of Radiology, Medstar Georgetown University Hospital, 110 Irving Street Northwest, Washington, DC 20010, USA
* Corresponding author.
E-mail address: aimorshi@utmb.edu

Magn Reson Imaging Clin N Am 29 (2021) 419–435
https://doi.org/10.1016/j.mric.2021.05.008
1064-9689/21/© 2021 Elsevier Inc. All rights reserved.

axis and gives rise to the proper hepatic artery, which bifurcates into the right and left hepatic arteries. There are 10 vascular variants of arterial anatomy described in Michel's classification.[2] This includes an accessory or replaced hepatic arteries, and common hepatic trunk arising from the superior mesenteric artery or the left gastric artery.[3]

Couinaud's liver segmental anatomy classification divides the liver into 8 anatomic sectors based on the identification of the three hepatic veins and the plane intersecting the portal vein bifurcation.[4] The liver is first divided into right and left hemilivers by the plane of the middle hepatic vein.[5] The right hemiliver is further divided into anterior and posterior based on the plane of the right hepatic artery. The left hemiliver is further divided into medial and lateral based on the plane connecting the left hepatic vein and the falciform ligament. The whole liver is divided into upper and lower segments at the plane intersecting the main portal vein bifurcation.

Volumetric calculation of each liver segment is obtained with 3D images obtained from source CT or MR examination. Evaluation of liver volumetry is important in presurgical planning for liver resection. To compensate for volume loss after a hepatic resection, adequate liver function can be maintained with 20% of the liver remnant in a liver without underlying liver disease. In the setting of cirrhosis, the required liver remnant should be at least 40% of the liver volume. And in the setting of the treated liver, a 30% liver remnant is required.[6]

IMAGING PROTOCOLS AND ADVANCED TECHNIQUES

The standard liver MR protocol includes T2-weighted (T2-W) single-shot fast spin-echo, T2-W fast spin-echo with fat suppression, in-phase, and opposed-phased sequences, diffusion-weighted imaging (DWI), and precontrast and postcontrast gradient recalled echo (GRE) T1-weighted (T1-W) imaging. The combination of sequences provides accurate lesion characterization. MR examinations of the abdomen are obtained with either extracellular or hepatobiliary gadolinium-based contrast agents (GBCA) with multiple phases obtained postgadolinium administration. The hemodynamics of extracellular GBCA is similar to that of CT-iodinated-contrast agents. Many institutions use extracellular agents for most routine cases with hepatobiliary agent being reserved for special cases, which can further characterize lesion based on their appearance on the hepatobiliary phase (HBP).[7,8]

Quantitative MR imaging is playing an increasing role beyond lesion characterization in the assessment of liver pathology and is expected to become more prevalent in daily practice.[9] MR sequences are used for the quantification of hepatic steatosis, fibrosis, and iron overload. Quantification of hepatic fat is achieved by measuring proton density fat fraction using chemical shift encoded techniques also known as Dixon techniques.[10] This allows the generation of water and fat only images in addition to the in-phase and opposed-phase series. The quantification of hepatic fibrosis with MR elastography evaluates liver parenchymal stiffness based on the speed of shear waves propagating through the liver.[11] Several MR imaging techniques have been developed for iron quantification, among them, the R2*/T2* relaxometry using multi-echo GRE sequence is gaining wide adoption.[12]

TECHNICAL ARTIFACTS AND PITFALLS
Respiratory Motion Artifact

Although the time of acquisition of MR sequences has been improving, respiratory motion remains a major challenge. Respiratory motion artifact is commonly encountered in breath-hold and non–breath-hold series in the daily radiology practice. It can lead to misinterpretation and missed lesions (**Fig. 1**). Multiple strategies have been used to minimize the effect of respiratory motion while imaging the liver. One of these strategies is faster acquisition time using techniques such as view sharing, parallel imaging, and compressed sensing, which allows for under 10 seconds acquisition time for 3D GRE sequences. This enables a shorter breath-hold for the patient while maintaining the same spatial resolution. One application for this technique is acquiring multiple arterial phases using fast T1 sequences, improving the chances of acquiring at least one motion-free late arterial sequence.[13,14]

Another strategy is the use of respiratory triggering or navigator-related techniques. The acquisition time for these techniques ranges from 80 to 100 seconds, thus precluding their use in dynamic multiphase liver imaging. The navigation techniques have been used for in-phase/opposed-phase, T2-W, and DWI sequences. Navigation series can also produce excellent delayed images, particularly during the HBP.[15,16]

A third type of strategy is the use of motion-resistant sequences such as free-breathing radial T1 3D GRE, which can be acquired during the delayed postcontrast phase or the HBP with an acquisition time in the range of 80 to 120 seconds.[17,18]

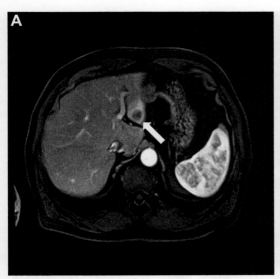 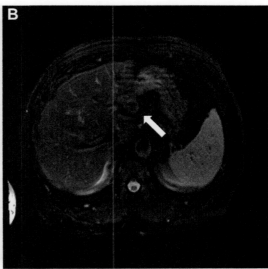

Fig. 1. A 67-year-old female with a history of colon cancer status postresection. Axial arterial phase MR imaging of the liver (*A*) showed a peripherally enhancing lesion in hepatic segment II (*arrow*). This lesion was not well visualized on the T2-W sequence (*B*) due to motion artifact.

Arterial Phase Timing

A major challenge in postgadolinium MR imaging is the optimum timing of postcontrast images, especially the first phase, the late arterial phase. Hypervascular liver lesions can be easily missed on too early or too late arterial phase timing.[19] An early arterial phase is recommended only when evaluation is directed at arterial anatomy. The optimal timing for evaluating arterially enhancing lesions is the late arterial phase. This is identified by brightly enhancing arteries, mildly enhancing portal veins, and no antegrade enhancement of hepatic veins. A commonly used method for acquiring optimal late arterial phase sequences is the bolus tracking method. It is performed by acquiring a tracking sequence for rapid sampling of the aorta at the level of the diaphragm with image acquisition being initiated automatically based on a specific signal threshold.[20] Predetermined delay is also used to allow for breath-holding and for the contrast to reach the target area. Newer sequences using view sharing techniques can allow the acquisition of multiple arterial phases in less than 15 seconds.[21]

Gadoxetate Disodium–Related Pitfalls

Gadoxetate disodium is a hepatobiliary agent. This agent-approved dose is 0.025 mmol/kg, which is a quarter of gadolinium-based extracellular agents. A diluted, power-injected contrast bolus with saline or using a slower injection rate results in better timing and minimizes motion artifact.[22] Another

pitfall associated with gadoxetate disodium is transient severe motion artifact resulting in severe degradation of the late arterial phase and potentially leading to a missed diagnosis. It is reported in up to 10% to 19.4% of patients receiving gadoxetate disodium along with symptoms of shortness of breath.[23] Methods to mitigate this artifact are similar to what was discussed with respiratory motion artifact including obtaining multiple arterial phases and faster acquisition.[13]

Pseudowashout

The transitional phase of contrast administration in the setting of hepatobiliary agents refers to the time between the portal venous phase (90 seconds) and the HBP (10–20 minutes). The HBP refers to a phase in which biliary excretion of the contrast is observed and is typically acquired at 20 minutes postcontrast administration. Here, the liver should be hyperintense to blood vessels. Pseudowashout is used to describe the hypointense appearance of focal lesions relative to the enhancing liver parenchyma on the transitional and HBP imaging when using gadoxetate disodium. These lesions typically do not demonstrate washout on the portal venous phase and falsely appear hypointense due to the progressively increased contrast uptake by the surrounding hepatocytes. This can be seen with rapid-filling hemangiomas and can represent a diagnostic challenge to the radiologist potentially leading to misdiagnosis as hepatocellular carcinoma (HCC; **Fig. 2**).[24] To mitigate this potential pitfall, washout

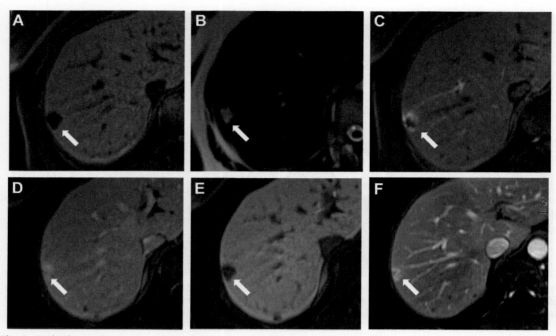

Fig. 2. Multiphasic MR imaging of the abdomen was performed with hepatobiliary contrast for characterization of a hepatic focal lesion. The lesions showed hypointense signal (*arrow*) on T1-weighted images (*A*) and hyperintense signal (*arrow*) on T2-weighted images (*B*). Arterial (*C*) and portal venous (*D*) phases showed progressive centripetal enhancement of the lesion (*arrows*). 20-minute delayed phase (*E*) showed hypointense signal relative to surrounding liver parenchyma (*arrow*). The signal characteristics and enhancement pattern of this lesion was consistent with hemangioma and the hypointense signal on HBP should not be confused with delayed washout seen with HCC. Follow-up MRI using extracellular agent 2 years later (*F*) showed stable size of this progressively enhancing lesion (*arrow*).

should be assessed only on the portal venous phase when using gadoxetate disodium, which is specified in the latest Liver Imaging Reporting and Data System (LI-RADS) recommendations.[25] Also, the T2-W images can assist in the characterization of hemangiomas, because of the relative hyperintensity.

Suboptimal Hepatobiliary Phase

As HBP imaging relies on intracellular contrast uptake by functioning hepatocytes, advanced cirrhosis and cholestasis can result in diminished contrast uptake in the hepatocytes and suboptimal HBP sequence.[26–28] The liver parenchyma appears iso/hypointense to the hepatic blood vessels with no contrast excretion into the biliary system and retained contrast within the spleen. Liver lesions can appear isointense to the suboptimally enhancing liver parenchyma leading to potential misdiagnosis. One proposed method to avoid this pitfall is delaying the HBP acquisition beyond 20 minutes.[29]

Subtraction-Related Pitfalls

Postgadolinium subtraction images can be generated to improve the sensitivity for the detection of

liver lesion enhancement.[30] Image misregistration occurs because of motion between two acquired sequences (**Fig. 3**). Radiologists need to identify this artifact to avoid mischaracterization of a non-enhancing lesion as an enhancing lesion based on the subtraction imaging. The benefit of subtraction is in the assessment of enhancement of lesions that are hyperintense on the precontrast T1-W imaging.

Diffusion Weighted Imaging-Related Artifacts

DWI images are usually acquired using T2-W echo-planar images. It is useful for the characterization of liver lesions and can help in detecting metastases that are not easily seen on T2-W or postcontrast sequences. The combination of DWI and apparent diffusion coefficient (ADC) maps may help in differentiating between hemangiomas and hepatic cysts from malignant lesions. The signal intensity of DWI depends on the water molecule diffusivity and intrinsic tissue T2 relaxation time. Lesions with a long T2 relaxation time will result in a high signal on DWI despite the absence of restricted water molecule diffusion.[31] This is described as T2 shine-through and can be identified by recognizing the high corresponding ADC value. T2 shine-through effect can be reduced using higher B-values for DWI images (B-1000 s/mm^2; **Fig. 4**). Another pitfall is the absence of diffusion restriction in the setting of necrosis or mucinous lesions that can resemble hepatic cysts on DWI images. A careful review of the patient's history, prior imaging, and the clinical context must be taken into consideration when interpreting images to avoid misdiagnosis. In addition, restricted diffusion can be seen with hemorrhage or inflammation/infection as they both feature limited mobility of water molecules.[32] This represents a diagnostic challenge for the radiologist as intralesional hemorrhage or abscess can demonstrate restricted diffusion, which can be potentially confusing in post-treatment scenarios. Thus, the assessment of locoregional response to treatment depends on residual arterial phase hyperenhancement rather than overall lesion size or diffusion restriction.

Heavily T2-W Sequence Pitfalls

Heavily T2-W sequences are acquired with a TE of at least 140 ms. Malignant hepatic lesions typically demonstrate a slight T2-W hyperintense signal. The degree of lesional signal hyperintensity decreases with prolonged TE to a point where it can appear as isointense to the surrounding parenchyma on heavily weighted T2 sequences. This results in obscured lesions that are usually well-depicted on shorter TE T2-W sequences. A benefit of the long TE T2-W sequence is in the characterization of cysts and

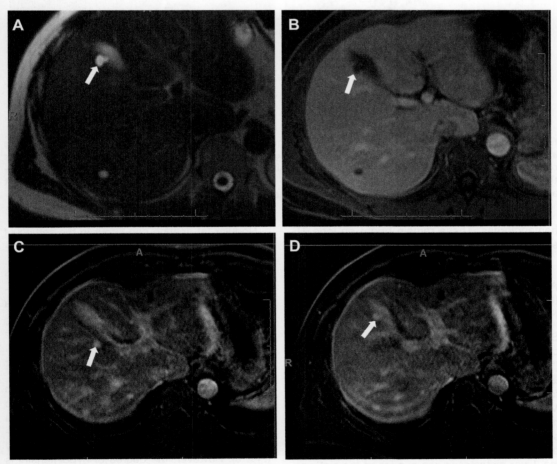

Fig. 3. A 52-year-old male underwent liver MR imaging for characterization of indeterminate focal lesions. T2-W sequence (*A*) showed a hyperintense lesion adjacent to the gallbladder (*arrows*) with gradual postcontrast enhancement (*B*). Subtraction images of the portal venous phase (*C*) show misregistration artifact with the lesion seen in a different location from prior sequences. Accurately registered delayed phase subtraction image (*D*) identifies the enhancing lesion at the correct location.

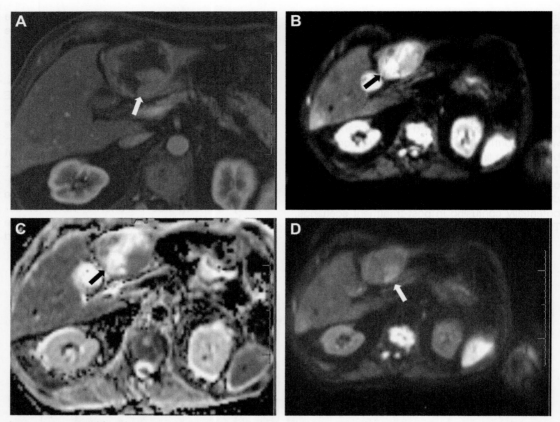

Fig. 4. A 79-year-old male with HCC. Postcontrast MR imaging (*A*) shows a peripherally enhancing mass (*white arrow*) with areas of central necrosis. DWI using B-50 images (*B*) shows high signal intensity of the central necrotic component (*black arrow*) with corresponding increased signal intensity on ADC map (*C*), consistent with T2 shine-through. A review of higher B-value DWI images (B-800) (*D*) shows low signal of the central necrotic component and diffusion restriction of the peripheral solid component (*white arrow*).

hemangiomas. These remain bright on long TE sequences.

PITFALLS RELATED TO METABOLIC CHANGES IN THE LIVER
Hepatic Steatosis–Related Pitfalls

Severe diffuse hepatic steatosis alters the signal characteristics of normal liver parenchyma (**Fig. 5**) and can obscure underlying focal hepatic lesions. In the setting of hepatic steatosis, on CT, focal lesions may become isointense to the liver. MR imaging is more sensitive than CT in detecting metastatic focal lesions in the setting of diffuse steatosis. This is assisted with the combination of in-phase/opposed-phase, DWI, and HBP imaging. Liver metastases can appear as hypointense to surrounding liver parenchyma on in-phase images and hyperintense to liver on the opposed-phase images due to severe drop in the signal of steatotic liver parenchyma.[33,34]

Nodular fat sparing can occur in the setting of diffuse hepatic steatosis. These can be misinterpreted as focal lesions or metastatic deposits. On MR imaging, they appear hyperintense relative to surrounding parenchyma on the T1 opposed-phase images. Focal fatty sparing can mimic a metastatic focal lesion and can lead to an overestimation of the lesion size. Assessment of the lesion on DWI or contrast-enhanced phases, especially HBP (if available), can aid in differentiation focal fat sparing from a true hepatic lesion.[35]

Focal steatosis is commonly encountered in cross-sectional imaging and can also mimic neoplastic processes when it accumulates in a nonuniform fashion. Focal fat can remain hypointense on HBP images thus simulating malignancy (**Fig. 6**). However, the degree of hypointensity is usually less than that of malignancy. Several other features can be used to confirm its benign nature, such as lack of diffusion restriction, drop in signal on chemical shift imaging, coursing vessels, and

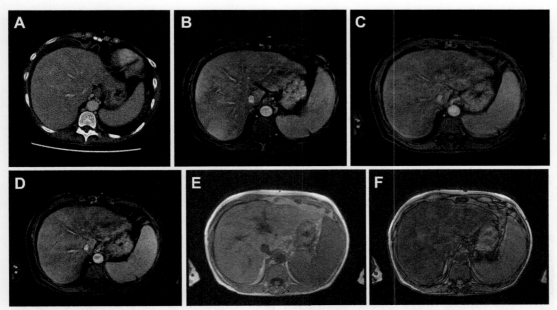

Fig. 5. A 64-year-old female with painless jaundice and elevated liver enzymes. Contrast-enhanced CT (*A*) showed diffuse narrowing of the hepatic veins and the intrahepatic IVC with perivenous hypoattenuating signal. Dynamic postcontrast MR imaging (*B–D*) showed a similar appearance of hepatic veins narrowing with surrounding low signal intensity and heterogeneous parenchymal enhancement. This appearance can mimic Budd–Chiari syndrome. In-phase (*E*) and opposed-phase (*F*) sequences demonstrated areas of signal intensity drop in opposed-phase images compared with in-phase images, consistent with the presence of hepatic steatosis. Liver biopsy later confirmed the diagnosis of steatohepatitis.

lack of mass effect.[36] Other patterns of steatosis such as geographic, subcapsular, perivascular, or nodular can, likewise, mimic other liver diseases and affect detection and characterization of focal liver lesions.[37] MR imaging with in-phase/opposed-phase imaging, DWI, and hepatobiliary contrast agents can be very useful in this context.

Iron Deposition–Related Pitfalls

Diffuse iron deposition in the setting of primary or secondary hemochromatosis results in alteration of normal parenchymal signal characteristics. This results in a signal loss in the setting of gradient-echo sequence and long TE series. For the in-phase/opposed-phase at 1.5 T magnet, a longer TE of 4.2 msec (in-phase) will result in signal loss compared with a TE of 2.1 msec (opposed-phase). T1 and T2 shortening occur because of the superparamagnetic properties of iron ions and results in loss of signal intensity of the affected organ proportional to the degree of iron deposition.[38] Nodular forms of iron deposition or sparing can be misinterpreted as focal hepatic lesions. The correct diagnosis can be reached by observing the signal characteristics on in-phase and opposed-phase images.

Focal metastatic lesions can erroneously mimic benign lesions in the setting of diffuse iron deposition. The liver parenchyma will demonstrate a diffuse decrease in T2 signal intensity, and a metastatic lesion can appear as T2 hyperintense relative to surrounding parenchyma even at long TE sequences, thus mimicking hemangiomas or cysts. Assessment of contrast-enhanced phases and DWI is essential for accurate diagnosis.

Nonuniform distribution of iron can be rarely identified and can mimic other diffuse infiltrative processes.[39] Iron can preferentially deposit surrounding the hepatic veins, thus giving the appearance of diffuse fatty change in the intervening liver parenchyma and perivenous fat sparing on CT (**Fig. 7**).

PITFALLS RELATED TO CIRRHOSIS AND CIRRHOSIS MIMICS

Cirrhosis is characterized pathologically with multiple regenerative nodules with surrounding fibrous tissue. It represents the end-stage disease of hepatic fibrosis and can be identified by multiple imaging criteria, including morphologic changes such as the nodular liver surface, signs of portal hypertension, atrophy of the right hepatic lobe,

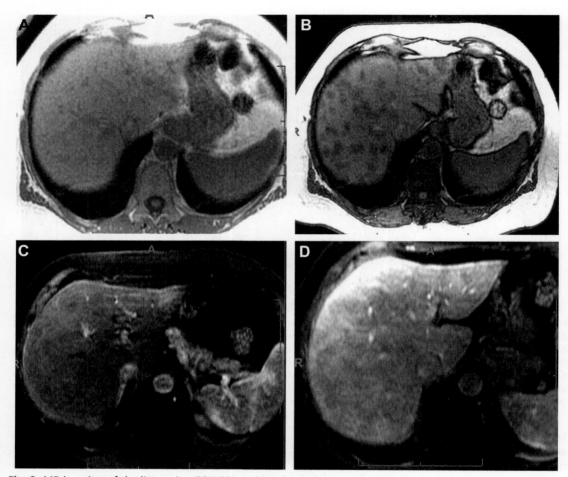

Fig. 6. MR imaging of the liver using EOVIST. In-phase (*A*) and opposed-phase (*B*) sequences demonstrate multifocal areas of drop in signal intensity on opposed-phase images consistent with focal steatosis. Transitional (*C*) and HBP (*D*) images show persistent hypointense signal of areas of focal steatosis. This appearance can mimic malignancy or mask the presence of a malignant lesion.

hypertrophy of caudate and left hepatic lobes, and expansion of gallbladder fossa. Noncirrhotic conditions can mimic cirrhosis and are therefore referred to as pseudocirrhosis. Awareness of the patient's history and recognition of pseudocirrhosis is important for accurate assessment of newly developed focal lesions.

Pseudocirrhosis has been described in patients with hepatic metastases who have been treated with chemotherapy. This leads to hepatic parenchymal distortion due to shrinkage of metastatic lesions and nodular regenerative hyperplasia due to chemotherapy-related hepatotoxic effects. Imaging findings include surface nodularity, segmental atrophy, and multifocal capsular retraction (**Fig. 8**). Accurate diagnosis depends on the clinical history and comparison to prior examination. In some patients, these findings have

resolved completely after the interruption of chemotherapy.[40]

Budd–Chiari syndrome characterized by hepatic venous obstruction not related to right heart strain can result in hepatic morphologic changes due to lobar redistribution that could be mistaken for cirrhosis. The affected segments will demonstrate atrophy with compensatory hypertrophy of the unaffected segments and caudate lobe. Enhancement pattern facilitates differentiation from cirrhosis as it is typically heterogeneous with delayed enhancement in the periphery and the tissues surrounding the hepatic veins.[41]

Chronic extrahepatic portal venous obstruction results in peripheral parenchymal atrophy with compensatory caudate and central hepatic hypertrophy. This can resemble cirrhosis but without the distinctive regenerative nodules, fibrosis, or

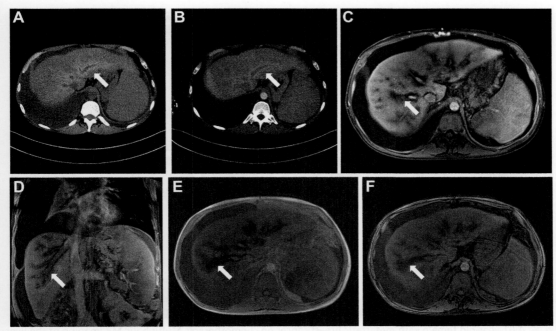

Fig. 7. A 25-year-old male presented with decompensated liver failure. Unenhanced CT (*A*) of the liver showed hypoattenuating parenchyma with perivenous sparing (*arrows*) that persisted on post-contrast phase (*B*). Axial (*C*) and coronal (*D*) postcontrast MR sequences showed hypointense signal surrounding the hepatic veins (*arrows*). In-phase sequence (*E*) showed increased perivenous signal drop (*arrows*) compared to opposed phase sequence (*F*). The intervening liver parenchyma did not demonstrate any significant drop in signal intensity on opposed phase images to suggest hepatic steatosis. This demonstrates an atypical pattern of iron deposition surrounding the hepatic veins and the patient was confirmed to have heterozygous hemochromatosis.

surface nodularity. Diagnosis depends on recognizing the direct signs of obstruction in addition to portal venous collaterals and mural calcifications, which suggest obstructive portal venopathy rather than cirrhosis.[42,43]

Confluent hepatic fibrosis is usually seen in patients with long-standing cirrhosis, particularly in the setting of alcoholic cirrhosis and biliary obstruction. It is characterized by peripheral parenchymal replacement by wedge-shaped thick fibrotic bands that cause overlying capsular retraction. In its early form, heterogeneous arterial phase hyperenhancement can be seen due to active inflammation and can mimic intrahepatic malignancies such as cholangiocarcinoma. On MR imaging, it demonstrates hypointense signal on T1-W sequences, mildly hyperintense signal on T2-W sequences, and progressive postcontrast enhancement on portal venous and delayed phases (**Fig. 9**). The typical appearance is wedge-shaped and extending from the porta hepatis to the liver capsule with progressive volume loss over time.[44]

MISINTERPRETED MALIGNANT LESIONS
Hypovascular Hepatocellular Carcinoma

Imaging plays a major role in the detection and diagnosis of HCC. The imaging diagnosis of HCC requires that an observation enhances in the late arterial phase of contrast administration. However, during the early phase of hepatocarcinogenesis, arterial supply is not sufficient to result in arterial phase hyperenhancement of approximately 10% to 20% of HCCs. Reviewing portal venous and delayed phases is important to recognize hypoenhancing masses that may represent early HCC (**Fig. 10**).[45,46] Regenerative and dysplastic nodules can also appear hypoenhancing on portal venous and delayed phases. LI-RADS was developed by the ACR to guide the characterization of liver lesions as HCC. LI-RADS does not depend only on arterial phase hyperenhancement as a major feature for HCC, it considers other features such as nonperipheral washout, enhancing capsule, and threshold growth.[47] If the observation is suspicious for hypovascular HCC, close monitoring or tissue sampling could confirm the diagnosis.

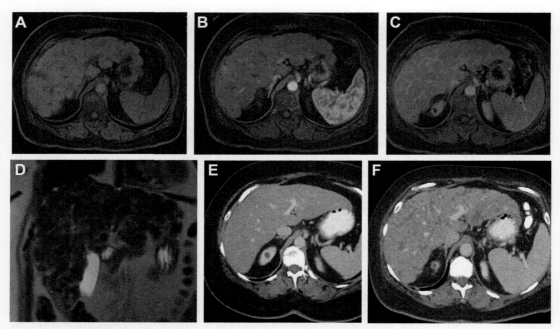

Fig. 8. A 61-year-old female with metastatic breast cancer on chemotherapy. Multiphasic MR imaging of the liver (*A–D*) shows nodular contour of the liver with heterogeneous enhancement pattern on the arterial (*B*) and delayed phases (*C*). A review of prior imaging shows no evidence of this nodular contour on a CT abdomen performed 1 year before the latest MR imaging (*E*). Another CT abdomen performed 8 months before the MR imaging shows milder contour nodularity (*F*). The comparison to prior examinations was essential in identifying the timeline of surface nodularity progression and, in addition to patient's history, helped correctly identify this as pseudocirrhosis.

Metastases with Atypical Enhancement

Hypovascular metastases are commonly encountered in the liver, originating in the breast, colon, pancreas, lung, or stomach. On MR imaging, they typically demonstrate hypointense signal on T1-W images and slightly hyperintense signal on T2-W images with hypoenhancement relative to surrounding liver parenchyma.[34] Some metastases exhibit delayed enhancement patterns due to contrast retention in fibrous and interstitial tissue. This can lead to misinterpretation as hemangioma. Clues to the accurate diagnosis include a history of primary malignancy, a continuous rim of enhancement, the lack of peripheral interrupted nodular enhancement with delayed filling, intermediate T2 signal intensity, and diffusion restriction.

Cystic Liver Metastases

The cystic appearance of liver metastases is rare. The cystic appearance can be due to necrosis, mucin overproduction, or as a response to treatment. Antiangiogenic therapy of some types of liver metastases can result in visualization of cystic lesions that were not appreciated before. On MR imaging, cystic metastases demonstrate hypointense signal on T1-W images and hyperintense

signal on T2-W sequences. They can be misinterpreted as simple or complex cysts.[48] Clues to the accurate diagnosis include clinical history, presence of enhancing septations, mural nodularity, and rim enhancement.

Coalescing Liver Metastases

Coalescing liver metastases present a diagnostic challenge because of the lack of normal background liver parenchyma for comparison. They can mimic diffuse steatosis or other diffuse liver diseases (**Fig. 11**). Clues to correct diagnosis are the presence of mass effect on blood vessels, contour nodularity, and capsular bulging in the absence of cirrhosis. On MR imaging, the liver may demonstrate increased T2 signal intensity without the typical decrease in signal intensity on opposed-phase images. Diffusion restriction is typically seen at higher b-value images unlike hepatic steatosis or cirrhosis.[33]

MISINTERPRETED BENIGN LESIONS
Hemangiomas Mimicking Hepatocellular Carcinoma

Hemangiomas are commonly seen in the liver. Typically, they demonstrate hypointense T1-W

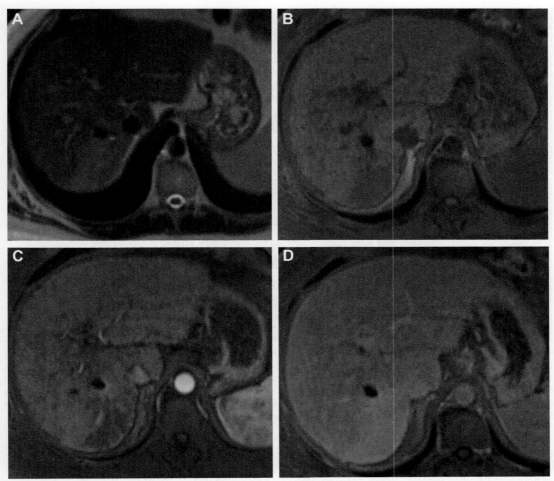

Fig. 9. A59-year-old patient with long-standing cirrhosis and prior TIPS procedure. Multiphasic MR imaging of the liver showed a segment VI peripheral wedge-shaped area of intermediate T2 signal (*A*), low T1 signal (*B*), and heterogeneous enhancement on the arterial phase (*C*). The lesion demonstrated progressive enhancement on venous and delayed phases (*D*). This lesion represents confluent hepatic fibrosis, and the heterogeneous arterial enhancement is attributed to active inflammation.

signal, intermediate T2-W signal between the CSF and spleen, and have progressive centripetal peripheral nodular interrupted enhancement. However, the rate of progressive enhancement is variable, and some hemangiomas can enhance completely by the time late arterial phase images are acquired, these are referred to as flash filling hemangiomas. This arterial hyperenhancement can be confused for HCC.[49] Clues to the accurate diagnosis include T2-W signal that is brighter than that of the spleen or HCC and persistent enhancement on the delayed phase similar to the blood pool.

As discussed earlier, hemangiomas may display pseudowashout on transitional and HBP imaging when using gadoxetate sodium, thus mimicking

HCC (see **Fig. 2**).[24] This pseudowashout appearance is more gradual compared with typical washout in HCC and the overall enhancement pattern will follow the blood pool.

Hemangiomas Mimicking Metastases

Sclerosed hemangiomas can mimic liver metastases. They have diverse enhancement patterns including no enhancement, heterogeneous enhancement, peripheral discontinuous, or continuous rim enhancement. On MR imaging, sclerosed hemangiomas may demonstrate decreased signal on T2-W images. Sclerosed hemangiomas with continuous rim enhancement can be misinterpreted as metastases and vice versa (**Fig. 12**).[50] Clues to accurate diagnosis of sclerosed

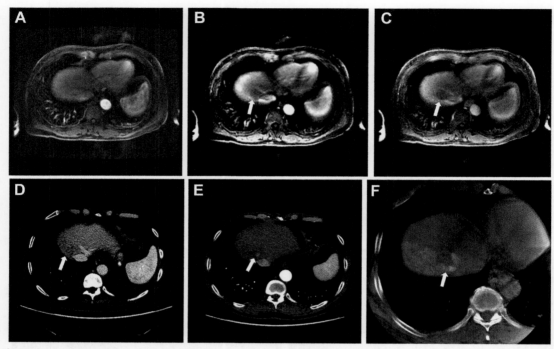

Fig. 10. A 66-year-old male with history of HCC. Multiphasic MRI of the liver showed no hyper-enhancing lesion on the arterial phase (*A*). On portal venous (*B*) and delayed (*C*) phases, a well-defined area of contrast washout is noted adjacent to the IVC (*arrows*). Follow-up CT after 3 months shows a hypo-enhancing mass (*arrow*) on arterial phase (*D*). Follow-up CT after 1-year shows development of focal arterial hyperenhancement (*arrow*) within the lesion (*E*). The lesion was managed as HCC and the patient underwent transarterial chemoembolization (*F*) that showed progressive enlargement of the arterially hyperenhancing component (*arrow*).

hemangioma include a progressive decrease in size over time, well-defined margins, and loss of previously enhancing regions. When encountering sclerosed hemangioma for the first time on imaging, it is prudent to recommend follow-up imaging or tissue biopsy, especially when there is a history of primary malignancy.[51]

Large Regenerative Nodules

Regenerative nodules typically develop in response to parenchymal damage and can be identified as masses on a background of the fibrotic liver. They are typically under 2 cm in size; however, giant nodules greater than 5 cm have been reported. On MR imaging, they appear hyperintense on T1-W images and iso or hypointense on T2-W images, unlike HCCs that classically appear moderately hyperintense on T2-W images. Subtraction images can only show true enhancement and are useful in differentiating between HCC and regenerative nodules.[52]

Siderotic Nodules

Siderotic nodules develop in the cirrhotic liver and represent cirrhosis-related nodules containing iron

molecules. On MR imaging, their appearance depends on the degree of iron accumulation and imaging parameters. Typically, they show decreased signal intensity on T2-W images and decreased signal intensity on gradient-echo sequences, which should not be misinterpreted as areas of washout.[53] They particularly standout on the in-phase sequence when compared with the opposed-phase sequence (**Fig. 13**).

Hepatic Radiation Injury

Radiation injury to the liver can result from radiation treatment to the liver, adjacent distal esophagus, lung bases, and pancreatic masses. Imaging changes are related to increased water content and fibrosis. On MR imaging, HBP imaging can show geographic hypoenhancement following the radiation contour during the HBP (**Fig. 14**).[54] Clues to the correct diagnosis include relevant clinical history, typical location within the radiation field, no mass effect on blood vessels, no diffusion restriction, and less conspicuous appearance on follow-up imaging.

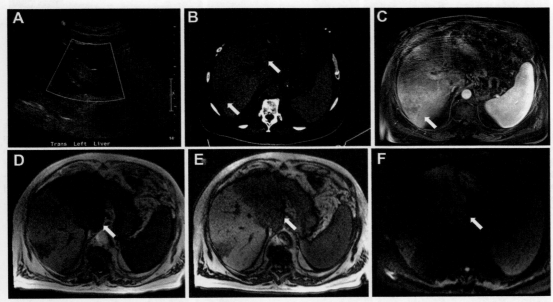

Fig. 11. A 78-year-old male presented with acute abdominal pain and elevated liver enzymes. Ultrasound (*A*) showed cirrhotic nodular liver morphology and perihepatic ascites. Unenhanced CT (*B*) showed geographic areas of hypoattenuation at the left and right hepatic lobes (*arrows*). MRI showed heterogeneous post contrast enhancement of the hepatic parenchyma (*arrow*) with motion artifact obscuring the left hepatic lobe (*C*). In-phase (*D*) and Opposed-phase (*E*) sequences showed low signal intensity of these geographic areas (*arrows*) involving the entirety of the left hepatic lobe (with no relative drop in signal between them) and a wedge-shaped area in the right hepatic lobe with restricted diffusion (*arrow*) on DWI sequence (*F*). Histopathological analysis demonstrated coalescing metastases from cholangiocarcinoma.

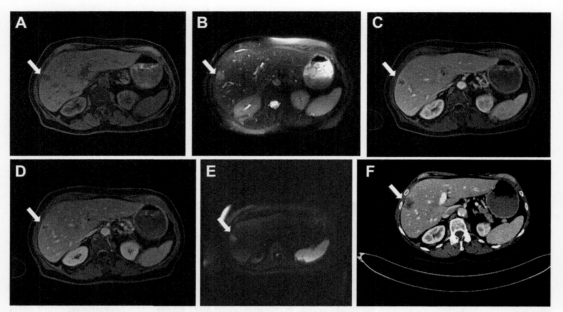

Fig. 12. A 70-year-old female with history of rectal cancer status post resection and chemoradiation. MRI of the liver was performed for evaluation of an indeterminate lesion detected on surveillance CT. It showed a 2 cm lesion at hepatic segment VIII (*arrows*) demonstrating T1 hypointense (*A*) and T2 intermediate signal (*B*). On post-contrast images, there is discontinuous peripheral enhancement (*arrow*) on the arterial phase (*C*) with progressive filling (*arrow*) on the delayed phase (*D*). This lesion was mistakenly characterized as sclerosed hemangioma despite the diffusion restriction (*arrow*) on DWI sequence (*E*). Follow up CT after 6 months (*F*) showed progressive enlargement and heterogenous enhancement pattern (*arrow*) worrisome for metastatic process. This lesion was biopsied and confirmed as metastatic adenocarcinoma.

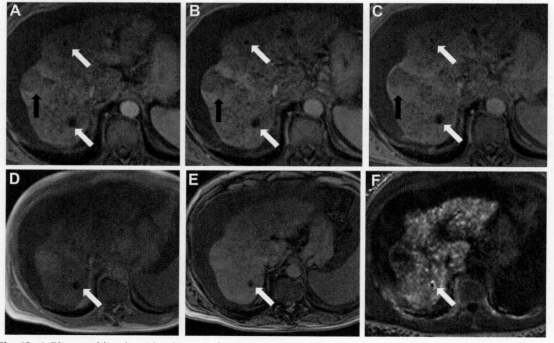

Fig. 13. A 70-year-old male with a history of HCC post–Y-90 radioembolization. Multiphasic MR imaging of the liver (*A–C*) shows numerous hypoenhancing focal lesions (*arrows*) and postradioembolization changes in segment VIII (*black arrow*). In-phase (*D*) and opposed-phase (*E*) show more prominent signal drop of these lesions on the in-phase sequence compared with opposed-phase sequence. R2* relaxometry (*F*) shows mild iron deposition within the dominant lesion in segment VII (*arrow*).

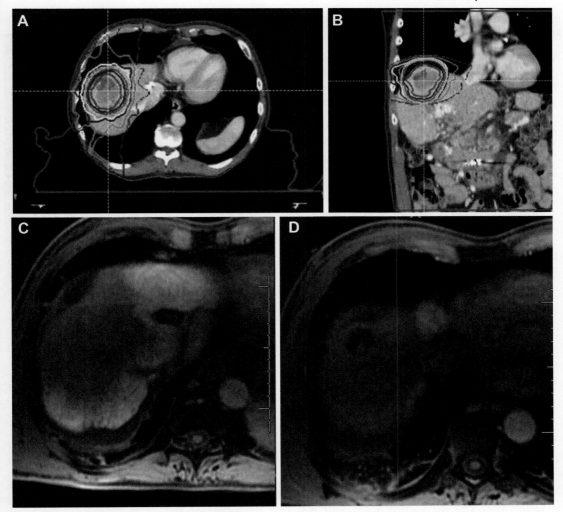

Fig. 14. A 68-year-old male status poststereotactic body radiation therapy to a hepatic dome HCC. Dose–volume histograms demonstrate the radiation field of the tumor (*A*, *B*). Post-treatment MR imaging using hepatobiliary contrast demonstrates diffuse parenchymal hypoenhancement surrounding the tumor on HBP (*C*, *D*) related to dysfunctional hepatocytes. This should be recognized on HBP as radiation-related changes and not to be confused with HCC recurrence.

SUMMARY

MR imaging of the liver is a powerful diagnostic tool that allows problem-solving indeterminate liver lesions. However, there are multiple technical artifacts and imaging pitfalls that are more pronounced in the chronically diseased liver. Knowledge and awareness of these pitfalls and artifacts and ways to mitigate them allow for more accurate and timely diagnosis.

CLINICS CARE POINTS

- Review of patient history and comparison to prior imaging and different imaging modalities help identify the correct pathology.

- Washout should be assessed only on the portal venous phase and not the hepatobiliary phase when using gadoxetate disodium, based on latest LI-RADS recommendations.
- Awareness of misregistration artifact on subtraction images is important to avoid mischaracterization of non-enhancing lesions.
- Reviewing portal venous and delayed phases is important to recognize hypoenhancing masses that may represent early or hypovascular HCC.

DISCLOSURE

The authors have nothing to disclose.

REFERENCES

1. Mathew RP, Venkatesh SK. Liver vascular anatomy: a refresher. Abdom Radiol 2018;43(8):1886–95.
2. Michels NA. Newer anatomy of the liver and its variant blood supply and collateral circulation. Am J Surg 1966;112(3):337–47.
3. Chernyak V, Fowler KJ, San UC, Claude D, Sirlin B. LI-RADS ® V2018 CT/MRI Manual Liver Anatomy Primary Author Contributing Authors. Available at: https://www.acr.org/-/media/ACR/Files/Clinical-Resources/LIRADS/Chapter-3–Liver-anatomy.pdf?la=en&hash=D98B467FF0340372D3B3501B0149B291.
4. Germain T, Favelier S, Cercueil JP, et al. Liver segmentation: Practical tips. Diagn Interv Imaging 2014;95(11):1003–16.
5. Botero AC, Strasberg SM. Division of the left hemiliver in man - Segments, sectors, or sections. Liver Transpl Surg 1998. https://doi.org/10.1002/lt.500040307.
6. Guiu B, Bize P, Gunthern D, et al. Portal vein embolization before right hepatectomy: Improved results using n-butyl-cyanoacrylate compared to microparticles plus coils. Cardiovasc Intervent Radiol 2013. https://doi.org/10.1007/s00270-013-0565-7.
7. LeBedis C, Luna A, Soto JA. Use of magnetic resonance imaging contrast agents in the liver and biliary tract. Magn Reson Imaging Clin N Am 2012. https://doi.org/10.1016/j.mric.2012.07.006.
8. Thian YL, Riddell AM, Koh DM. Liver-specific agents for contrast-enhanced MRI: Role in oncological imaging. Cancer Imaging 2013. https://doi.org/10.1102/1470-7330.2013.0050.
9. Curtis WA, Fraum TJ, An H, et al. Quantitative MRI of Diffuse Liver Disease: Current Applications and Future Directions. Radiology 2019;290(1):23–30.
10. Reeder SB, Cruite I, Hamilton G, et al. Quantitative assessment of liver fat with magnetic resonance imaging and spectroscopy. J Magn Reson Imaging 2011. https://doi.org/10.1002/jmri.22580.
11. Venkatesh SK, Yin M, Ehman RL. Magnetic resonance elastography of liver: Technique, analysis, and clinical applications. J Magn Reson Imaging 2013. https://doi.org/10.1002/jmri.23731.
12. Sirlin CB, Reeder SB. Magnetic resonance imaging quantification of liver iron. Magn Reson Imaging Clin N Am 2010. https://doi.org/10.1016/j.mric.2010.08.014.
13. Yoo JL, Lee CH, Park YS, et al. The short breath-hold technique, controlled aliasing in parallel imaging results in higher acceleration, can be the first step to overcoming a degraded hepatic arterial phase in liver magnetic resonance imaging: A prospective randomized control study. Invest Radiol 2016. https://doi.org/10.1097/RLI.0000000000000249.
14. Ogawa M, Kawai T, Kan H, et al. Shortened breath-hold contrast-enhanced MRI of the liver using a new parallel imaging technique, CAIPIRINHA (controlled aliasing in parallel imaging results in higher acceleration): a comparison with conventional GRAPPA technique. Abdom Imaging 2015;40(8):3091–8.
15. Inoue Y, Hata H, Nakajima A, et al. Optimal techniques for magnetic resonance imaging of the liver using a respiratory navigator-gated three-dimensional spoiled gradient-recalled echo sequence. Magn Reson Imaging 2014. https://doi.org/10.1016/j.mri.2014.05.013.
16. Ogasawara G, Inoue Y, Matsunaga K, et al. Evaluation of a respiratory navigator-gating technique in Gd-EOB-DTPA-enhanced magnetic resonance imaging for the assessment of liver tumors. Eur J Radiol 2016. https://doi.org/10.1016/j.ejrad.2016.04.003.
17. Azevedo RM, de Campos ROP, Ramalho M, et al. Free-Breathing 3D T1-Weighted Gradient-Echo Sequence With Radial Data Sampling in Abdominal MRI: Preliminary Observations. Am J Roentgenol 2011;197(3):650–7.
18. Reiner CS, Neville AM, Nazeer HK, et al. Contrast-enhanced free-breathing 3D T1-weighted gradient-echo sequence for hepatobiliary MRI in patients with breath-holding difficulties. Eur Radiol 2013;23(11):3087–93.
19. Yacoub JH, Elsayes KM, Fowler KJ, et al. Pitfalls in liver MRI: Technical approach to avoiding misdiagnosis and improving image quality. J Magn Reson Imaging 2019;49(1):41–58.
20. Hussain HK, Londy FJ, Francis IR, et al. Hepatic arterial phase MR imaging with automated bolus-detection three-dimensional fast gradient-recalled-echo sequence: Comparison with test-bolus method. Radiology 2003. https://doi.org/10.1148/radiol.2262011593.
21. Ikram NS, Yee J, Weinstein S, et al. Multiple arterial phase MRI of arterial hypervascular hepatic lesions: improved arterial phase capture and lesion enhancement. Abdom Radiol 2017;42(3):870–6.
22. Polanec SH, Bickel H, Baltzer PAT, et al. Respiratory motion artifacts during arterial phase imaging with gadoxetic acid: Can the injection protocol minimize this drawback? J Magn Reson Imaging 2017. https://doi.org/10.1002/jmri.25657.
23. Pietryga JA, Burke LMB, Marin D, et al. Respiratory motion artifact affecting hepatic arterial phase imaging with gadoxetate disodium: Examination recovery with a multiple arterial phase acquisition. Radiology 2014;271(2):426–34.
24. Doo KW, Lee CH, Choi JW, et al. "Pseudo washout" sign in high-flow hepatic hemangioma on gadoxetic acid contrast-enhanced mri mimicking hypervascular tumor. Am J Roentgenol 2009;193(6). https://doi.org/10.2214/AJR.08.1732.
25. Tang A, Bashir MR, Corwin MT, et al. Evidence supporting LI-RADS major features for CT- and MR imaging-based diagnosis of hepatocellular

carcinoma: A systematic review. Radiology 2018. https://doi.org/10.1148/radiol.2017170554.

26. Verloh N, Haimerl M, Rennert J, et al. Impact of liver cirrhosis on liver enhancement at Gd-EOB-DTPA enhanced MRI at 3 tesla. Eur J Radiol 2013. https://doi.org/10.1016/j.ejrad.2013.05.033.

27. Kanki A, Tamada T, Higaki A, et al. Hepatic parenchymal enhancement at Gd-EOB-DTPA-enhanced MR imaging: Correlation with morphological grading of severity in cirrhosis and chronic hepatitis. Magn Reson Imaging 2012. https://doi.org/10.1016/j.mri.2011.11.002.

28. CT/MRI LI-RADS v2018 | American College of Radiology. Available at: https://www.acr.org/Clinical-Resources/Reporting-and-Data-Systems/LI-RADS/CT-MRI-LI-RADS-v2018. Accessed March 19, 2021.

29. Liang M, Zhao J, Xie B, et al. MR liver imaging with Gd-EOB-DTPA: The need for different delay times of the hepatobiliary phase in patients with different liver function. Eur J Radiol 2016. https://doi.org/10.1016/j.ejrad.2015.12.015.

30. An C, Rhee H, Han K, et al. Added value of smooth hypointense rim in the hepatobiliary phase of gadoxetic acid-enhanced MRI in identifying tumour capsule and diagnosing hepatocellular carcinoma. Eur Radiol 2017;27(6):2610–8.

31. Taouli B, Koh DM. Diffusion-weighted MR imaging of the liver. Radiology 2010. https://doi.org/10.1148/radiol.09090021.

32. Lall C, Bura V, Lee TK, et al. Diffusion-weighted imaging in hemorrhagic abdominal and pelvic lesions: restricted diffusion can mimic malignancy. Abdom Radiol 2018. https://doi.org/10.1007/s00261-017-1366-2.

33. Kanematsu M, Kondo H, Goshima S, et al. Imaging liver metastases: Review and update. Eur J Radiol 2006;58(2):217–28.

34. Sica GT, Ji H, Ros PR. CT and MR Imaging of Hepatic Metastases. Am J Roentgenol 2000;174(3):691–8.

35. Elsayes KM, Shaaban AM. Specialty imaging: pitfalls and classic signs of the abdomen and Pelvis E-Book. Amsterdam (Netherlands): Elsevier Health Sciences; 2014. Available at: https://books.google.com/books?id=0yIVCwAAQBAJ.

36. Rinella ME, McCarthy R, Thakrar K, et al. Dual-echo, chemical shift gradient-echo magnetic resonance imaging to quantify hepatic steatosis: Implications for living liver donation. Liver Transpl 2003;9(8):851–6.

37. Venkatesh SK, Hennedige T, Johnson GB, et al. Imaging patterns and focal lesions in fatty liver: a pictorial review. Abdom Radiol 2017;42(5):1374–92.

38. Queiroz-Andrade M, Blasbalg R, Ortega CD, et al. MR imaging findings of iron overload. Radiographics 2009;29(6):1575–89.

39. Horowitz JM, Nikolaidis P, Chen ZME, et al. Iron deposition surrounding the hepatic veins of cirrhotic patients on MRI. J Magn Reson Imaging 2011;33(3):598–602.

40. Kang SP, Taddei T, McLennan B, et al. Pseudocirrhosis in a pancreatic cancer patient with liver metastases: A case report of complete resolution of pseudocirrhosis with an early recognition and management. World J Gastroenterol 2008. https://doi.org/10.3748/wjg.14.1622.

41. Buckley O, O'Brien J, Snow A, et al. Imaging of Budd-Chiari syndrome. Eur Radiol 2007. https://doi.org/10.1007/s00330-006-0537-2.

42. Glatard AS, Hillaire S, D'Assignies G, et al. Obliterative portal venopathy: Findings at CT imaging. Radiology 2012;263(3):741–50.

43. Vilgrain V, Lagadec M, Ronot M. Pitfalls in liver imaging. Radiology 2016;278(1):34–51.

44. Brancatelli G, Baron RL, Federle MP, et al. Focal confluent fibrosis in cirrhotic liver: Natural history studied with serial CT. Am J Roentgenol 2009. https://doi.org/10.2214/AJR.07.2782.

45. Takayasu K, Arii S, Sakamoto M, et al. Clinical implication of hypovascular hepatocellular carcinoma studied in 4,474 patients with solitary tumour equal or less than 3 cm. Liver Int 2013. https://doi.org/10.1111/liv.12130.

46. Hanna RF, Aguirre DA, Kased N, et al. Cirrhosis-associated Hepatocellular Nodules: Correlation of Histopathologic and MR Imaging Features. Radio-Graphics 2008;28(3):747–69.

47. Elsayes KM, Kielar AZ, Chernyak V, et al. p>LI-RADS: a conceptual and historical review from its beginning to its recent integration into AASLD clinical practice guidance</p>. J Hepatocell Carcinoma 2019;6:49–69.

48. Del Poggio P, Buonocore M, Méndez-Sánchez N. Cystic tumors of the liver: A practical approach. World J Gastroenterol 2008;21(1423):3616–20.

49. Elsayes KM, Chernyak V, Morshid AI, et al. Spectrum of pitfalls, pseudolesions, and potential misdiagnoses in cirrhosis. Am J Roentgenol 2018;211(1):87–96.

50. Cheng HC, Tsai SH, Chiang JH, et al. Hyalinized liver hemangioma mimicking malignant tumor at MR imaging. Am J Roentgenol 1995;165(4):1016–7.

51. Elsayes KM, Menias CO, Morshid AI, et al. Spectrum of pitfalls, pseudolesions, and misdiagnoses in non-cirrhotic liver. Am J Roentgenol 2018;211(1). https://doi.org/10.2214/AJR.18.19820.

52. Hussain SM, Zondervan PE, Ijzermans JNM, et al. Benign versus malignant hepatic nodules: MR imaging findings with pathologic correlation. Radiographics 2002. https://doi.org/10.1148/radiographics.22.5.g02se061023.

53. Brancatelli G, Federle MP, Ambrosini R, et al. Cirrhosis: CT and MR imaging evaluation. Eur J Radiol 2007;61(1):57–69.

54. Seidensticker M, Seidensticker R, Mohnike K, et al. Quantitative in vivo assessment of radiation injury of the liver using Gd-EOB-DTPA enhanced MRI: tolerance dose of small liver volumes. Radiat Oncol 2011;6(1):40.

Magnetic Resonance Imaging of Liver Transplant

Roberto Cannella, MD[a,b], Anil Dasyam, MD[c], Frank H. Miller, MD[d],
Amir A. Borhani, MD[c,d],*

KEYWORDS

- Liver transplantation • Living liver donor transplantation • Orthotopic liver transplantation
- Magnetic resonance imaging • Complications

KEY POINTS

- Understanding different surgical techniques and normal postoperative anatomy is crucial for radiologic evaluation of liver transplant.
- Contrast-enhanced MR angiography has similar accuracy to Doppler ultrasound for diagnosis of vascular complications.
- Hepatic artery thrombosis, if not treated, can rapidly progress to biliary ischemia and necrosis, manifesting as multifocal nonanastomotic biliary strictures and intrahepatic bilomas.
- MR with administration of hepatobiliary contrast agent improves the sensitivity for the diagnosis of biliary leaks and allows for direct visualization of active leak.
- Recurrent hepatocellular carcinoma and post-transplant lymphoproliferative disorder should be considered in the differential diagnosis of post-transplant liver masses.

INTRODUCTION

Liver transplantation (LT) is the curative treatment of choice for patients with end-stage liver disease, fulminant liver failure, and early-stage hepatocellular carcinoma (HCC), with expanding indications for other liver malignancies in select candidates.[1] Given the shortage of cadaveric allografts, constantly increasing demand, and regional/national restrictions for organ allocation, there has been increased interest in use of living liver donors in past decade. According to the Organ Procurement and Transplantation Network (OPTN), 8896 LTs were performed in the United States in 2019, comprising 8372 deceased donor and 524 living donor LTs (LDLTs).[2] The survival rates for both techniques remain high, with 1-year, 3-year, and 5-year survival rates of 91.2%, 82.8%, and 75.1%, respectively, for deceased donor LTs, and 92.3%, 88.4%, and 87.4%, respectively, for LDLTs.[2]

Complications post-LT usually have silent or nonspecific clinical presentation. Imaging plays a pivotal role for early detection of these

[a] Section of Radiology - Department of Biomedicine, Neuroscience and Advanced Diagnostics (BiND), University Hospital "Paolo Giaccone", Via del Vespro 129, Palermo 90127, Italy; [b] Department of Health Promotion, Mother and Child Care, Internal Medicine and Medical Specialties (PROMISE), University of Palermo, Via del Vespro, 129, Palermo 90127, Italy; [c] Department of Radiology, Abdominal Imaging Division, University of Pittsburgh School of Medicine, 200 Lothrop Street, UPMC Presbyterian Suite 200, Pittsburgh, PA 15213, USA; [d] Department of Radiology, Body Imaging Section, Northwestern University Feinberg School of Medicine, 676 N Saint Clair Street, Chicago, IL 60611, USA
* Corresponding author. Northwestern University Feinberg School of Medicine, 676 N Saint Clair Street, Arkes Pavillion, Suite 800, Chicago, IL 60611.
E-mail address: Amir.Borhani@northwestern.edu

Magn Reson Imaging Clin N Am 29 (2021) 437–450
https://doi.org/10.1016/j.mric.2021.05.010
1064-9689/21/© 2021 Elsevier Inc. All rights reserved.

Liver Transplantation: Anatomy Deceased Donor

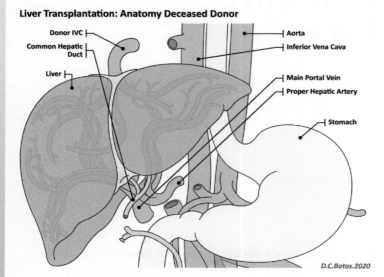

Fig. 1. Schematic illustration showing usual anastomoses in setting of deceased donor LT. (Courtesy of Mr David Botos (dcb.radiology@northwestern.edu))

complications in order to preserve graft function and to minimize morbidity and mortality. MR imaging increasingly is utilized for these indications due to its superior contrast resolution and capability of studying vascular, parenchymal, and biliary structures in a single setting. Knowledge of the surgical techniques and familiarity with the spectrum of complications after LT are of upmost importance when interpreting these studies.

This article reviews normal postoperative anatomy and discusses the role of MR imaging in the postoperative assessment of liver transplant and its complications.

SURGICAL TECHNIQUES AND POSTSURGICAL ANATOMY
Deceased Donor Liver Transplantation

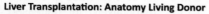

Deceased donor LT currently is the most performed liver transplant procedure in the United States and worldwide. In adult patients, the entire donor liver is implanted. Four anastomoses typically are arranged for reconstruction of hepatic artery, portal vein, venous outflow, and biliary system (**Fig. 1**).[3]

The hepatic artery anastomosis usually is done in an end-to-end fashion, most commonly

Liver Transplantation: Anatomy Living Donor

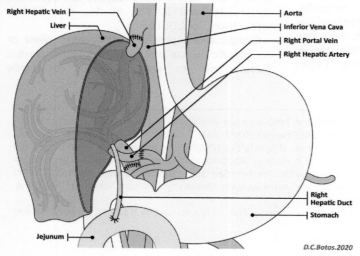

Fig. 2. Schematic illustration showing usual anastomoses in setting of right lobe LDLT. (Courtesy of Mr David Botos (dcb.radiology@northwestern.edu))

between the common hepatic artery of the donor and the proper hepatic artery of the recipient.[4,5] Vascular reconstruction or arterial grafts may be necessary in cases of variant vascular anatomy or underlying abnormalities of the vessels.[6] The portal vein anastomosis typically is done in an end-to-end fashion between the donor and recipient main portal veins. In patients with extensive portal vein thrombosis, an interposition graft can be used between the donor main portal vein and the recipient superior mesenteric vein.[3,5,6] The outflow reconstruction usually is done using the piggyback technique in which the donor inferior vena cave (IVC) is anastomosed with the common stump of recipient hepatic veins[4,5]—this technique is preferred because it does not require interruption of flow through donor IVC during the surgery.[7] Outflow anastomosis also can be performed with the conventional bicaval technique, in which the retrohepatic IVC of the recipient is removed and exchanged for the retrohepatic IVC of the donor in an end-to-end fashion.[4,5]

Biliary reconstruction usually is done via an end-to-end duct-to-duct anastomosis between the donor and the recipient extrahepatic ducts (choledochocholedochostomy), avoiding additional intestinal surgery and preserving the sphincter of Oddi function to minimize enteric reflux into the biliary system.[3] Both donor and recipient gallbladders, if present, are removed. In selected patients with underlying biliary pathologies (such as primary sclerosing cholangitis or biliary atresia) or unfavorable anatomy (such as short extrahepatic duct), the donor common bile duct or common hepatic duct is anastomosed with a loop of jejunum (choledochojejunostomy), typically performed in Roux-en-Y fashion.[3,4]

Living Donor Liver Transplantation

LDLT is a complex procedure in which the liver of a healthy subject is divided anatomically. A part of the donor's liver then serves as the allograft and is implanted. The surgical approach and selection process of which part of the liver to be harvested are influenced by size/age of the recipient, donor vascular/biliary anatomy, and multiple other donor-related and recipient-related factors. The right lobe is the preferred lobe to harvest in adult LDLT, allowing a larger graft volume.[8] The left lobe or the left lateral segment typically is used for pediatric LDLTs due to the smaller size.[9] Despite technical complexity and potential risks to the healthy donor, there are several advantages to this technique, including reduce in waiting time and associated mortality in patients with nonprioritized conditions, improved preprocedural planning, improved graft selection, and more robust and wider inclusion of patients who otherwise would not be candidates, or prioritized, for deceased donor LT.[10]

For right lobe LDLT, the liver is transected along Cantlie line, the vertical oblique plane across the gallbladder fossa coursing 1 cm posterior to the middle hepatic veins (**Fig. 2**).[11] Right portal vein, right hepatic artery, and right hepatic vein are transected and anastomosed with the recipient main portal vain, main hepatic artery, and IVC, respectively. Anatomic variants in the donor affect the number and type of vascular anastomoses that may be observed on postoperative MR imaging. Biliary anastomosis is performed either via duct-to-duct anastomosis or via choledochojejunostomy, depending on the surgeon's preference and underlying biliary anatomy. Depending on

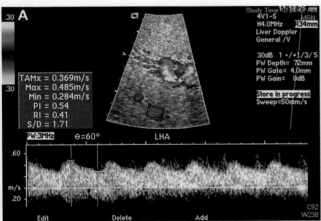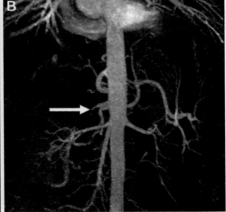

Fig. 3. (*A*) Spectral Doppler in a 57-year-old man with history of orthotopic LT 10 months earlier shows dampening of arterial waveforms with diminished resistive indices. (*B*) Frontal maximum intensity projection from subsequent MR angiography showed abrupt cutoff of proper hepatic artery (*arrow*) consistent with occlusive thrombosis. Subsequent catheter angiography confirmed the finding (not shown).

the branching pattern of donor biliary tree, 1 or more biliary anastomoses may be created.[9]

The plane of resection for harvesting left lobe graft is anterior to the middle hepatic vein.[12] The exact location of resection plane is dictated by what is deemed to be the safest and by recipient's size (in cases of pediatric recipients).[13] A transumbilical approach, with resection along the fissure for ligamentum teres, is used in cases of left lateral segment LDLT.[12,14]

VASCULAR COMPLICATIONS

Vascular complications occur in 7% to 13% of transplant recipients.[15] They range from minor clinically inconsequential complications to devastating ones resulting in graft failure and subsequent morbidity and mortality. Imaging plays a crucial role in diagnosis of vascular complications, due to lack of specific clinical and laboratory markers. In many instances, patients are asymptomatic with no clinical or laboratory abnormalities. Doppler ultrasound is the first-line imaging modality for assessment of vascular patency. Spectral Doppler allows for evaluation of flow dynamics and waveforms in major vessels, which helps with early detection of vascular stenosis.[15–19] In many institutions, Doppler ultrasound is performed routinely in immediate and early postoperative settings to screen for, and to exclude, early vascular complications. Contrast-enhanced computed tomography (CT) and MR imaging are

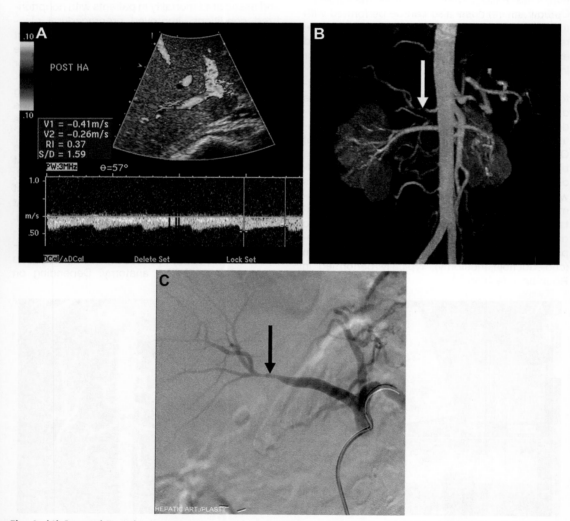

Fig. 4. (*A*) Spectral Doppler in a 30-year-old man with history of right lobe LDLT 4 months earlier shows dampening of arterial waveforms with markedly diminished resistive indices. (*B*) Frontal maximum intensity projection from MR angiography showed severe narrowing at the level of arterial anastomosis (*arrow*). (*C*) Subsequent catheter angiography confirmed the hepatic artery stenosis (*arrow*). Patient underwent angioplasty.

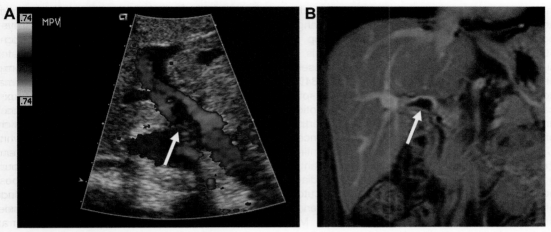

Fig. 5. (A) Color Doppler in a patient with history of orthotopic LT shows nonocclusive thrombus (*arrow*) in main portal vein. (B) Coronal contrast-enhanced T1-weighted MR image on portal venous phase depicts the thrombus (*arrow*) in the postanastomotic main portal vein.

performed as second-line tests to confirm and better delineate the vascular abnormalities detected by ultrasound and to evaluate for associated parenchymal or biliary complications.[19]

Hepatic Artery Complications

Arterial complications include hepatic artery stenosis, thrombosis, and pseudoaneurysm formation. Hepatic artery occlusive thrombosis is the most feared complication, accounting for approximately 50% of all arterial complications, and affects 4% to 12% of transplanted patients.[20,21] The hepatic artery is the sole blood supply of

biliary epithelium in the transplanted liver.[22] Hepatic artery thrombosis quickly can lead to biliary ischemia and necrosis, manifesting as nonanastomotic biliary strictures and intrahepatic bilomas, which can lead to graft failure.[22] Early recognition of hepatic artery thrombosis, therefore, is of upmost importance and may allow salvage of graft. Management includes endovascular treatments (thrombectomy and stenting), re-exploration, and/or arterial reconstruction.[21] Several surgical and nonsurgical risk factors can attribute to hepatic artery thrombosis. Those include acute rejection, prolonged cold ischemic time, differences in caliber of donor and recipient arteries, blood type

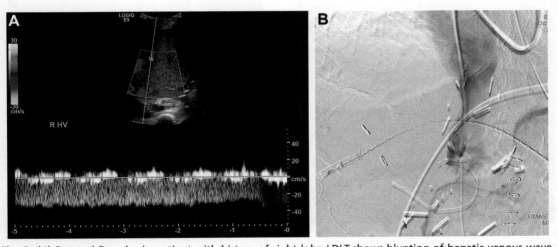

Fig. 6. (A) Spectral Doppler in patient with history of right lobe LDLT shows blunting of hepatic venous waveforms with loss of phasicity. (B) Frontal projection from subsequent catheter cavogram showed severe narrowing at the level of retrohepatic IVC and piggyback anastomosis. Note nonopacification of hepatic vein and lower IVC during the cavogram.

incompatibility, and recipient preexisting vascular abnormalities.[23–25] Contrast-enhanced MR angiography has been shown to have high (up to 100%) sensitivity for detection of thrombosis or significant stenosis of major allograft vessels, although the specificity is lower (74%–84%) compared with CT.[26,27] Quality of MR angiography can be affected by patient-related factors (motion and body habitus), pulse sequence, and expertise of the facility in MR imaging. Contrast-enhanced CT angiography may be performed to confirm the arterial thrombosis whereas conventional angiography remains the reference standard for diagnosing arterial complications.[19,28] Abrupt cutoff of the hepatic artery observed on early arterial-phase MR imaging or contrast-enhanced MR angiography is suggestive of hepatic artery thrombosis (**Fig. 3**).[19,26]

Hepatic artery stenosis is the second most common vascular complications, reported in 5% to 11% of all transplant recipients.[29] Hepatic artery stenosis usually manifests within the first 3 months after LT at the site of arterial anastomosis and may progress to hepatic artery thrombosis, if untreated.[22] Stricture can be appreciated on MR angiography and arterial-phase MR images as a focal area of luminal narrowing (**Fig. 4**).[30] MR imaging, however, has lower sensitivity for detection of mild-to-moderate stenosis compared with more severe stenosis. There is a possibility of overestimation of degree of stenosis, due to slow flow, and false positivity by susceptibility artifacts from surgical clips.[26–28,31] In select cases, when vascular findings are equivocal, further confirmation with CT angiography or conventional angiography may be considered.

Hepatic artery pseudoaneurysm is an uncommon, but potentially life-threating complication due to its high risk of rupture, occurring in approximately 2% of transplanted patients.[32] Pseudoaneurysms could be a complication of prior arterial interventions or could be mycotic in origin.[33] The anastomosis site is the most common location. MR imaging shows a T1-hypointense and T2-hypointense rounded structure abutting the hepatic artery, with enhancement pattern paralleling that of arteries.[18,23] MR imaging has lower sensitivity for detection of small pseudoaneurysms, due to its inherently inferior spatial resolution compared to CT and angiography.

Portal Vein Complications

Complications related to the portal veins, which include thrombosis and stenosis, are uncommon (1%–2% of all LTs).[21] Portal vein thrombosis, most commonly originating in the extrahepatic portal vein, is attributed to slow flow, pretransplant portomesenteric venous thrombosis, and hypercoagulable states.[24] On MR imaging, acute-phase bland portal vein thrombosis usually has high signal on T1-weighted and T2-weighted images.[34] Postcontrast MR images are highly accurate for the detection of portal vein thrombosis.[19]

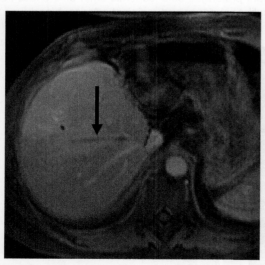

Fig. 7. Axial contrast-enhanced T1-weighted MR images on portal venous phase in a patient with history of right LDLT shows thrombosis of a branch of right hepatic vein (*arrow*) with associated perfusion abnormality.

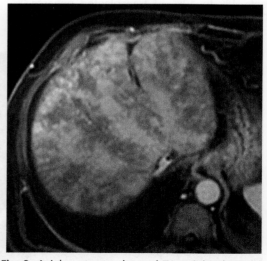

Fig. 8. Axial contrast-enhanced T1-weighted MR image on portal venous phase in a patient with history of orthotopic LT shows markedly heterogenous enhancement of liver parenchyma. Major allograft vessels were patent. Subsequent transjugular biopsy showed sinusoidal obstruction.

Bland thrombus appears as a nonenhancing filling defect in the vein on portal venous and delayed phases (**Fig. 5**). Balanced steady-state free precession imaging also may be helpful, especially in patients who cannot receive contrast material. Chronic portal vein thrombosis may be associated with development of collateral vessels and cavernous transformation of the portal vein.[23]

Portal vein stenosis is characterized by severe reduction of the portal vein caliber at the level of the anastomosis. Effect of this narrowing on flow dynamics, and hence its clinical significance, is better evaluated by Doppler ultrasound. Apparent narrowing at the level of venous anastomosis commonly is encountered in cases of discrepancy between size of the donor and recipient portal veins.[18] This phenomenon is more common in LDLT.

Inferior Vena Cava, Hepatic Vein, and Other Outflow Complications

IVC and hepatic veins complications are rare, accounting for fewer than 2% of patients.[28] These complications include stenosis at the anastomotic levels and thrombosis of the hepatic veins or IVC (**Fig. 6**). Type of outflow reconstruction, mismatch between the donor and recipient vessels, LDLT, and presence of large perihepatic collections are considered risk factors for IVC complications.[35] MR imaging findings of thrombosis include lack of contrast enhancement in the hepatic veins (**Fig. 7**) or IVC with associated congestion and heterogeneous (mosaic pattern) enhancement of the hepatic parenchyma during portal venous and delayed phases.[23,30,36] Outflow obstruction may happen at the level of sinusoids and postsinusoidal venules, as a consequence of rejection, resulting in sinusoidal obstruction syndrome. MR imaging shows mosaic enhancement of liver on postcontrast phases and heterogeneous parenchymal signal on T2-weighted imaging (**Fig. 8**).

BILIARY COMPLICATIONS

Biliary complications are the most frequent complications after LT, accounting for approximately 14% to 30% of patients, and are major causes of graft dysfunction and morbidity.[37,38] They include strictures, bile leaks, bilomas, biliary ischemia, stone/cast formation, recurrent cholangiopathy, and infections. Surgical technique, prior stent placement, hepatic artery thrombosis, and infections are major known risk factors associated with biliary complications.[38] Clinical and laboratory markers often are nonspecific, which hinders prompt diagnosis. MR imaging, including MR cholangiopancreatography (MRCP), is the most accurate noninvasive methods for the assessment of the biliary system.[19,38,39] MRCP is based on multiplanar acquisition of heavily T2-weighted (fluid-sensitive) sequences allowing accurate visualization of the biliary tree and assessment of complications.[37] Administration of hepatobiliary contrast agents may be helpful when evaluation of the biliary system is required. Gadoxetate disodium (trade names Eovist and Primovist; Bayer HealthCare, Whippany, New Jersey), which currently is the most commonly used hepatobiliary agent, has 50% hepatic uptake and excretion into the biliary system, which allows acquiring hepatobiliary images (approximately 20 minutes following administration of contrast). Contrast-filled bile ducts, during hepatobiliary phase, appear markedly hyperintense on T1-weighted images. In patients with impaired liver function and biliary obstruction, longer delay time may be needed to achieve hepatobiliary phase. Extracellular contrast agents are preferred, however, over hepatobiliary agents for vascular (especially arterial) imaging, due to lower contrast volume and high incidence of transient respiratory motion with the latter.[40] In the authors' opinion, the choice of contrast agent should be an active decision based on the indication and specifics of the individual patient.

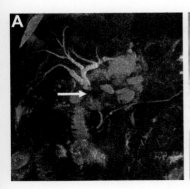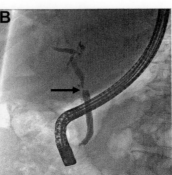

Fig. 9. (*A*) Coronal maximum intensity projection from 3-dimensional MRCP in a 60-year-old man with history of orthotopic LT 1 week earlier shows marked narrowing at the level of duct-to-duct biliary anastomosis (*arrow*), with associated intrahepatic biliary ductal dilatation. (*B*) Coronal projection from endoscopic retrograde cholangiography confirmed the stricture (*arrow*). Patient underwent balloon dilatation and stenting.

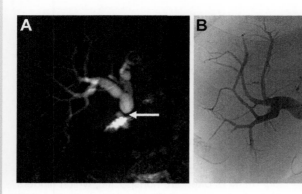

Fig. 10. (*A*) Coronal thick-slab 2-dimensional MR cholangiography in a 57-year-old man with history of orthotopic LT 10 months earlier shows marked narrowing at the level of biliary-enteric anastomosis (*arrow*), with associated intrahepatic biliary ductal dilatation. (*B*) Coronal projection from percutaneous transhepatic cholangiography confirmed the stricture (*arrow*).

Biliary Strictures

Biliary strictures, the most frequent biliary complications, can be divided into anastomotic and non-anastomotic types.[41] Anastomotic strictures, a result of scarring and fibrotic changes at the biliary anastomosis, usually manifest in the first year post-LT.[38,41] MRCP, which has high sensitivity for detection of this type of stricture, shows short-segment abrupt narrowing at the level of biliary anastomosis with associated marked upstream dilatation (**Figs. 9 and 10**).[39,41] Biliary stones or sludge frequently are present in patients with long-standing strictures.[39] Transient mild narrowing at the level of the anastomosis may be noted in first few weeks following LT, presumably related to the bile duct edema.[42] Correlation between MR findings and laboratory markers is important in order to exclude a persistent mechanical obstruction.

Nonanastomotic strictures are associated most commonly with hepatic artery thrombosis and associated biliary ischemia (**Fig. 11**).[39] Because the hepatic artery is the sole blood supply to the biliary ducts, its thrombosis rapidly can lead to irreversible biliary ischemia and necrosis. Other causes of nonanastomotic strictures are recurrent cholangitis, chronic rejection, and recurrence of primary sclerosis cholangitis.[42] On MR imaging, nonanastomotic strictures often are multifocal and characterized by alternating segments of stenosis and dilatation, predominantly affecting the intrahepatic bile ducts.[23,41] Concomitant bilomas as well as biliary sludge and cast frequently are seen in this setting (**Fig. 12**).[37,38] Diffusion-weighted imaging may show hyperintensity in, and around, the bile ducts, likely related to the inflammatory and ischemic changes.[43]

Orphan bile ducts are biliary radicles near the cut surface of the liver (in setting of LDLT), which are not draining into central bile ducts. These ducts may become dilated and mimic stricture (**Fig. 13**). Their typical location next to the cut surface and absence of biliary dilatation elsewhere help with the diagnosis.

The combination of gadoxetate disodium–enhanced MR imaging and MRCP improves the accuracy for detection of both anastomotic and nonanastomotic biliary strictures, with reported sensitivity and specificity of 79% and 96% to 100%, respectively.[44] It is important to fully evaluate the hepatic arteries whenever biliary ischemia is suspected.

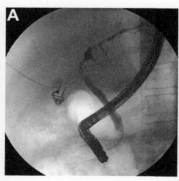
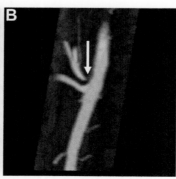

Fig. 11. (*A*) Frontal projection endoscopic retrograde cholangiography in a 59-year-old man with history of orthotopic LT shows marked irregularity of intrahepatic bile ducts and nonfilling of the right hepatic duct, secondary to severe stricture, suggestive of ischemic cholangiopathy. (*B*) Sagittal maximum intensity projection from MR angiography shows severe stenosis of celiac axis (*arrow*).

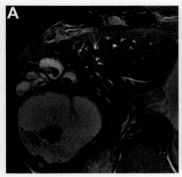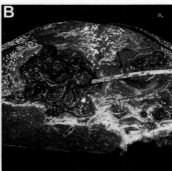

Fig. 12. (*A*) Axial T2-weighted MR image in a patient with remote history of orthotopic LT shows multiple intrahepatic bilomas, containing stones and sludge in the right lobe in setting of ischemic cholangiopathy and biliary necrosis. (*B*) Gross specimen following allograft hepatectomy demonstrates multiple bilomas.

Bile Leaks

Bile leaks are major complications of LT resulting in morbidity and mortality. Large leaks lead to biloma formation, which are at further risk of superinfection and sepsis.[38] Biliary leaks occur most commonly at the anastomotic site. Nonanastomotic leaks typically are seen in setting of underlying biliary ischemia and hepatic artery thrombosis. The indirect sign of biliary leaks on MR imaging is the presence of perigraft bilomas, which are markedly hyperintense on T2-weighted and hypointense on T1-weighted imaging, in vicinity of the site of biliary anastomosis or hepatectomy margins (in cases of LDLT). Differentiation of bilomas from other intraperitoneal fluid collections, however, is difficult, due to overlap in their imaging findings. As an alternative to hepatobiliary scintigraphy, off-label use of MR hepatobiliary agents allows for functional evaluation and direct visualization of site of active bile leak. On hepatobiliary phase images, they present as extraluminal contrast adjacent to the site of leak with layering of contrast in the adjacent biloma.[45] Gadoxetate disodium–enhanced MR imaging in combination with MRCP improves the sensitivity and specificity for detection of biliary leaks after LT, with reported sensitivity and specificity of 76% and 100%,

respectively.[46] In patients with slow flow leak or in patients with impaired liver function, a delay longer than 20 minutes might be necessary to depict the leak.[45,46]

Biliary Cast and Stones

Biliary stones, cast, and sludge are other abnormalities frequently encountered after LT.[37,47] Biliary cast syndrome, characterized by precipitation of biliary cast in the biliary tree, is seen more often in the first 6 months after LT. Proposed etiologies include sloughing of biliary epithelium (as a result of acute rejection or prolonged cold), alteration of the bile milieu, biliary infection, and use of biliary stents.[48] These complications are more common in patients with biliary strictures due to stasis of bile. MRCP has high sensitivity for the detection of stones.[38,41] Assessment of their signal intensity on T1-weighted images can increase the specificity because many of these abnormalities are hyperintense on this sequence (**Fig. 14**).[47] These entities should be differentiated from pneumobilia, frequently present in patients with choledochojejunostomy. Pneumobilia typically has nondependent distribution and shows hypointensity on all sequences. Hemobilia, defined as presence of blood in the bile ducts, is

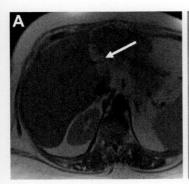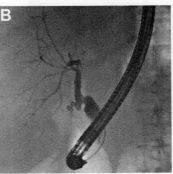

Fig. 13. (*A*) Axial T2-weighted MR image in a patient with history of lobe LDLT showed dilated ducts adjacent to the cut surface of the liver (*arrow*). (*B*) Coronal projection from endoscopic retrograde cholangiography showed normal right hepatic ducts without opacification of the dilated radicles, confirming orphan ducts adjacent to the hepatectomy margin.

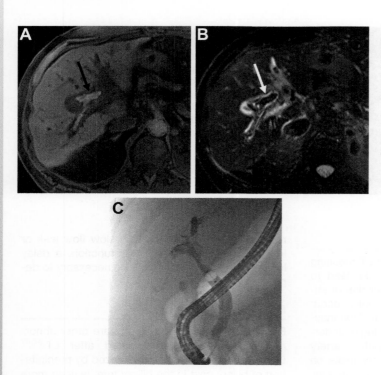

Fig. 14. (*A*) Axial precontrast T1-weighted and (*B*) axial fat-suppressed T2-weighted MR images in a patient with history of orthotopic LT show filling defects in the right hepatic ducts, showing markedly increased T1 ([*A*] *arrow*) and low T2 signal ([*B*] *arrow*) suggestive of biliary cast. Subsequent endoscopic retrograde cholangiogram (*C*) showed sludge and cast in the bile ducts.

another consideration that could be seen as a complication of recent bile duct procedures or liver biopsy.[28,38] Familiarity with the type of biliary reconstruction and knowing the clinical history help with differential diagnosis.

POST-TRANSPLANT MALIGNANCIES
Recurrent Hepatocellular Carcinoma

Approximately 25% of patients with HCC have recurrence within 5 years after LT.[49] The liver is

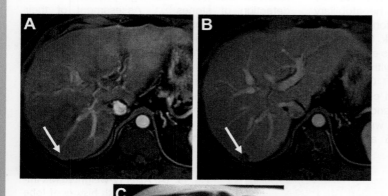

Fig. 15. (*A*) Axial arterial T1-weighted, (*B*) axial portal venous T1-weighted, and (*C*) axial T2-weighted MR images in a patient with history of orthotopic LT for HCC show a new lesion in segment VII (*arrows*) consistent with recurrence in the allograft. The lesion shows rim arterial phase hyperenhancement, washout, and moderate T2 hyperintensity.

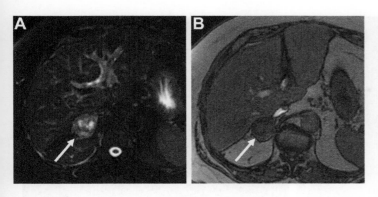

Fig. 16. (*A*) Axial fat-suppressed T2-weighted MR image in a 71-year-old man with history of hepatocellular cell carcinoma status postorthotopic LT 2 years earlier shows heterogeneous right adrenal mass (*arrow*). (*B*) Axial opposed-phase T1-weighted image shows absence of intralesional fat. The mass was new since the prior examination from 1 year earlier, consistent with adrenal metastasis.

the most common site of post-transplant recurrence (**Fig. 15**).[49] Other sites of recurrence are abdominal lymph nodes, lungs, bones, and other abdominal organs (**Fig. 16**). Major risk factors for recurrence include original tumor size greater than 3 cm, macrovascular invasion, and presence of viable tumor after locoregional treatments.[49] Other histopathologic risk factors are higher tumor grade, microvascular invasion, microsatellite nodules.

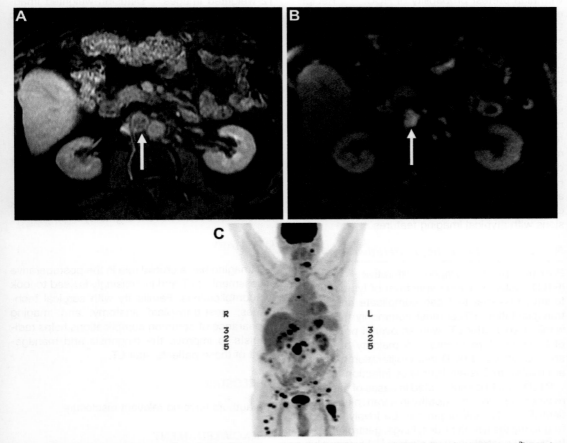

Fig. 17. (*A*) Axial portal venous phase T1-weighted and (*B*) axial diffusion-weighted (B value 500 s/mm²) MR images in a patient with history of orthotopic LT for HCC 2 years earlier show a new enlarged aortocaval lymph node (*arrow*). Biopsy was consistent with monomorphic PTLD. (*C*) Coronal maximum intensity projection from staging PET/CT shows extensive nodal involvement.

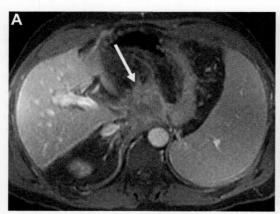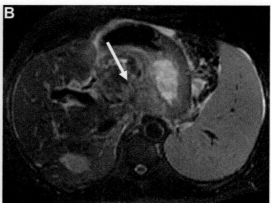

Fig. 18. (*A*) Axial contrast-enhanced T1-weighted and (*B*) axial fat-suppressed T2-weighted MR images show large enhancing gastric mass (*arrow*) with extension along the gastrohepatic ligament. Patient had orthotopic LT 15 years earlier. Biopsy showed gastric adenocarcinoma.

The Liver Imaging Reporting and Data System (LI-RADS) has been designed to achieve the highest specificity for diagnosis of HCC in populations with high pretest probability of HCC.[50,51] Recipients of LT with history of HCC are considered an LI-RADS high-risk population, irrespective of the status of the allograft.[52] HCC recurrence may present as single hepatic lesion or, less commonly, as multiple hepatic lesions. MR imaging features of HCC recurrence in the allograft are similar to the ones in native liver. A recent study, however, showed that HCC recurrences after LT were more likely to present with atypical imaging features (such as rim arterial phase hyperenhancement and targetoid appearance) on gadoxetate disodium–enhanced MR imaging compared with HCC occurring in native livers.[53] Tumor markers and history of other malignancies should be considered to guide the differential diagnosis of lesions with atypical imaging features.

Post-transplant Lymphoproliferative Disorder

Post-transplant lymphoproliferative disorder (PTLD) includes a wide spectrum of lymphoproliferative diseases that can complicate any organ transplantation. PTLD most commonly manifests within 1 year after LT, with an overall prevalence of 2.2% in LT recipients.[54] A majority of PTLDs are characterized by B-cell proliferation and they are related to Epstein-Barr virus infection.[54]

PTLD should be suspected in cases of new solid masses or lymphadenopathy in a transplanted patient (**Fig. 17**). Any organ can be involved, most frequently the lymph nodes, lungs, gastrointestinal tract, and central nervous system.[54] Liver involvement by PTLD may be in form of multiple hypovascular focal lesions or diffuse infiltrative pattern. Periportal involvement with enlarged regional

lymph nodes may be observed.[41] PTLD lesions usually are hypointense on T1-weighted sequences and have mild to moderate signal on T2-weighted images.[54] Diffusion-weighted imaging can be helpful for better depiction of hepatic lesion and lymph nodes. On postcontrast imaging, the lesions are hypoenhancing in all phases, which could allow to differentiate from recurrent HCC.[41]

Other Malignancies

LT recipients have higher risk for development of de novo malignancies, compared with general population (**Fig. 18**).[55] Also, patients who had LT for non-HCC malignancies (such as neuroendocrine neoplasm) are at particular risk for tumor recurrence, both in the allograft and in other sites. Careful evaluation of the liver and extrahepatic organs is necessary on surveillance imaging to look for recurrent or de novo malignancy.

SUMMARY

MR imaging has a crucial role in the postoperative assessment of LT and increasingly is used to look for complications. Familiarity with surgical techniques, post-transplant anatomy, and imaging appearance of common complications helps radiologists to improve the diagnosis and management of these patients after LT.

DISCLOSURE

The authors have no relevant disclosure.

ACKNOWLEDGMENT

The authors wish to thank David C. Botos, the visual communications specialist at Northwestern University, for his help with medical illustrations.

REFERENCES

1. Hughes CB, Humar A. Liver transplantation: current and future. Abdom Radiol (NY) 2020;46(1):2–8.

2. U.S. Department of Health & Human Services. Organ procurement and transplantation network: national data. Available at: https://optn.transplant.hrsa.gov/data/view-data-reports/national-data/#. Accessed October 2020.

3. Eghtesad B, Kadry Z, Fung J. Technical considerations in liver transplantation: what a hepatologist needs to know (and every surgeon should practice). Liver Transpl 2005;11:861–71.

4. Di Martino M, Rossi M, Mennini G, et al. Imaging follow-up after liver transplantation. Br J Radiol 2016;89:20151025.

5. Baheti AD, Sanyal R, Heller MT, et al. Surgical techniques and imaging complications of liver transplant. Radiol Clin North Am 2016;54:199–215.

6. Chupetlovska KP, Borhani AA, Dasyam AK, et al. Post-operative imaging anatomy in liver transplantation. Abdom Radiol (NY) 2021;46(1):9–16.

7. Mehrabi A, Mood ZA, Fonouni H, et al. A single-center experience of 500 liver transplants using the modified piggyback technique by Belghiti. Liver Transpl 2009;15:466–74.

8. Belghiti J, Kianmanesh R. Surgical techniques used in adult living donor liver transplantation. Liver Transpl 2003;9:S29–34.

9. Broelsch CE, Whitington PF, Emond JC, et al. Liver transplantation in children from living related donors. Surgical techniques and results. Ann Surg 1991; 214:428–39.

10. Berumen J, Hemming A. Liver transplantation for hepatocellular carcinoma. Abdom Radiol (NY) 2018; 43:185–92.

11. Hecht EM, Kambadakone A, Griesemer AD, et al. Living donor liver transplantation: overview, imaging technique, and diagnostic considerations. AJR Am J Roentgenol 2019;213(1):54–64.

12. de Ville de Goyet J, di Francesco F, Sottani V, et al. Splitting livers: Trans-hilar or trans-umbilical division? Technical aspects and comparative outcomes. Pediatr Transplant 2015;19:517–26.

13. Horvat N, Marcelino ASZ, Horvat JV, et al. Pediatric liver transplant: techniques and complications. Radiographics 2017;37:1612–31.

14. Carollo V, Cannella R, Sparacia G, et al. Optimizing liver division technique for procuring left lateral segment grafts - new anatomical insights. Liver Transpl 2020;27(2):281–5.

15. Delgado-Moraleda JJ, Ballester-Vallés C, Marti-Bonmati L. Role of imaging in the evaluation of vascular complications after liver transplantation. Insights Imaging 2019;10:78.

16. Crossin JD, Muradali D, Wilson SR. US of liver transplants: normal and abnormal. Radiographics 2003; 23:1093–114.

17. Tamsel S, Demirpolat G, Killi R, et al. Vascular complications after liver transplantation: evaluation with Doppler US. Abdom Imaging 2007;32:339–47.

18. Itri JN, Heller MT, Tublin ME. Hepatic transplantation: postoperative complications. Abdom Imaging 2013; 38:1300–33.

19. Caiado AH, Blasbalg R, Marcelino AS, et al. Complications of liver transplantation: multimodality imaging approach. Radiographics 2007;27:1401–17.

20. Pareja E, Cortes M, Navarro R, et al. Vascular complications after orthotopic liver transplantation: hepatic artery thrombosis. Transplant Proc 2010;42:2970–2.

21. Duffy JP, Hong JC, Farmer DG, et al. Vascular complications of orthotopic liver transplantation: experience in more than 4,200 patients. J Am Coll Surg 2009;208:896–905.

22. Bhargava P, Vaidya S, Dick AA, et al. Imaging of orthotopic liver transplantation: review. AJR Am J Roentgenol 2011;196:WS15–38.

23. Craig EV, Heller MT. Complications of liver transplant. Abdom Radiol (NY) 2019;46(1):43–67.

24. Kimura Y, Tapia Sosa R, Soto-Trujillo D, et al. Liver transplant complications radiologist can't miss. Cureus 2020;12:e8465.

25. Horrow MM, Huynh ML, Callaghan MM, et al. Complications after liver transplant related to preexisting conditions: diagnosis, treatment, and prevention. Radiographics 2020;40:895–909.

26. Glockner JF, Forauer AR, Solomon H, et al. Three-dimensional gadolinium-enhanced MR angiography of vascular complications after liver transplantation. AJR Am J Roentgenol 2000;174:1447–53.

27. Kim BS, Kim TK, Jung DJ, et al. Vascular complications after living related liver transplantation: evaluation with gadolinium-enhanced three-dimensional MR angiography. AJR Am J Roentgenol 2003;181: 467–74.

28. Singh AK, Nachiappan AC, Verma HA, et al. Postoperative imaging in liver transplantation: what radiologists should know. Radiographics 2010;30:339–51.

29. Frongillo F, Grossi U, Lirosi MC, et al. Incidence, management, and results of hepatic artery stenosis after liver transplantation in the era of donor to recipient match. Transplant Proc 2013;45:2722–5.

30. Yen LH, Sabatino JC. Imaging complications of liver transplantation: a multimodality pictorial review. Abdom Radiol (NY) 2019. https://doi.org/10.1007/s00261-019-02270-2.

31. Girometti R, Como G, Bazzocchi M, et al. Post-operative imaging in liver transplantation: state-of-the-art and future perspectives. World J Gastroenterol 2014;20:6180–200.

32. Fistouris J, Herlenius G, Bäckman L, et al. Pseudoaneurysm of the hepatic artery following liver transplantation. Transplant Proc 2006;38:2679–82.

33. St Michel DP, Goussous N, Orr NL, et al. Hepatic artery pseudoaneurysm in the liver transplant

recipient: a case series. Case Rep Transplant 2019; 2019:9108903.

34. Jha RC, Khera SS, Kalaria AD. Portal vein thrombosis: imaging the spectrum of disease with an emphasis on MRI features. AJR Am J Roentgenol 2018;211:14–24.

35. Ye Q, Zeng C, Wang Y, et al. Risk factors for hepatic venous outflow obstruction in piggyback liver transplantation: the role of recipient's pattern of hepatic veins drainage into the inferior vena cava. Ann Transplant 2017;22:303–8.

36. Lee HJ, Kim KW, Mun HS, et al. Uncommon causes of hepatic congestion in patients after living donor liver transplantation. AJR Am J Roentgenol 2009; 193:772–80.

37. Valls C, Alba E, Cruz M, et al. Biliary complications after liver transplantation: diagnosis with MR cholangiopancreatography. AJR Am J Roentgenol 2005; 184:812–20.

38. Girometti R, Cereser L, Como G, et al. Biliary complications after orthotopic liver transplantation: MRCP findings. Abdom Imaging 2008;33:542–54.

39. Boraschi P, Donati F, Pacciardi F, et al. Biliary complications after liver transplantation: assessment with MR cholangiopancreatography and MR imaging at 3T device. Eur J Radiol 2018;106:46–55.

40. Furlan A, Close ON, Borhani AA, et al. Respiratory-motion artefacts in liver MRI following injection of gadoxetate disodium and gadobenate dimeglumine: an intra-individual comparative study in cirrhotic patients. Clin Radiol 2017;72:93.e1–6.

41. Camacho JC, Coursey-Moreno C, Telleria JC, et al. Nonvascular post-liver transplantation complications: from US screening to cross-sectional and interventional imaging. Radiographics 2015;35: 87–104.

42. Novellas S, Caramella T, Fournol M, et al. MR cholangiopancreatography features of the biliary tree after liver transplantation. AJR Am J Roentgenol 2008; 191:221–7.

43. Wang J, Liu JJ, Liang YY, et al. Could diffusion-weighted imaging detect injured bile ducts of ischemic-type biliary lesions after orthotopic liver transplantation? AJR Am J Roentgenol 2012;199: 901–6.

44. Kinner S, Schubert TB, Said A, et al. Added value of gadoxetic acid-enhanced T1-weighted magnetic resonance cholangiography for the diagnosis of post-transplant biliary complications. Eur Radiol 2017;27:4415–25.

45. Alegre Castellanos A, Molina Granados JF, Escribano Fernandez J, et al. Early phase detection of bile leak after hepatobiliary surgery: value of Gd-EOB-DTPA-enhanced MR cholangiography. Abdom Imaging 2012;37:795–802.

46. Kantarcı M, Pirimoglu B, Karabulut N, et al. Non-invasive detection of biliary leaks using Gd-EOB-DTPA-enhanced MR cholangiography: comparison with T2-weighted MR cholangiography. Eur Radiol 2013;23:2713–22.

47. Borhani AA, Dasyam AK, Papachristou G, et al. Radiologic features of pancreatic and biliary complications following composite visceral transplantation. Abdom Imaging 2015;40:1961–70.

48. Ayoub WS, Esquivel CO, Martin P. Biliary complications following liver transplantation. Dig Dis Sci 2010;55:1540–6.

49. Kim YS, Lim HK, Rhim H, et al. Recurrence of hepatocellular carcinoma after liver transplantation: patterns and prognostic factors based on clinical and radiologic features. AJR Am J Roentgenol 2007; 189:352–8.

50. Tang A, Fowler KJ, Chernyak V, et al. LI-RADS and transplantation for hepatocellular carcinoma. Abdom Radiol (NY) 2018;43:193–202.

51. Cunha GM, Tamayo-Murillo DE, Fowler KJ. LI-RADS and transplantation: challenges and controversies. Abdom Radiol (NY) 2021;46(1):29–42.

52. American College of Radiology. CT/MRI Liver imaging reporting and data system v2018 core. Available at: https://www.acr.org/Clinical-Resources/Reporting-and-Data-Systems/LI-RADS/CT-MRI-LI-RADS-v2018. Accessed October, 2020.

53. Kim M, Kang TW, Jeong WK, et al. Gadoxetic acid-enhanced magnetic resonance imaging characteristics of hepatocellular carcinoma occurring in liver transplants. Eur Radiol 2017;27:3117–27.

54. Borhani AA, Hosseinzadeh K, Almusa O, et al. Imaging of posttransplantation lymphoproliferative disorder after solid organ transplantation. Radiographics 2009;29:981–1002.

55. Chandok N, Watt KD. Burden of de novo malignancy in the liver transplant recipient. Liver Transpl 2012; 18:1277–89.

Artificial Intelligence in Imaging of Chronic Liver Diseases
Current Update and Future Perspectives

Carl F. Sabottke, MD[a],*, Bradley M. Spieler, MD[b], Ahmed W. Moawad, MD[c],
Khaled M. Elsayes, MD, PhD[d]

KEYWORDS

- Artificial intelligence • Deep learning • Machine learning • Radiomics • Chronic liver disease
- Cirrhosis • Hepatic steatosis • Hepatic fibrosis

KEY POINTS

- There is promising potential for artificial intelligence models that target chronic liver disease evaluation to decrease the need for invasive procedures such as biopsy or catheterization to measure hepatic venous pressure gradient.
- Multiple convolutional neural network architectures such as U-nets and fully convolutional networks have been demonstrated to have success for segmentation of liver parenchyma and lesions such as hepatocellular carcinoma.
- Artificial intelligence models of liver fibrosis often benefit when applied in the context of elastography-based evaluation.
- Ultrasound-based assessment of hepatic steatosis with artificial intelligence has demonstrated excellent performance albeit in studies with relatively small datasets.

INTRODUCTION

Chronic liver disease (CLD) has multiple potential etiologies which include alcoholic liver disease, nonalcoholic fatty liver disease (NAFLD), chronic viral hepatitis, genetic causes such as alpha-1 antitrypsin deficiency or hereditary hemochromatosis, and autoimmune variants.[1] Because hepatocellular carcinoma (HCC) is one of the most clinically important sequelae of CLD, there has been interest in the use of artificial intelligence (AI) algorithms for HCC detection and treatment analysis.[2] However, AI algorithms also have clinical utility for evaluation of CLD independent of HCC assessment,[3] and, to give these topics due

attention, we focus this review specifically on AI techniques for liver disease assessment that are not related directly to HCC evaluation. Instead, we focus here on a review of AI techniques that aim to assess stages of CLD while obviating the need for invasive or resource-intensive procedures, such as catheterization to measure hepatic venous pressure gradient (HVPG) when assessing for portal hypertension[4] or biopsy and magnetic resonance elastography (MRE) to assess fibrosis.[5] We also address how AI techniques have been proposed for sonographic evaluation of hepatic steatosis as an alternative to biopsy or MRI proton density fat fraction (PDFF).[6,7]

---

[a] Department of Medical Imaging, University of Arizona College of Medicine, 1501 N. Campbell, P.O. Box 245067, Tucson, AZ 85724-5067, USA; [b] Department of Radiology, Louisiana State University Health Sciences Center, 1542 Tulane Avenue, Rm 343, New Orleans, LA 70112, USA; [c] Department of Imaging Physics, The University of Texas, MD Anderson Cancer Center, Unit 1472, P.O. Box 301402, Houston, TX 77230-1402, USA; [d] Department of Abdominal Imaging, The University of Texas, MD Anderson Cancer Center, 1400 Pressler St, Houston, TX 77030, USA
* Corresponding author.
E-mail addresses: csabottke@email.arizona.edu; cfs121090@gmail.com

Magn Reson Imaging Clin N Am 29 (2021) 451–463
https://doi.org/10.1016/j.mric.2021.05.011
1064-9689/21/© 2021 Elsevier Inc. All rights reserved.

In this review of AI in the evaluation of CLD, a wide variety of machine learning and deep learning techniques are discussed under the umbrella of AI along with comparison with radiomics algorithms.[8] Deep learning architectures used for liver segmentation include U-nets[9] and fully convolutional networks (FCNs),[10] whereas the VGG-19 convolutional neural network (CNN) architecture has been used for portal hypertension assessment.[11] Recent trends have favored a shift to deep learning with CNNs, but investigations have also included analysis of support vector machines (SVMs),[12] as well as other machine learning techniques that do not rely on artificial neural networks.[13] We discuss these techniques in 4 contexts: liver segmentation, evaluation of portal hypertension, assessment of liver fibrosis, and assessment of hepatic steatosis.

DISCUSSION
Liver Segmentation

When using AI systems targeting hepatocellular disease, liver segmentation is often a critical initial or intermediate step in the image processing pipeline to localize analysis to the appropriate regions of interest (ROIs). Liver segmentation analysis can be applied to the entire liver or used to specifically target lesions within the liver. AI-based segmentation of liver parenchyma and liver tumors can then be used for additional analysis, such as the assessment of imaging characteristics related to tumor response to various locoregional therapies.[14,15]

The importance of liver segmentation is further underscored by the 2017 Medical Image Computing & Computer Assisted Intervention (MICCAI) conference hosting the Liver Tumor Segmentation (LiTS) Challenge.[16] This challenge received 61 valid submissions for liver and LiTS based on a public training dataset of 131 computed tomography (CT) scans and 70 additional CT scans were reserved as testing data. The Dice score was used as one of the primary metrics for evaluating segmentation accuracy, which in this case would be the amount of overlap between the AI-generated segmentation boundaries compared with manually generated segmentations.[17,18] For pixelated images with 2 such segmentations, the Dice score calculation can be described as multiplying the number of overlapping pixels between the segmentations by 2 while dividing by the total number of pixels in each segmentation.[18] For the whole liver segmentation task within LiTS, the top Dice score per case was 0.963. Of the 61 model entries, 18 were able to achieve a Dice score per case of greater than 0.9. Meanwhile, liver tumor segmentation was more difficult for the models in this challenge with the highest Dice score per case only achieving 0.702.[16]

Aside from the 201 segmented CT scans in the LiTS dataset, additional public datasets available for training AI models of liver segmentation include the Combined CT-MR Healthy Abdominal Organ Segmentation (CHAOS) Challenge data, which includes 40 MRI cases and 40 CT cases with liver and other organ segmentations for patients without known underlying disease.[19] Thirty liver segmentation CT cases were also released when MICCAI hosted a 2007 liver segmentation challenge a decade before the more recent LiTS challenge.[20] There are also 22 segmented CT cases with varying presence of liver lesions available through the Research Institute against Digestive Cancer (IRCAD) in the 3D-IRCADb-01 and 3D-IRCADb-02 datasets.[21] Additionally, the Imaging Methods Assessment and Reporting (IMAR) project hosts 4 CT cases with liver segmentations via MIDAS.[22] These datasets are summarized in **Table 1**.

Table 1
Summary of public datasets available with 3D volumes of CT and MRIs that include liver segmentation data

Dataset Name	Affiliation	Content
Liver Tumor Segmentation Challenge (LiTS)	MICCAI 2017	201 segmented CT volumes
Segmentation of the Liver Competition 2007 (SLIVER07)	MICCAI 2007	30 segmented CT volumes
Combined Healthy Abdominal Organ Segmentation (CHAOS)	IEEE International Symposium on Biomedical Imaging 2019	40 segmented CT volumes and 40 segmented MRI volumes
3D-IRCADb-01 and 3D-IRCADb-02	IRCAD	22 segmented CT volumes
MIDAS	IMAR	4 segmented CT volumes

Both public datasets and local datasets have been used to generate multiple variants of segmentation models for the whole liver and liver lesions. For AI-based segmentation, U-nets are currently one of the most frequently used neural network model architectures.[9] Indeed, 95% of the LiTS challenge models used this architecture. Importantly, given the frequent clinical use of both CT scans and MRI for liver imaging, Wang and colleagues[23] have shown that transfer learning can be used to adapt a liver segmentation AI model trained on 1 cross-sectional imaging modality to another using a very limited in size second training dataset for the second modality compared with the first. This demonstration involved first training a U-net on 300 spoiled gradient-echo MRI sequences before subsequently training on 10 CT scans to adapt an MRI liver segmentation model into a CT liver segmentation model. Their model achieved a Dice score of 0.94 on a 230

CT scan validation dataset. Meine and colleagues[24] have also studied U-net–based liver segmentation and, based on their hardware constraints (an NVIDIA GeForce GTX 1080 GPU with 8 GiB memory), they determined that a model using three 2-dimensional U-nets trained on orthogonal slices outperformed both single slice orientation 2-dimensional U-net models and 3-dimensional U-net models. **Fig. 1** shows an example of U-net–based segmentation of liver parenchyma and tumor for a CT volume extracted from the LiTS dataset.

Aside from the U-net architecture, the whole liver segmentation modeling of Lu and colleagues[25] used 3-dimensional CNNs to generate a liver probability map that could then be refined with a graph cut technique. FCNs, which are architecturally similar to U-nets, have been used by Vorontsov and colleagues[26] for segmentations of suspected liver metastases in colorectal cancer patients.

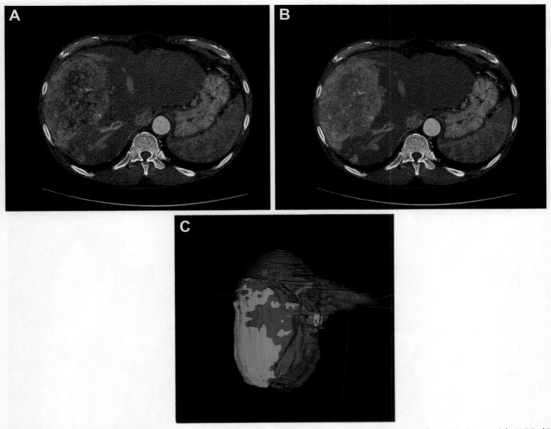

Fig. 1. Example of liver segmentation. (*A*) Contrast-enhanced CT scan of the abdomen for a patient with HCC. (*B*) Voxel-level segmentation of the liver (*red*) and tumor (*green*) in every slice is an essential step for further analysis in any AI-related task. In this example, segmentation was done using the U-Net architecture with training on the LiTS dataset. Segmentation showed a DSC of 0.90 of liver parenchyma segmentation, and DSC of 0.76 in tumor segmentation. (*C*). Three-dimensional volume rendering of the segmentation is used for qualitative assessment of segmentation accuracy and can be used for treatment planning or feature analysis.

Christ and colleagues[27] used a cascade of FCNs on 3D-IRCADb to first segment the liver with 1 FCN and then segment lesions based only on liver ROIs with a second FCN. FCNs have also been used for a combination of liver segmentation and metastatic lesion detection by Ben-Cohen and associates.[28] Meanwhile, for the specific problem of liver tumor segmentation for multiphase CT studies, Sun and colleagues[29] developed multichannel FCNs in which FCNs are trained on separate CT phases and then fused to generate segmentation predictions. More distinctly, Ibragimov and colleagues[30] have also used a combination of CNNs with Markov random fields for segmentation of the portal vein in liver stereotactic body radiation therapy planning. In this case, the Markov random fields were used to smooth the CNN segmentation outputs, and the portal vein was targeted for segmentation rather than the liver or an intrahepatic lesion.

Radiologic Assessment of Portal Circulation

Although Ibragimov and colleagues designed their portal vein segmentation model in the context of stereotactic body radiation therapy planning, we can speculate that an AI analysis of portal vein morphology may have further applications in the clinical assessment of CLD. Portal hypertension is a key clinical sequela of cirrhosis that in turn can lead to complications such, as variceal bleeding or ascites.[31] The HVPG is essentially the gold standard for evaluating portal hypertension and represents the gradient between the portal vein and the hepatic veins. The HVPG is calculated as the difference between wedged hepatic venous pressure and free hepatic venous pressure. An HVPG of greater than 6 mm Hg represents portal hypertension, and an HVPG of greater than 10 mm Hg is seen to represent clinically significant portal hypertension.[4] **Fig. 2** shows an example of portal hypertension in a cirrhotic patient who underwent transjugular intrahepatic portosystemic shunting with the caveat that the hepatic atrial pressure gradient was measured during the procedure rather than HVPG.[32] However, to avoid the requirement of an invasive procedure to measure portal vein pressure gradients, there has been interest in multiple surrogate approaches for estimating

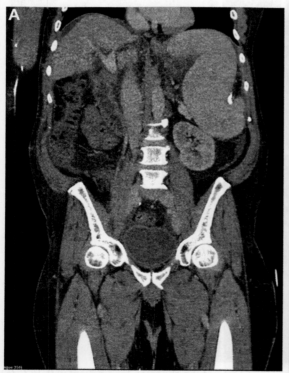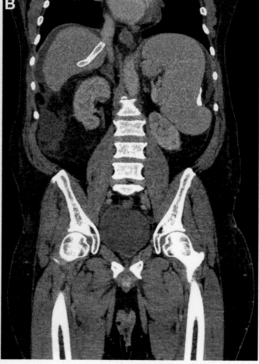

Fig. 2. Example case of patient with cirrhosis and portal hypertension before and after a transjugular intrahepatic portosystemic shunt procedure. (*A*) Preprocedure coronal slice of the abdomen and pelvis with a prominent portal vein. (*B*) Postprocedure coronal slice with shunt visible. The portal vein pressure was measured as 28 mm Hg during the procedure with a calculated portosystemic gradient before transjugular intrahepatic portosystemic shunt of 18 mm Hg. The postprocedure portosystemic gradient was measured as 11 mm Hg. The pressure gradient measured for this procedure was hepatic atrial pressure gradient rather than the hepatic venous pressure gradient.

portal hypertension. One such surrogate approach is ultrasound (US)-based transient elastography.[33–35] A meta-analysis and systematic review of transient elastography by Kim and colleagues[36] showed that transient elastography had a sensitivity of 0.85 and a specificity of 0.71 compared with HVPG for detecting clinically significant portal hypertension (HVPG of >10 mm Hg) with an overall correlation estimate of 0.75.

Another surrogate approach involves using Doppler US examination for the assessment of portal hemodynamics and estimation of portal vein velocity.[37] In a study of 236 cirrhotic patients, Kondo and colleagues[38] found that a lower mean portal vein trunk velocity (< 12.8 cm/s) was associated with an increased risk of decompensation. In 76 cirrhotic patients, Kim and colleagues[39] found that the damping index of the Doppler hepatic vein waveform correlated with an increase in the HVPG.

Single energy CT scans allow for the detection of findings correlated with portal hypertension, such as liver surface nodularity or varices.[40,41] More recently, however, Wang and colleagues[42] used dual energy spectral CT scans to investigate the correlation between iodine concentrations of the portal vein and portal venous pressure. They studied 45 patients with liver cirrhosis who received a dual energy spectral CT scan within 3 days before a percutaneous transhepatic portal vein puncture procedure, which allowed for the direct measurement of portal vein pressure. A portal vein iodine concentration of 58.27 mg/mL was used as a threshold for estimation of clinically significant portal hypertension (>10 mm Hg HVPG), and this threshold was found to have a 94% sensitivity and 69% specificity.[42]

For MR-based assessment of portal hypertension, Palaniyappan and colleagues[43] measured the HVPG in 30 patients and compared these measurements with MR-based quantification of liver T1 relaxation time, splenic artery velocity, and superior mesenteric artery velocity. A multiple linear regression model consisting of liver T1 signal relaxation time and splenic artery velocity achieved a correlation of 0.9 with the measured HVPG.[43] Levick and colleagues[44] studied 19 patients with HVPG measurements and compared this assessment of portal hypertension with iron-corrected T1 relaxation time in the liver and spleen. In their study, iron-corrected T1 relaxation time in the spleen had a correlation with HVPG of 0.69, whereas the iron-corrected T1 relaxation time in the liver, perhaps surprisingly, had a weaker correlation with HVPG of 0.4. Splenic iron-corrected T1 relaxation time was able to achieve an area under the receiver operator characteristic (AUROC) of 0.92 for both

portal hypertension (HVPG of >5 mm Hg) and clinically significant portal hypertension (HVPG of >10 mm Hg).[44]

For gadoxetate disodium–enhanced MR, the portal vein hyperintensity sign has been described as the portal vein appearing hyperintense to liver parenchyma on delayed hepatobiliary phase imaging.[45] Asenbaum and colleagues[46] studied MR features in 178 patients with HVPG measurements, and 74 of these patients had a positive portal vein hyperintensity sign. The median HVPG was 17 mm Hg for patients with positive portal vein hyperintensity sign and the median HVPG was 8.5 mm Hg for patients without portal vein hyperintensity sign. The interquartile range was 13 to 21 mm Hg in positive portal vein hyperintensity sign cases and 5 to 16 mm Hg in negative portal vein hyperintensity sign cases.[46]

For MRE, Navin and colleagues[47] compared 41 patients with noncirrhotic portal hypertension with 41 patients with cirrhotic portal hypertension and found that the liver stiffness measurement (LSM) was significantly lower in the noncirrhotic portal hypertension group (mean LSM of 8.7 kPa for cirrhotic portal hypertension vs 3.4 kPa for noncirrhotic portal hypertension). They also found that the ratio of splenic stiffness measurement to LSM ratio was significantly higher in the noncirrhotic portal hypertension patients.[47] Wagner and colleagues[48] compared MRE results with HVPG measurements across 34 patients with CLD and found that the LSMs had a correlation of 0.486 with HVPG.

Given limitations in existing noninvasive methods for assessment of portal hypertension, this lead to interest in using AI to assess for portal hypertension, which has been recently investigated by Liu and colleagues.[49] Liu and colleagues used CT data from the CHESS1701 cohort and MRI data from the CHESS1802 cohort for patients who had scans performed within 14 days of transjugular catheterization, which allowed for HVPG measurement. They performed analysis on 679 patients with CT images and 271 patients with MR images and analyzed both liver and spleen images with CNNs. For their CT-based model, they reported an AUROC of 0.912 for the detection of clinically significant portal hypertension in their validation dataset (136 cases) and an AUROC of 0.933 for their testing dataset (136 cases). For MRI-based models, they reported AUROC of 0.924 in the validation dataset (55 cases) and 0.940 in the testing dataset (54 cases). Their CT-based CNN used 64 × 64 pixel patches of liver and spleen ROIs as model inputs. For their MRI-based CNN, they used a VGG-19 model architecture with 224 × 224 pixel inputs.[49]

Another potential benefit of AI in CLD is through the detection of esophageal varices. Esophageal varix formation is a direct and potentially lethal result of portal hypertension.[50] As a consequence, all patients with cirrhosis are screened for esophageal variceal formation with esophagogastroduodenoscopy, a common invasive procedure that is seldomly associated with complications.[51] Dong and associates[52] used a random forest algorithm as both a tool for detection and risk of bleeding assessment, achieving an AUROC of 0.84 and 0.82 for the detection of varices in their respective testing and validation datasets, as well as an AUROC of 0.74 and 0.75 for the elucidation of varices requiring treatment for their respective training and validation datasets. This work showcases the potential for AI in the reduction of unnecessary costs and rare risks associated with esophagogastroduodenoscopies, particularly in that large esophageal varices are detected by esophagogastroduodenoscopy in less than half of cirrhotic patients undergoing screening, which suggests the possibility of implementing a more refined process for patient selection before esophagogastroduodenoscopy screening.[53]

Liu and colleagues[54] have also worked to develop a radiomics signature for portal hypertension assessment using the CHESS1701 cohort. They used CT images to develop a radiomic signature for clinically significant portal hypertension based on a training dataset of 222 patients. The ROIs were extracted from portal venous phase CT scans in the liver at the porta hepatis level and in the spleen at the level of the splenic hilum by segmenting the liver and spleen in these axial CT slices. Radiomic features were extracted with least absolute shrinkage and selection operator regression, which led to the selection of 7 liver features and 4 spleen features for use in a radiomics signature. They then calculated the concordance index (C-index) using 163 patients to form 4 validation cohorts. The C-index is a generalization of AUROC that helps to account for situations with censored data.[55] For the largest validation cohort (105 cases), the C-index was 0.889 for their radiomic signature for detecting an HVPG of greater than 10 mm Hg. The C-index was 0.800 in validation cohort 2 (26 cases), 0.917 in cohort 3 (16 cases), and 0.827 in cohort 4 (16 cases).[54] Thus, this CT radiomic signature's performance for detecting clinically significant portal hypertension seems to underperform the CNN approach of Liu and colleagues.[49] However, it is also worth noting that the CNN approach of Liu and colleagues, which achieved a 0.924 AUROC for their MR validation dataset and a 0.94 AUROC for their testing dataset, has similar reported AUROCs to the 0.92

AUROC reported by Levick and colleagues[44] for their 19 case analysis of predicting portal hypertension with splenic iron corrected T1 relaxation time. Thus, although neural network and radiomics-based approaches for noninvasive estimation of portal hypertension show promise, there is a need for more research into optimizing these approaches and their potential to act as surrogate mechanisms for estimating clinically significant portal hypertension.

Fibrosis Assessment

The progression of fibrosis in CLD does not occur at a constant rate over time; rather, it is a nonlinear progression that differs in accordance with stage, such as the METAVIR score.[56–58] As a result, the longitudinal assessment of fibrosis using typical clinical disease progression models can be difficult, particularly given a high degree of overlap in perceived stage of fibrosis and relevancy to different etiologies.[59] Machine learning models, however, have the capability to expand longitudinal data analysis through a heightened capacity with respect to the integration of various predicting metrics of fibrosis. A recent multivariate analysis using boosted survival tree–based models that analyzed more than 11,000 cirrhotic patients over a span of 7 years demonstrated higher AUROC measurements at all timepoints with longitudinal modeling; however, less complex cross-sectional models, although outperformed, showed comparable accuracy.[60] Wei and colleagues[61] also displayed great diagnostic potential through their gradient boosting prediction model, which bested noninvasive laboratory-based liver fibrosis scores in the categorization of cirrhotic versus noncirrhotic livers as well the acuity of fibrosis in both hepatitis B and C cohorts. Given that progression to fibrosis in the setting of hepatitis B may be suppressed and even reversed in its early stages, the detection of an early stage of fibrosis can be pivotal for patient outcomes. A recent application of artificial neural networks using a standard backpropagation technique involving clinical data including serum biomarkers showed better performance than logistic regression, and an AUC of 0.809 versus 0.756, respectively, for the prediction of liver fibrosis reversal in hepatitis B patients undergoing antiviral treatment.[62]

Although multiple staging systems for liver fibrosis exist, including the METAVIR score,[63] New Inuyama classification,[64] the Knodell score,[65] the Ishak score (modified Knodell score),[66] the Scheuer system,[67] the Batts-Ludwig system,[68] and the Laennec staging system,[69] the fibrosis component of the METAVIR score or its histologic equivalent proposed by the Korean Study Group for the Pathology of Digestive Diseases[70] has been used as the comparison standard for multiple AI models of liver fibrosis.[71–74] The METAVIR score consists of an activity score (intensity of necroinflammatory lesions graded from A0 to A3 based on a spectrum of no activity to severe activity) and a fibrosis score, which is graded as F0 (no fibrosis), F1 (portal fibrosis without septa), F2 (few septa), F3 (numerous septa without cirrhosis), and F4 (cirrhosis).[63] Lee and colleagues[71] developed a CNN using a total of 3446 patients to assess for liver fibrosis based on B-mode US images in comparison with the METAVIR classifications. The CNN was trained to classify US images into 4 classes with F2 and F3 combined into a single merged class. On an external test dataset of 572 patients, they achieved AUROC of 0.866 for the identification of fibrosis stage F2 or greater and an AUROC of 0.857 for identification of cirrhosis (stage F4).[71] Choi and colleagues[72] developed a deep learning system for CT-based fibrosis classification that involved a U-net for liver segmentation followed by a subsequent CNN for the F0 to F4 classification of fibrosis. On a test dataset of 891 patients, they achieved 79.4% accuracy and an AUROC of 0.96 for the identification of fibrosis stage F2 or greater and an AUROC of 0.95 for the identification of stage F4 fibrosis (cirrhosis).[72]

Yasaka and colleagues[75] used deep learning to compare hepatobiliary phase MR images with fibrosis classifications based on the New Inuyama classification system. The New Inuyama fibrosis classification stages are F0 (no fibrosis), F1 (fibrous portal expansion), F2 (bridging fibrosis), F3 (bridging fibrosis with architectural distortion), and F4 (cirrhosis).[64] There were 534 patients who were assigned to a training group and 100 were assigned to the test group for the development of a CNN on 350 × 350 pixel cropped MR images resized to 80 × 80 pixels for model development. The model achieved AUROCs of 0.85, 0.84, and 0.84 for New Inuyama stages F2, F3, and F4, respectively.[75]

Radiomics has also been used for fibrosis assessment in addition to the work performed with deep learning and CNNs. Park and colleagues[76] developed a radiomics fibrosis index for gadoxetic acid-enhanced MRI, which achieved an AUROC of 0.90 for the identification of fibrosis stage F2 or greater and 0.91 for identification of cirrhosis (stage F4, fibrosis graded per Korean Study Group for the Pathology of Digestive Diseases) in their test dataset of 107 patients. Consequently, although not necessarily directly comparable, this radiomics-based approach seems to outperform the CNN approach of Yasaka and colleagues for the identification of cirrhosis on MRI.

Deep learning and radiomics have also been used for fibrosis classification for US imaging- and MR-based elastography. Treacher and colleagues[77] used a dataset of 326 patients who underwent US shear wave elastography (SWE) and found that a CNN was unable to predict the measured shear wave velocity (SWV) based on US B-mode images alone ($r^2 = 0.01$ in a mean square error analysis), suggesting that the US elastography technique provides unique clinical information not inherently embedded in the liver echotexture. Brattain and colleagues[78] compared multiple automated machine learning techniques with the assessment of a METAVIR score of F2 or greater based on US SWE using a dataset of 328 patients. They found that CNNs performed best in this classification task, achieving an AUROC of 0.89, compared with a random forest model, which had an AUROC of 0.83 and a SVM with and AUROC of 0.82. They also compared outcomes with a nonmachine learning estimate that simply involved computing the median of the mean liver stiffness across 10 ROIs, and this simplified technique only achieved an AUROC of 0.74.[78] Gatos and colleagues[74] analyzed the benefit of automatic temporal stability preprocessing of CNN inputs of US SWE in 200 cases and compared the results of METAVIR score-based fibrosis classification accuracy with and without this temporal stability preprocessing. Without temporal stability masking, their CNN model achieved an AUROC of 0.94 for the identification of F4 stage fibrosis; the AUROC improved to 0.97 with temporal stability masking.[74] Wang and colleagues[73] achieved similar success with a CNN analysis of manually selected ROI inputs from US SWE in a dataset of 398 patients. The CNN classification was compared with the METAVIR score and achieved an AUROC of 0.97 for identification of cirrhosis (F4) and an AUROC of 0.99 for identification of stage F3 or greater.[73]

For MR elastography, the mean shear stiffness values calculated based on ROIs can be compared directly with histologic fibrosis classification.[5,79,80] Chang and colleagues[80] stratified their patients based on chronic hepatitis B (CHB) infection and assigned a higher mean shear stiffness value cutoff for fibrosis staging for patients without CHB. Using a threshold of 2.57 kPa, they achieved a sensitivity of 92.0% and specificity of 92.2% for identifying fibrosis with a METAVIR score of F2 or greater in patients with CHB (138 patients), and a threshold of 2.9 kPa achieved 90.0% sensitivity and 100% specificity for patients without CHB. For the 332 CHB patients used to compute the 2.57 kPa cutoff, the AUROC for stage F2 or greater fibrosis was 0.97, and for the 84 patients without CHB used to compute the 2.90 kPa cutoff, the AUROC was 0.96 for a stage F2 or greater classification.[80] Given the ability of MRE to predict histologic fibrosis stage accurately without AI assistance, He and colleagues[81] instead investigated the ability of an SVM to predict MRE stiffness values of less than or greater than 3 kPa without the direct use of MRE data, but instead a combination of nonelastography MR images and clinical data. Their model achieved greater accuracy than the effort of Treacher and colleagues to reproduce US SWV without B-mode US and a CNN,[77] but their SVM model was still only able to achieve 75% accuracy with an AUROC of 0.80 on an external validation dataset of 84 patients.[81] Meanwhile, Murphy and

colleagues investigated artificial neural networks as an alternative to multimodel direct inversion[82] for the estimation of stiffness based on MRE data and achieved promising results in simulations compared with multimodel direct inversion.[83]

Hepatic Steatosis

Given that epidemiologic analysis suggests a 25.2% global prevalence of NAFLD, which has a 40.8% risk of progression to fibrosis,[84] US assessment of hepatic steatosis has received great interest as a potential screening tool.[85] We visualize this in **Fig. 3** with a case of nonalcoholic steatohepatitis imaged via CT scan (**Fig. 3**A), B-mode US (**Fig. 3**B), and SWE (**Fig. 3**C, D). Cao and

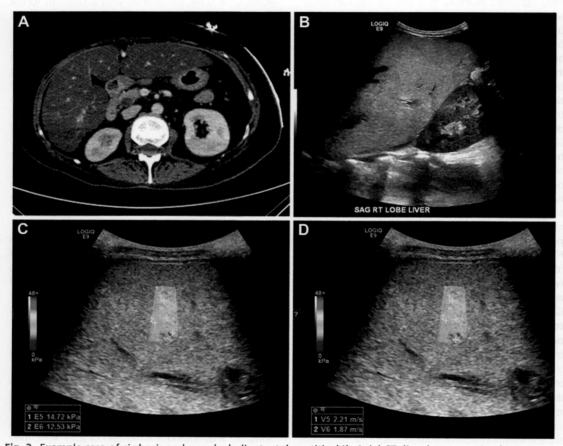

Fig. 3. Example case of cirrhosis and nonalcoholic steatohepatitis. (*A*). Axial CT slice demonstrating hypoattenuation of the liver compatible with hepatic steatosis along with surface contour nodularity and left hepatic lobe hypertrophy consistent with cirrhosis. (*B*) B-mode US image showing increased parenchymal echotexture of the liver compared with the right kidney with poor delineation of periportal fat planes consistent with fatty infiltration. (*C*) SWE image showing sample measurements of shear pressure (median shear pressure of 13.69 kPa). (*D*) SWE image showing sample measurements of shear wave velocity (mean shear velocity of 2.09 m/s). Liver biopsy reported bridging fibrosis and 70% to 80% of hepatic parenchyma exhibiting mixed steatosis. nonalcoholic steatohepatitis grading for biopsy reported 3/3 steatosis, 2/3 lobular inflammation, and 2/3 portal inflammation, consistent with cirrhosis and steatohepatitis.

colleagues[87] used a CNN to predict the Hamaguchi score[86] for NAFLD as assessed by physicians. Their deep learning method achieved an AUROC of 0.96 on their dataset of 240 patients. However, it has been noted that this study has a suboptimal reference standard in the US-based Hamaguchi score and does not use an external validation or testing dataset.[88]

Byra and colleagues[89] used an Inception-ResNet-v2 CNN to generate features from US images that were subsequently used by an SVM for comparison with steatosis estimates obtained via biopsy in a dataset of 55 obese patients and predictions of greater than 5% hepatocytes with steatosis. They also compared CNN input features combined with an SVM to the use of a gray-level co-occurrence matrix input features for an SVM and found a significantly greater AUROC for CNN-based features compared with gray-level co-occurrence matrix features (0.977 vs 0.893). However, they did not find that their combination of a CNN and SVM outperformed the hepatorenal index, because this simple computation (the mean brightness of a liver ROI divided by the mean brightness for an ROI placed within the right kidney)[90] achieved an AUROC of 0.959.[89] Biswas and colleagues[91] analyzed a dataset of 63 patients and assessed performance for CNN and SVM models to predict biopsy assessment of fatty liver disease using US images. They found that their CNN model outperformed the SVM model and was able to achieve 1.0 AUROC compared with 0.79 for SVM.[91] Saba and colleagues[92] investigated a variety of features in conjunction with artificial neural networks for 63 patients to assess for fatty liver disease and reported a 97.6% accuracy with a combination of geometric, Fourier, Gupta, Gabor, Haralick, and discrete cosine transform features.[92] Acharya and colleagues[93] assessed decision trees and fuzzy classifiers in 100 cases using wavelet, spectral, and texture input features and achieved maximum accuracy of 93.3% for their decision tree models compared with 86.7% for the fuzzy classifiers. Yet, despite impressive reported performance in many of these studies, concerns have been still raised about limited dataset sizes, which have lacked large external validation or testing datasets.[88]

Recent work by Han and colleagues[94] expanded on preceding applications of CNNs in US imaging with respect to the analysis of 2-dimensional greyscale B-mode images using 2 different 1-dimensional CNNs. Driven by a proposed loss of data in the process of image reconstruction, which can lead to diagnostic challenges for the radiologist in the interpretation of tissue echogenicity at US imaging, the investigators used a standardized approach to region of interest placement, which could be applied independent of time gain compensation. One CNN distinguished normal liver from NAFLD (>5% fat fraction) with an AUROC of 0.98 and 0.95 for the detection of NAFLD with and without time gain compensation, respectively. A second CNN achieved Pearson correlation coefficients of 0.85 and 0.80 between the estimated fat fraction and that derived from MRI-PDFF without and with time gain compensation, while having a notably high correlation with MRI-PDFF fat fractions of less than or equal to 18%. Although the CNN underperformed with respect to the estimation of fat fraction in subjects with an MRI-PDFF of more than 18%, this work is most impactful in its capability of fat quantification without the necessity of a phantom for the purposes of calibration, thereby elucidating the potential for a refined assessment of fat fraction through the deep learning analysis of radiofrequency data. The team's methods could provide a more facile framework for future deep learning techniques in fat quantification via US imaging.

SUMMARY

AI has much to offer the medical community for quantitative assessment of the liver. AI-driven segmentation has many uses for partitioning the liver and often can be used as an initial step in more sophisticated analysis pipelines, which can include tumor localization and stereotactic body radiation therapy planning. AI-based assessment of portal hypertension offers opportunities to decrease the need for invasive measurement via catheterization and can capture clinically useful prognostic information. The AI assessment of steatosis and fibrosis also offer valuable prognostic information without the need for a biopsy. However, a caveat for steatosis and fibrosis is that MRI-PDFF and MRE are also able to accurately characterize these pathologies. Nevertheless, in the cases of fibrosis and steatosis, AI offers an opportunity for potential use of less resource-intensive modalities with US-based assessment.

Concerns have been raised previously that some of these initial AI investigations do not have optimal dataset sizes or partitions[88] and not all components of recently disseminated checklist guidelines such as CLAIM, CONSORT-AI, and SPIRIT-AI are satisfied as applicable.[95–97] Consequently, further research is needed to appreciate the full potential of deep learning and other AI techniques for the evaluation of CLD and its sequelae. Nevertheless, there is great potential for AI to offer prognostic information and reduce the need for invasive or resource-intensive procedures.

CLINICS CARE POINTS

- AI has developing potential to reduce the need for invasive procedures such as biopsy for the evaluation of CLD.

- Segmentation techniques such as U-nets and FCNs can assist with automating liver analysis pipelines by identifying regions of liver parenchyma and liver lesions such as HCC.

- CNN models for portal hypertension have achieved AUROCs of greater than 0.92, yet these AI models are not yet definitively superior to non-AI MRI–based techniques as alternatives to direct measurement of portal vein pressure via catheterization.

- AI assessment of liver fibrosis has been explored both with and without elastography with superior performance obtained with supplemental elastography data.

- AI assessment of hepatic steatosis has focused on US examination with some models assessed on small datasets able to achieve perfect or near-perfect performance for steatosis identification.

DISCLOSURE STATEMENT

The authors have nothing to disclose.

REFERENCES

1. Sharma ANS. Chronic liver disease [Updated 2020 Feb 28]. In: StatPearls [Internet]. StatPearls Publishing; 2020. Available: https://www.ncbi.nlm.nih.gov/books/NBK554597/. Accessed: December 14, 2020.

2. Pérez MJ, Grande RG. Application of artificial intelligence in the diagnosis and treatment of hepatocellular carcinoma: a review. World J Gastroenterol 2020;26(37):5617–28.

3. Zhou LQ, Wang JY, Yu SY, et al. Artificial intelligence in medical imaging of the liver. World J Gastroenterol 2019;25(6):672–82.

4. Suk KT a. Hepatic venous pressure gradient: clinical use in chronic liver disease. Clin Mol Hepatol 2014;20(1):6–14.

5. Huwart L, Peeters F, Sinkus R, et al. Liver fibrosis: non-invasive assessment with MR elastography. NMR Biomed 2006;19(2):173–9.

6. Tang A, Tan J, Sun M, et al. Nonalcoholic fatty liver disease: MR imaging of liver proton density fat fraction to assess hepatic steatosis. Radiology 2013; 267(2):422–31.

7. Lee H, Jun DW, Kang BK, et al. Estimating of hepatic fat amount using MRI proton density fat fraction in a real practice setting. Med (United States). 2017;96(33). https://doi.org/10.1097/MD.0000000000007778.

8. Hu W, Yang H, Xu H, et al. Radiomics based on artificial intelligence in liver diseases: where we are? Gastroenterol Rep 2020;8(2):90–7.

9. Ronneberger O, Fischer P, Brox T. U-net: convolutional networks for biomedical image segmentation. Lecture Notes in computer Science (including Subseries Lecture Notes in artificial intelligence and lecture notes in bioinformatics), 9351. Springer Verlag; 2015. p. 234–41.

10. Long J, Shelhamer E, Darrell T. Fully convolutional networks for Semantic segmentation. 2015 IEEE Conference on Computer Vision and Pattern Recognition (CVPR). 2015. p. 3431-40. doi: 10.1109/CVPR.2015.7298965.

11. Simonyan K, Zisserman A. Very deep convolutional networks for large-scale image recognition. In: 3rd International conference on learning representations, ICLR 2015 - conference track Proceedings. International conference on learning representations. San Diego: ICLR; 2015.

12. Bhavsar H, Panchal MH. A review on support vector machine for data classification, 1, 2012.

13. Choy G, Khalilzadeh O, Michalski M, et al. Current applications and future impact of machine learning in radiology. Radiology 2018;288(2):318–28.

14. Morshid A, Elsayes KM, Khalaf AM, et al. A machine learning model to predict hepatocellular carcinoma response to transcatheter arterial chemoembolization. Radiol Artif Intell 2019;1(5):e180021.

15. Spieler B, Sabottke C, Moawad AW, et al. Artificial intelligence in assessment of hepatocellular carcinoma treatment response. Abdom Radiol (NY) 2021. doi: 10.1007/s00261-021-03056-1. Epub ahead of print. Erratum in: Abdom Radiol (NY). 2021. PMID: 33786653.

16. Bilic P, Christ PF, Vorontsov E, et al. The liver tumor segmentation benchmark (LiTS). arXiv 2019. Available: http://arxiv.org/abs/1901.04056. Accessed: December 2, 2020.

17. Dice LR. Measures of the amount of ecologic association between species. Ecology 1945;26(3):297–302.

18. Taha AA, Hanbury A. Metrics for evaluating 3D medical image segmentation: analysis, selection, and tool. BMC Med Imaging 2015;15(1):29.

19. Kavur AE, Selver MA, Dicle O, et al. CHAOS - combined (CT-MR) Healthy abdominal organ segmentation challenge data 2019. https://doi.org/10.5281/ZENODO.3431873.

20. Ginneken B, Heimann T, Styner M. 3D segmentation in the clinic: a grand challenge. 2007.

21. 3Dircadb | IRCAD France. 2009. Available: https://www.ircad.fr/research/3dircadb/. Accessed December 2, 2020.

22. MIDAS - Collection Livers and liver tumors with expert hand segmentations. Available: http://insight-

journal.org/midas/collection/view/38. Accessed December 2, 2020.

23. Wang K, Mamidipalli A, Retson T, et al. Automated CT and MRI liver segmentation and biometry using a generalized convolutional neural network. Radiol Artif Intell 2019;1(2):180022.

24. Meine H, Chlebus G, Ghafoorian M, et al. Comparison of U-net-based convolutional neural networks for liver segmentation in CT. arXiv 2018. Available: http://arxiv.org/abs/1810.04017. Accessed December 2, 2020.

25. Lu F, Wu F, Hu P, et al. Automatic 3D liver location and segmentation via convolutional neural network and graph cut. Int J Comput Assist Radiol Surg 2017;12(2):171–82.

26. Vorontsov E, Cerny M, Régnier P, et al. Deep Learning for Automated Segmentation of Liver Lesions at CT in Patients with Colorectal Cancer Liver Metastases. Radiol Artif Intell 2019;1(2):180014.

27. Ferdinand Christ P, Ezzeldin Elshaer MA, Ettlinger F, et al. Automatic liver and lesion segmentation in CT using cascaded fully convolutional neural networks and 3D conditional random fields. Available: http://ircad.fr/research/3d-ircadb-01. Accessed December 2, 2020.

28. Ben-Cohen A, Diamant I, Klang E, et al. Fully convolutional network for liver segmentation and lesions detection. 2016.

29. Sun C, Guo S, Zhang H, et al. Automatic segmentation of liver tumors from multiphase contrast-enhanced CT images based on FCNs. Artif Intell Med 2017;83:58–66.

30. Ibragimov B, Toesca D, Chang D, et al. Combining deep learning with anatomical analysis for segmentation of the portal vein for liver SBRT planning. Phys Med Biol 2017;62(23):8943–58.

31. De Franchis R, Primignani M. Natural history of portal hypertension in patients with cirrhosis. Clin Liver Dis 2001;5(3):645–63.

32. La Mura V, Abraldes JG, Berzigotti A, et al. Right atrial pressure is not adequate to calculate portal pressure gradient in cirrhosis: a clinical-hemodynamic correlation study. Hepatology 2010; 51(6):2108–16.

33. Kumar A, Khan NM, Anikhindi SA, et al. Correlation of transient elastography with hepatic venous pressure gradient in patients with cirrhotic portal hypertension: a study of 326 patients from India. World J Gastroenterol 2017;23(4):687–96.

34. Jung KS, Kim SU. Clinical applications of transient elastography. Clin Mol Hepatol 2012;18(2):163–73.

35. Sandrin L, Fourquet B, Hasquenoph JM, et al. Transient elastography: a new noninvasive method for assessment of hepatic fibrosis. Ultrasound Med Biol 2003;29(12):1705–13.

36. Kim G, Kim MY, Baik SK. Transient elastography versus hepatic venous pressure gradient for diagnosing portal hypertension: a systematic review and meta-analysis. Clin Mol Hepatol 2017;23(1): 34–41.

37. Maruyama H, Yokosuka O. Ultrasonography for noninvasive assessment of portal hypertension. Gut Liver 2017;11(4):464–73.

38. Kondo T, Maruyama H, Sekimoto T, et al. Impact of portal hemodynamics on Doppler ultrasonography for predicting decompensation and long-term outcomes in patients with cirrhosis. Scand J Gastroenterol 2016;51(2):236–44.

39. Kim MY, Baik SK, Park DH, et al. Damping index of Doppler hepatic vein waveform to assess the severity of portal hypertension and response to propranolol in liver cirrhosis: a prospective nonrandomized study. Liver Int 2007;27(8):1103–10.

40. Smith AD, Branch CR, Zand K, et al. Liver surface nodularity quantification from routine CT images as a biomarker for detection and evaluation of cirrhosis. Radiology 2016;280(3):771–81.

41. de Franchis R. Non-invasive (and minimally invasive) diagnosis of oesophageal varices. J Hepatol 2008;49(4):520–7.

42. Wang J, Gao F, Shen JL. Noninvasive assessment of portal hypertension using spectral computed tomography. J Clin Gastroenterol 2019;53(9):e387–91.

43. Palaniyappan N, Cox E, Bradley C, et al. Non-invasive assessment of portal hypertension using quantitative magnetic resonance imaging. J Hepatol 2016;65(6):1131–9.

44. Levick C, Phillips-Hughes J, Collier J, et al. Non-invasive assessment of portal hypertension by multi-parametric magnetic resonance imaging of the spleen: a proof of concept study. PLoS One 2019;14(8):e0221066.

45. Lee NK, Kim S, Kim GH, et al. Significance of the "Delayed hyperintense portal vein sign" in the hepatobiliary phase MRI obtained with Gd-EOB-DTPA. J Magn Reson Imaging 2012;36(3):678–85.

46. Asenbaum U, Ba-Ssalamah A, Mandorfer M, et al. Effects of Portal Hypertension on Gadoxetic Acid–Enhanced Liver Magnetic Resonance. Invest Radiol 2017;52(8):462–9.

47. Navin PJ, Gidener T, Allen AM, et al. The role of magnetic resonance elastography in the diagnosis of noncirrhotic portal hypertension. Clin Gastroenterol Hepatol 2019;18(13). https://doi.org/10.1016/j.cgh.2019.10.018.

48. Wagner M, Hectors S, Bane O, et al. Noninvasive prediction of portal pressure with MR elastography and DCE-MRI of the liver and spleen: preliminary results. J Magn Reson Imaging 2018;48(4):1091–103.

49. Liu Y, Ning Z, Örmeci N, et al. Deep convolutional neural network-aided detection of portal hypertension in patients with cirrhosis. Clin Gastroenterol Hepatol 2020;18(13). https://doi.org/10.1016/j.cgh.2020.03.034.

50. Garcia-Tsao G, Abraldes JG, Berzigotti A, et al. Portal hypertensive bleeding in cirrhosis: risk stratification, diagnosis, and management: 2016 practice guidance by the American Association for the study of liver diseases. Hepatology 2017;65(1):310–35.

51. Ahlawat R, Hoilat GJ, Ross AB. Esophagogastroduodenoscopy. StatPearls Publishing; 2020. Available: http://www.ncbi.nlm.nih.gov/pubmed/30335301. Accessed December 8, 2020.

52. Dong TS, Kalani A, Aby ES, et al. Machine Learning-based Development and Validation of a Scoring System for Screening High-Risk Esophageal Varices. Clin Gastroenterol Hepatol 2019;17(9):1894–901.e1.

53. Chalasani N, Imperiale TF, Ismail A, et al. Predictors of Large Esophageal Varices in Patients With Cirrhosis. Am J Gastroenterol 1999;94(11):3285–91.

54. Liu F, Ning Z, Liu Y, et al. Development and validation of a radiomics signature for clinically significant portal hypertension in cirrhosis (CHESS1701): a prospective multicenter study. EBioMedicine 2018;36:151–8.

55. Uno H, Cai T, Pencina MJ, et al. On the C-statistics for evaluating overall adequacy of risk prediction procedures with censored survival data. Stat Med 2011;30(10):1105–17.

56. Zeremski M, Dimova RB, Pillardy J, et al. Fibrosis Progression in Patients with Chronic Hepatitis C Virus Infection. J Infect Dis 2016;214(8):1164–70.

57. Masugi Y, Abe T, Tsujikawa H, et al. Quantitative assessment of liver fibrosis reveals a nonlinear association with fibrosis stage in nonalcoholic fatty liver disease. Hepatol Commun 2018;2(1):58–68.

58. Axley P, Mudumbi S, Sarker S, et al. Patients with stage 3 compared to stage 4 liver fibrosis have lower frequency of and longer time to liver disease complications. PLoS One 2018;13(5):e0197117.

59. Duarte-Rojo A, Altamirano JT, Feld JJ. Noninvasive markers of fibrosis: key concepts for improving accuracy in daily clinical practice. Ann Hepatol 2012;11(4):426–39.

60. Konerman MA, Beste LA, Van T, et al. Machine learning models to predict disease progression among veterans with hepatitis C virus. PLoS One 2019;14(1):e0208141.

61. Wei R, Wang J, Wang X, et al. Clinical prediction of HBV and HCV related hepatic fibrosis using machine learning. EBioMedicine 2018;35:124–32.

62. Wei W, Wu X, Zhou J, et al. Noninvasive evaluation of liver fibrosis reverse using artificial neural network model for chronic hepatitis B patients. Comput Math Methods Med 2019;2019. https://doi.org/10.1155/2019/7239780.

63. Bedossa P, Poynard T. An algorithm for the grading of activity in chronic hepatitis C. Hepatology 1996;24(2):289–93.

64. Ichida F, Tsuji T, Omata M, et al. New Inuyama classification; new criteria for histological assessment of chronic hepatitis. Int Hepatol Commun 1996;6(2):112–9.

65. Knodell RG, Ishak KG, Black WC, et al. Formulation and application of a numerical scoring system for assessing histological activity in asymptomatic chronic active hepatitis. Hepatology 1981;1(5):431–5.

66. Ishak K, Baptista A, Bianchi L, et al. Histological grading and staging of chronic hepatitis. J Hepatol 1995;22(6):696–9.

67. Scheuer PJ. Classification of chronic viral hepatitis: a need for reassessment. J Hepatol 1991;13(3):372–4.

68. Batts KP, Ludwig J. Chronic hepatitis: an update on terminology and reporting. Am J Surg Pathol 1995;19(12):1409–17.

69. Kim SU, Oh HJ, Wanless IR, et al. The Laennec staging system for histological sub-classification of cirrhosis is useful for stratification of prognosis in patients with liver cirrhosis. J Hepatol 2012;57(3):556–63.

70. Yu E. [Histologic grading and staging of chronic hepatitis: on the basis of standardized guideline proposed by the Korean Study Group for the Pathology of Digestive Diseases]. Taehan Kan Hakhoe Chi 2003;9(1):42–6.

71. Lee JH, Joo I, Kang TW, et al. Deep learning with ultrasonography: automated classification of liver fibrosis using a deep convolutional neural network. Eur Radiol 2020;30(2):1264–73.

72. Choi KJ, Jang JK, Lee SS, et al. Development and validation of a deep learning system for staging liver fibrosis by using contrast agent–enhanced CT images in the liver. Radiology 2018;289(3):688–97.

73. Wang K, Lu X, Zhou H, et al. Deep learning radiomics of shear wave elastography significantly improved diagnostic performance for assessing liver fibrosis in chronic hepatitis B: a prospective multicentre study. Gut 2019;68(4):729–41.

74. Gatos I, Tsantis S, Spiliopoulos S, et al. Temporal stability assessment in shear wave elasticity images validated by deep learning neural network for chronic liver disease fibrosis stage assessment. Med Phys 2019;46(5):2298–309.

75. Yasaka K, Akai H, Kunimatsu A, et al. Liver fibrosis: deep convolutional neural network for staging by using gadoxetic acid–enhanced hepatobiliary phase MR images. Radiology 2018;287(1):146–55.

76. Park HJ, Lee SS, Park B, et al. Radiomics analysis of gadoxetic acid–enhanced MRI for staging liver fibrosis. Radiology 2019;290(3):380–7.

77. Treacher A, Beauchamp D, Quadri B, et al. Deep learning convolutional neural networks for the estimation of liver fibrosis severity from ultrasound texture. doi:10.1117/12.2512592.

78. Brattain LJ, Telfer BA, Dhyani M, et al. Objective liver fibrosis estimation from shear wave elastography. In:

Proceedings of the Annual International conference of the IEEE Engineering in medicine and Biology Society, EMBS, Vol 2018-July. Institute of Electrical and Electronics Engineers Inc.; 2018. p. 3472–6.

79. Mitsuka Y, Midorikawa Y, Abe H, et al. A prediction model for the grade of liver fibrosis using magnetic resonance elastography. BMC Gastroenterol 2017; 17(1):133.

80. Chang W, Lee JM, Yoon JH, et al. Liver fibrosis staging with MR elastography: comparison of diagnostic performance between patients with chronic hepatitis B and those with other etiologic causes. Radiology 2016;280(1):88–97.

81. He L, Li H, Dudley JA, et al. Machine learning prediction of liver stiffness using clinical and T2-weighted MRI radiomic data. Am J Roentgenol 2019;213(3):592–601.

82. Silva AM, Grimm RC, Glaser KJ, et al. Magnetic resonance elastography: evaluation of new inversion algorithm and quantitative analysis method. Abdom Imaging 2015;40(4):810–7.

83. Murphy MC, Manduca A, Trzasko JD, et al. Artificial neural networks for stiffness estimation in magnetic resonance elastography. Magn Reson Med 2018; 80(1):351–60.

84. Younossi ZM, Koenig AB, Abdelatif D, et al. Global epidemiology of nonalcoholic fatty liver disease—meta-analytic assessment of prevalence, incidence, and outcomes. Hepatology 2016;64(1):73–84.

85. Ferraioli G, Monteiro LBS. Ultrasound-based techniques for the diagnosis of liver steatosis. World J Gastroenterol 2019;25(40):6053–62.

86. Hamaguchi M, Kojima T, Itoh Y, et al. The severity of ultrasonographic findings in nonalcoholic fatty liver disease reflects the metabolic syndrome and visceral fat accumulation. Am J Gastroenterol 2007;102(12):2708–15.

87. Cao W, An X, Cong L, et al. Application of deep learning in quantitative analysis of 2-dimensional ultrasound imaging of nonalcoholic fatty liver disease. J Ultrasound Med 2020;39(1):51–9.

88. Park HJ, Park B, Lee SS. Radiomics and deep learning: Hepatic applications. Korean J Radiol 2020;21(4):387–401.

89. Byra M, Styczynski G, Szmigielski C, et al. Transfer learning with deep convolutional neural network for liver steatosis assessment in ultrasound images. Int J Comput Assist Radiol Surg 2018;13(12): 1895–903.

90. Webb M, Yeshua H, Zelber-Sagi S, et al. Diagnostic value of a computerized hepatorenal index for sonographic quantification of liver steatosis. Am J Roentgenol 2009;192(4):909–14.

91. Biswas M, Kuppili V, Edla DR, et al. Symtosis: a liver ultrasound tissue characterization and risk stratification in optimized deep learning paradigm. Comput Methods Programs Biomed 2018;155:165–77.

92. Saba L, Dey N, Ashour AS, et al. Automated stratification of liver disease in ultrasound: an online accurate feature classification paradigm. Comput Methods Programs Biomed 2016;130:118–34.

93. Acharya UR, Sree SV, Ribeiro R, et al. Data mining framework for fatty liver disease classification in ultrasound: a hybrid feature extraction paradigm. Med Phys 2012;39(7):4255–64.

94. Han A, Byra M, Heba E, et al. Noninvasive diagnosis of nonalcoholic fatty liver disease and quantification of liver fat with radiofrequency ultrasound data using one-dimensional convolutional neural networks. Radiology 2020;295(2):342–50.

95. Mongan J, Moy L, Kahn CE. Checklist for Artificial Intelligence in Medical Imaging (CLAIM): a guide for authors and reviewers. Radiol Artif Intell 2020;2(2): e200029.

96. Liu X, Cruz Rivera S, Moher D, et al. CONSORT-AI extension. Nat Med 2020;26(September):1364–74.

97. Cruz Rivera S, Liu X, Chan AW, et al. Guidelines for clinical trial protocols for interventions involving artificial intelligence: the SPIRIT-AI extension. Lancet Digit Heal 2020;2(10):e549–60.

Moving?

Make sure your subscription moves with you!

To notify us of your new address, find your **Clinics Account Number** (located on your mailing label above your name), and contact customer service at:

Email: journalscustomerservice-usa@elsevier.com

800-654-2452 (subscribers in the U.S. & Canada)
314-447-8871 (subscribers outside of the U.S. & Canada)

Fax number: 314-447-8029

Elsevier Health Sciences Division
Subscription Customer Service
3251 Riverport Lane
Maryland Heights, MO 63043

*To ensure uninterrupted delivery of your subscription, please notify us at least 4 weeks in advance of move.

Printed and bound by CPI Group (UK) Ltd, Croydon, CR0 4YY

08/05/2025

01864694-0009